Fundamentals of Perioperative Management

Fundamentals of Perioperative Management

Dr David Green MB, FRCA, MBA

Dr Max Ervine BMSc (Hon), BDS, MBChB, FFARCSI, FRCA

Dr Stuart White FRCA, BSc, MA
Department of Anaesthetics,
Intensive Care and Pain Relief
King's College Hospital
London

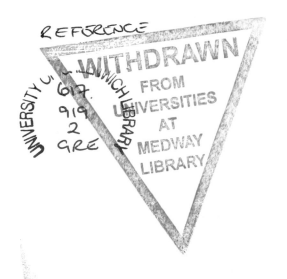

GMM

LONDON   SAN FRANCISCO

GMM

Greenwich Medical Media
4th Floor, 137 Euston Road,
London
NW1 2AA

© 2003

870 Market Street, Ste 720
San Francisco
CA 94109, USA

ISBN   1841101354   SRB

First published 2003

www.greenwich-medical.co.uk

Distributed by Plymbridge Distributors, UK and in the USA by JAMCO Distribution.

Typeset by Charon Tec Pvt. Ltd, Chennai, India

Printed by Hong Kong Graphics and Printing Ltd, China

Contents

1

Introduction

'From inability to let well alone; from too much zeal for the new and contempt for what is old; from putting knowledge before wisdom, science before art, and cleverness before common sense; from treating patients as cases, and from making the cure of the disease more than the endurance of the same, Good Lord deliver us.' Robert Hutchison (*BMJ* 1953, i, 671).

The new paradigm of medical education

In the recent changes to the medical school curriculum, the GMC has stressed the need for the integration of basic and clinical science. The 'core curriculum' should be system based, its component parts being the combined responsibility of basic scientists and clinicians integrating their contributions to a common purpose, thus eliminating the rigid pre-clinical/clinical divide and the exclusive departmentally based course. Competency-based clinical training is now emphasised and student progression though the course is partly determined by the testing of 'skills', such as putting up a drip, taking a psychiatric history, examining a lump and performing basic life support (BLS). These are tested through the medium of objective structured clinical examinations (OSCEs). While it is admirable that a student should be able to put up a drip, it is equally important that they understand the scientific background to intravenous (i.v.) therapy.

The emphasis on *Knowledge, Skills and Attitudes* seems to us to be tipped in favour of skills and attitudes rather than knowledge. Many textbooks reflect this imbalance and present the student with lists of differential diagnoses and lists of 'things to do'. The physiological, pathological and pharmacological basis of therapy is accepted as given. However, formal teaching and assessment of clinical pharmacology and therapeutics (CPT) and, especially, physiology is virtually non-existent in the clinical years. Added to this, there may be no formal testing of CPT in the final examination. The emphasis of the final clinical year (year 5) in many medical schools is now in 'shadowing' pre-registration house officers (PRHOs) and 'learning the trade' rather than increasing or at least consolidating background knowledge. We feel that this background knowledge is absolutely crucial to sound clinical management. How can you manage a patient's postoperative fluids, if you do not even know what is in a bag of 'normal saline' or what the normal daily Na^+ requirement is? Some students are not even sure of the concentration of oxygen in the air. Then how can they manage a hypoxic respiratory patient, who needs a minimal increase in inspired oxygen concentration?

Who is this book aimed at?

This book is aimed at the recent graduate and medical student in the new curriculum and accepts that the traditional post-graduate year of the PRHO is now effectively year 6 of medical school. For this reason, it is even more important to include the background CPT and physiology that is often missing from the clinical years.

We also feel that there is a clear need for graduate anaesthetic and surgical trainees to have a concise, one-stop reference for the key points of perioperative management. Currently, trainees in surgery have no obvious texts to go to. Training days on perioperative management are being run in some hospitals to make-up for the deficiency of good texts, and are often run by anaesthetists for surgery trainees. The latter seems particularly keen that such a book should provide authoritative coverage of CPT and physiology and include topics such as oxygen delivery and perioperative nutrition.

SHOs in anaesthesia are now expected to spend at least 3 months in the high-dependency unit (HDU) and intensive care unit (ICU). Thus, they need to know about the basic patient management in this situation, but more particularly be aware (as do SHOs in surgery) of those patients who represent a failure of ward-based management and need the benefits of HDU/ICU treatment at an early stage. SHOs in surgery and accident and emergency should also benefit from this experience. We also appreciate that there is a need for the first one or two SHO years to be more broadly based with flexibility for change between specialties before reaching the specialist registrar (SpR) stage. Thus, there must be a core curriculum for SHOs too. We hope to instil in the reader that, perhaps more than in any other branch of medicine, management of the patient in the perioperative period requires a team approach.

The hierarchy of learning

The quotation at the beginning of this chapter encapsulates many of the principles that underpin this book. The process by which patients are managed in the perioperative period (and elsewhere) deserves consideration. The main management route often seems to be initiated by a perceived deviation from normality in a symptom, sign or test, e.g. breathlessness, abnormal preoperative blood pressure (BP), blood glucose, serum K^+ or postoperative fall in urine output or alteration in arterial oxygen saturation (SpO_2). It is interesting to analyse the route by which this data is assimilated by the PRHO or SHO and then translated into suitable therapy.

Rackow noted a hierarchy from Data to Wisdom, the latter representing the pinnacle of excellence in management.

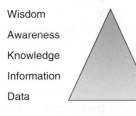

- *Data:* The simple collection of values, such as BP or urine output, usually by machine or non-medical staff, e.g. a monitor or a nurse on the ward.

- *Information:* The presentation and interpretation of that *Data*, e.g. a BP of 70/50 is a low reading in an 80-year old (but not in a 3-month old). This interpretation is again often made by non-medical staff.

- *Knowledge:* The ability to act competently and appropriately upon this *Information* compatible with the status of the clinician (e.g. a PRHO would not be expected to be as well informed as the consultant).

- *Awareness:* The ability to rationalise and bring judgement to that knowledge, such as when to call for more senior help.

- *Wisdom:* The ability to distinguish between effectiveness (i.e. doing the right job) and efficiency (i.e. doing the job right). In the former case, the appropriate treatment is given and in the latter an inappropriate treatment is given, but done efficiently. For example, the effective use of health care is the performance of a timely operation on a man with early prostate cancer to effect a cure. Efficient use is the performance of 50 varicose vein operations, because the waiting list for these operations is over a nominal government target.

How do these concepts affect medical management? Firstly, let us take a simple case. A PRHO has sent off a sample for preoperative haemoglobin (Hb) estimation.

Data
The Hb is found in the automated laboratory to be 8.5 g/dl and is printed out on the results form and returned to the ward. This, as yet, has no impact on patient management, as it is only one of a mountain of data that is processed by the laboratory.

Information
The form is now seen on the ward and the *Data* is interpreted by the PRHO. The Hb is noted to be low, i.e. below the normal lower limit (it should be noted that the normal range is arbitrary, and 8.5 g/dl just represents

a figure more than two standard deviations below the mean). This result is now in the public domain and needs to be acted upon.

Knowledge
The question is what do we do about this *Information*? This needs *Knowledge* of normal values and the implications of a reduced Hb on oxygen transport and so on. It is clearly a low value, needs to be investigated and likely reasons found for the low reading.

Awareness
Beyond *Knowledge*, this case is knowing that in most cases, there is no need to transfuse patients who are undergoing minor procedures with an Hb of 8.5 g. In other words, the operation may not need to be postponed, despite the fact that the patient needs to be investigated.

Wisdom
In medicine, this is often tacit or implicit experience of the real world and what has happened in previous cases in the experience of the clinician or may be the result of *an evidence-based approach* based on recent meta-analyses or large trials. Thus, much of this 'wisdom' or clinical judgement is not actually written down, but is passed down 'from generation to generation'. It comes from years of experience. So, in this case, the consultant anaesthetist working with his consultant surgical colleague will probably agree to do the operation, whereas the SHO and SpR will push for postponement.

The challenge is to codify and record this *Wisdom* so that the organisation 'learns' from previous successes (and failures). The emphasis on guidelines and protocols reflects these attempts. However, many experienced clinicians will maintain that all patients are individuals and medicine, as a holistic art as well as a science, does not always lend itself to such compartmentalisation.

A much more complex example might be the interpretation of a low BP, e.g. 70/50 in a 75-year old postoperative patient. Often, the *Data* side is simply a column on a chart, i.e.

it never reaches consciousness, especially, if it is the middle of the night! Once it becomes *Information*, then it should be clear to the PRHO that this is a low reading. What other *Data* is being recorded in the patient? Urine output is found to be only 20 ml/h or less for the last 3 h. Hmmm! What about fluid input and output? As more and more *Data* is gathered to become *Information* on the patient, *Knowledge* is now needed for correlation. For example, if the patient lost a lot of blood perioperatively, how much was replaced and what other fluids were given? How do we assess fluid status in this patient? Does the fact that the patient is a 75-year old and a known hypertensive with left-ventricular dysfunction make the assessment of fluid status different from a fit 32-year old? Can we learn anything from analysing the urine osmolality and Na^+ concentration? Did the PRHO realise that the patient had an epidural in place and was receiving relatively large doses of local anaesthetics and opioids? *Awareness* of all these other factors is needed before management can be finalised.

It should be clear that even looking at these two simple and common examples, a background knowledge beyond lists of differential diagnoses or 'things to do' is needed before the patient can be appropriately managed. This book attempts to provide the fifth year medical student through to the SHO background information, knowledge and awareness to appropriately manage common postoperative problems. *Wisdom* will eventually come when experience is married to sound clinical judgement, but unfortunately is beyond the scope of this textbook!

Conclusion

This book, therefore, attempts to provide sufficient data, information and knowledge to allow the process of awareness and wisdom to develop and, hopefully, to optimise perioperative management.

2

Accidents and complications of anaesthesia and surgery

2

The aims of this chapter are to

- describe the recommendations of the National Confidential Enquiry into Perioperative Deaths (NCEPOD),

- highlight the common complications that occur in the perioperative period.

Objectives

After reading this chapter, you should be able to

- understand that perioperative morbidity and mortality can result from sub-optimal medical care,

- recognise what complications can occur after surgery,

- focus on the lessons to be learnt from NCEPOD reports,

- modify and improve your practice to include appropriate guidelines that help to reduce complications,

- understand how team work and good communication can improve outcome.

Introduction

Perioperative accidents and complications all occur too commonly. They are often the result of

- inadequate preoperative preparation,

- equipment failure,

- 'person failure' (inadequate knowledge and inadequate expertise),

- inadequate postoperative care.

These factors often occur in combination and can result in a series of events that have an adverse, even fatal, outcome for the patient. All the factors are avoidable. This book emphasises the importance of preoperative and postoperative care, but these are inconsequential if, for instance, the surgeon is operating beyond his capabilities or the anaesthetist fails to recognise a life-threatening intra-operative event.

The NCEPOD is a registered charity, whose aim is to review clinical practice and identify potentially remediable factors in the practice of anaesthesia, surgery and other invasive medical procedures. NCEPOD looks at the quality of the delivery of care, rather than the cause of death. The recommendations made in the annual reports are based on peer review of the data, questionnaires and other records submitted. NCEPOD does not produce any kind of comparison between clinicians. The Royal Colleges, Faculties and Associations nominate members of the NCEPOD Steering Group. The enquiries were started in 1988. Since 1 April 1999, NCEPOD has come under the aegis of the National Institute for Clinical Excellence (NICE), who provides the majority of the organisation's funding. A separate enquiry is conducted in Scotland, the Scottish Audit of Surgical Mortality (SASM). The enquiry collects data on all deaths occurring in hospital within 30 days of a surgical procedure, and a sample of the total number of reported deaths is selected for detailed review (normally 10%). The review process includes relevant consultant surgeons and the NCEPOD clinical co-ordinators and advisory group reviews anaesthetists responding to a questionnaire on each sample case and the returned questionnaires. Complete report summaries may be found in the NCEPOD website: http://www.ncepod.org.uk.

The seven key issues

The seven key issues have recurred throughout the 12 reports of NCEPOD (Table 2.1).

1. Training and skills
Patients expect to be treated and managed by fully trained and competent staff. They assume that trainees are taught appropriately

Table 2.1 **Recurring themes in NCEPOD reports**

Theme	Remedial action required
Training and skills	Medical skills should be matched according to the patients' needs
Decision-making and consultation	Improved interdisciplinary and intradisciplinary teamwork
Clinical experience, education and audit	All staff should participate in audit, M+M meetings and continued professional development
Essential services and facilities	Hospitals providing emergency services should offer 24-h operating facilities, and be able to provide ICU and HDU care
Clinical issues	Perioperative optimisation is essential in the sick or elderly Thrombo-embolic prophylaxis should be routine Practice guidelines should be employed
Medical records and data collection	Both should be improved
Post-mortem examinations	The number of examinations should be increased

2

and supervised when necessary. Surgeons and anaesthetists, in particular, must work together as a team and fully involve other specialties and paramedical staff as appropriate. Their skills should always be appropriate to the physiological and pathological status of the patient.

2. Decision-making and consultation

A team approach, involving frequent and effective communication between senior surgeons, anaesthetists and physicians, is required for more complex cases, particularly concerning the care of the elderly and cancer patients, who have poor physical status and high-perioperative mortality and morbidity. In these patients, a commitment to provide appropriate postoperative care, including high-dependency or intensive care support, must be provided. Patients and their relatives need to recognise the limits of surgery in advanced malignant disease. Operation may not be in the best interests of the patient,

though this is a decision that should be made jointly by consultant surgeons and anaesthetists.

Consultant anaesthetists, surgeons and hospital managers should plan the administration and management of emergency admissions for operation, in order to minimise out-of-hours operating. A theatre arbitrator should be nominated to decide the relative priority of emergency theatre cases.

3. Clinical experience, education and audit

Local audit meetings are essential to good clinical practice and all staff must participate. Audit activities must be fully supported by Trusts. Much can be learnt from regular interdepartmental morbidity and mortality (M + M) meetings. It is a professional responsibility to audit one's own practice and seek ways to improve surgical and anaesthetic management. Effective audit, as part of

7

clinical governance, aids the maintenance of professional credibility and public support.

4. Essential services and facilities
All hospitals admitting emergency surgical patients must be of sufficient size to provide 24-h operating rooms, a fully staffed emergency surgery list, and other critical care services on a single site, if possible. The absence of an ICU and HDU is common. This is detrimental to patient care, as it places unreasonable pressure on surgeons and anaesthetists in their decision-making, impeding the flexible and graduated use of expensive critical care resources. There should be sufficient, fully staffed, daytime theatre and recovery facilities to ensure that no elderly patient requiring an urgent operation waits for more than 24 h, once fit for surgery. This also includes weekends.

5. Clinical issues
Multidisciplinary optimisation of a patient's condition is required prior to anaesthesia and surgery. This may include both the preoperative use of critical care facilities and the management of co-morbidities by appropriate consultant medical specialists. The elderly, who constitute a large proportion of the workload, are often subject to poor fluid management and analgesia. In this group, clinically unsuspected gastrointestinal complications are commonly found at post-mortem to be the cause, or contribute to the cause, of death following surgery. Certain clinical problems (those over 90 years of age, those with aortic stenosis, those who need radical pelvic surgery, those who need transfer to neuro-surgical units and those for emergency vascular operations) merit special attention by consultant anaesthetists and consultant surgeons.

More research into and awareness of thrombo-embolism is needed, as it remains a major cause of death after surgery.

Enforceable standards of practice need to be developed for the management of many common, acute conditions (e.g. head injuries, aortic aneurysm, colorectal cancer and gastrointestinal bleeding).

6. Medical records and data collection
NCEPOD has repeatedly highlighted the need to improve the recording and management of patient data. Trusts and hospitals must establish systems to ensure that all patients' medical records are always available to clinicians throughout the perioperative period. The inability to trace patients' notes after their death prevents surgeons and anaesthetists from completing returns to NCEPOD, and is unacceptable.

7. Post-mortem examinations
Efforts should be made to increase the number of post-mortem examinations. Despite clinicians' scepticism, at least 49% of post-mortems demonstrate significant, new and unexpected findings. Post-mortems are an important form of quality control.

Common complications and problems in the perioperative period

These may be subdivided into preoperative, operative and postoperative groups. Several problems are common to all three groups. Others begin in one group and progress throughout the continuum of treatment.

Preoperative problems and complications
These are covered in more depth in Chapter 4, but include:

- failure to take necessary medications;
- taking unnecessary medications, or medications that are hazardous in the perioperative period;
- smoking;
- inadequate patient assessment;
- inadequate consent for operation, including discussion with relatives;
- dehydration and malnutrition;
- hypertension;
- anaemia.

Intra-operative problems and complications

Anaesthesia
Hypotension, hypertension, dysrhythmia, hypoxia, awareness, hypothermia, transfusion reactions and problems with fluid management.

Embolism (Chapter 7)
Thrombus, air and tissue may embolise from any part of the circulation and result in hypoxia (pulmonary embolism (PE)), ischaemia (arterial embolism), myocardial or cerebral infarction. Particular care should be taken in patients with right-to-left cardiac shunts, because venous emboli bypass the filtrative effect of the pulmonary circulation and enter the arterial tree.

Neuro-endocrine stress reaction
For detailed information see Chapter 15.

Haemorrhage
For detailed information see Chapter 7.

Sepsis
For detailed information see Chapter 13.

Surgery
Problems include tissue maceration, iatrogenic damage, failure to remove all swabs, operating on the wrong organ/wrong side, expected complications of type of surgery, unexpectedly difficult surgery and equipment failure.

Postoperative problems and complications

This section may be subdivided into early (within 24 h of surgery), intermediate (24–72 h) and late (more than 72 h). Obviously, there is significant overlap in the timing of these complications (Table 2.2).

Early complications

Pain (Chapter 10)
Despite the administration of intra-operative analgesia, patients may emerge from their anaesthesia in considerable pain. This may occur for a variety of reasons:

- Insufficient analgesia has been administered.

- Inadequate analgesia has been administered for that patient or for that operation.

- Analgesia has not been administered early enough before emergence. This is especially true if a short-acting (e.g. fentanyl) or ultra-short-acting (e.g. remifentanil) analgesic has been administered.

- Analgesia has not been administered effectively (e.g. failed epidural and missed epidural segment).

- Psychological reasons (some patients expect to wake in pain, especially if this has happened before).

- Specific surgical reasons (e.g. urinary retention, bowel spasm (in which case an antispasmodic may be useful), ureteric spasm and shoulder tip pain after laparoscopy).

Nausea and vomiting (Chapter 18)
This occurs in up to a third of patients postoperatively and is more common in overweight, female patients after gastrointestinal or gynaecological surgery, who have previously had nausea and vomiting after surgery or are prone to travel sickness. It may persist into the later postoperative stages, in which case other causes such as bowel obstruction and ileus should be sought.

Ischaemia (Chapters 6, 7 and 10)
This may occur globally in an anaemic, hypotensive, hypoxic patient, or locally, due to pressure on tissues (e.g. bed pressure sores, tight bandages or plastering) or poor perfusion (elevated limbs, oedematous or macerated tissue).

Anaemia (Chapter 7)
The patient may be mildly anaemic before surgery. Blood loss may have occurred during surgery. Haemorrhage may be ongoing.

2

9

Table 2.2 Common perioperative complications of anaesthesia and surgery

Preoperative	Intra-operative	Postoperative
Medication problems	Anaesthesia	Early
Failure to take those necessary	Hypo/hypertension	Ischaemia
Taking those that are unnecessary	Dysrhythmia	Anaemia
Taking those that are potentially	Hypoxia	Hypotension
hazardous	Hypothermia	Hypoxia
	Awareness	Pain
	Transfusion reactions	
	Fluid management	
Smoking	Surgery	Intermediate
Inadequate patient assessment	Tissue maceration	Pain
Co-existent medical problems	Iatrogenic damage	Nausea and vomiting
Angina	Expected/unexpected	Constipation/ileus/
Hypertension	complications	diarrhoea
Diabetes	Equipment failure	Hypoxia
Inadequate consent for	Embolism	Myocardial ischaemia
operation	Neuro-endocrine stress	DVT/PE
Dehydration	reaction	Oliguria
Malnutrition and obesity	Reperfusion injury	Infection
Anaemia	Haemorrhage	Haemorrhage
	Sepsis	Acute confusional state
		Late
		Wound dehiscence
		Abscess
		Pressure sores/mobility
		Malnutrition
		Psychological problems

Hypotension (Chapters 6, 7 and 10)
This is a common occurrence and may be due to residual anaesthesia, epidural anaesthesia, hypovolaemia, myocardial ischaemia, PE and rewarming (i.e. relative hypovolaemia).

Hypoxia (Chapter 16)
All patients should be given supplemental oxygen in the early postoperative period. An obstructed airway and hypoventilation are the commonest causes. Obstruction of the airway may be due to excessive somnolence (excess anaesthesia, excess analgesia, hypocarbia, hypothermia, hypoglycaemia and cerebral ischaemia), laryngospasm or a foreign body (tongue, swab/pack and vomit). Hypoventilation may be caused by excessive somnolence or paralysis.

Intermediate complications

Pain
Pain may continue to occur for the above reasons (see under Early complications), but in addition may be caused by movement, coughing, vomiting, lax administration of analgesia, non-use of regular analgesia (such that breakthrough pain occurs between haphazard dosage of analgesics), change over from epidural analgesia or patient-controlled analgesia to oral analgesia, tissue ischaemia or constipation.

Hypoxia
Hypoxia may occur secondary to atelectasis (retained secretions), bronchopneumonia, pneumothorax, aspiration pneumonia, return

of rapid eye movement (REM) sleep (72 h), left-ventricular failure with pulmonary oedema and PE. It is more common in smokers.

Myocardial infarction (Chapter 15)
This may occur at any time, but incidence appears to peak at day 3, possibly due to a combination of increased blood hypercoagulability and hypoxia (coincident on the return of REM sleep). Left-ventricular failure may ensue, particularly if the patient is hypervolaemic and hypoproteinaemic as a result of malnutrition.

Deep vein thrombosis and PE (Chapter 7)
This was considered by NCEPOD to be an easily preventable perioperative complication. PE should be suspected in any patient experiencing a sudden onset of breathlessness or hypoxia, chest pain, dysrhythmia or collapse.

Infection (Chapter 13)
Infections may be preventable by use of scrupulous intrapersonal and interpersonal hygiene, together with good clinical patient care. Infections are treatable by the same factors, combined with the rational use of narrow spectrum antibiotics.

Oliguria (Chapters 6 and 18)
This may be caused by pre-renal (hypovolaemia), renal (ischaemia, infarct and nephrotoxins) or postrenal (ureteric obstruction, clot and prostatic hypertrophy) factors.

Constipation/ileus (Chapter 18)
Ileus is very common after bowel surgery. Persistent ileus may be due to biochemical disarray or persistent bowel disease and infection. Constipation is also common and is often related to not eating, cessation of smoking or drugs that cause GI hypomotility (e.g. opioids).

Diarrhoea (Chapter 18)
Diarrhoea is less common than constipation and may be caused by infection, biochemical abnormalities, constipation or bowel motilients.

Haemorrhage (Chapter 7)
Haemorrhage may occur at any time postoperatively. If it occurs after a period of stability, infection or displacement of haemostatic mechanisms (clot, sutures and staples) may be suspected.

Acute confusional state (Chapter 19)
The differential diagnosis of this condition is large, but includes hypoxia, cerebral ischaemia, biochemical abnormalities, infection, drugs (administration and omission), alcohol withdrawal and uraemia.

Late complications

All of the above
This includes problems presented in early and intermediate complications.

Wound dehiscence
This may be due to poor surgical technique, pre-operative malnutrition, coughing, vomiting, wound infection or fluid discharge through the wound.

Abscess formation
The formation of an abscess should be expected if the patient has an unexplained swinging temperature and a raised white cell count (WCC).

Pressure sores
This is especially common in the obese patient (Chapter 11).

Malnutrition
The patient may well be malnourished prior to surgery. Postoperative malnutrition occurs as a result of failure to feed patient adequately, in chronic diseases and infection, excessive vomiting, malabsorption and after gut-shortening surgery.

Psychological dysfunction
Acute confusional state may persist. Disfiguring surgery and terminal disease are particularly associated with depression. Interference with drug administration may be associated with re-manifestation

of an underlying psychiatric disorder (e.g. schizophrenia).

Patients rarely die intra-operatively, when compared to the numbers that die in the postoperative period. The rapid diagnosis and effective treatment of the complications listed above considerably reduce the mortality and morbidity rates of those patients who have survived an operation. As suggested by NCEPOD, the use of nationwide or Trust-wide guidelines, for instance for the prevention of DVT, together with aspects of clinical governance (audit and risk management) will inevitably reduce perioperative complications and adverse outcomes for patients.

3

Principles of pharmacology, autonomic physiology and circulatory control relevant to the perioperative period

Aims

■ To review the basic principles of pharmacology, autonomic physiology and circulatory control and their relevance to the use of drugs in the perioperative period.

Objectives

After reading this chapter, you should be able to

■ understand the terms pharmacokinetics and pharmacodynamics and explain their significance for drugs used in the perioperative period;

■ explain the significance of drug ionisation, lipid solubility and the principles of drug movement across membranes;

■ define and calculate from relevant information: volume of distribution, clearance and half life of a commonly used perioperative drug such as cimetidine;

■ explain the principles and importance of bioavailability, how it is measured and its relevance to the use of drugs in the perioperative period when bioavailability may be altered due to changes in gut motility;

■ understand the principles and purpose of hepatic metabolism and renal excretion of drugs, and changes that may occur in the perioperative period resulting from the effects of drugs and changes in volume status;

■ define the main receptor types and explain what is meant by an agonist, antagonist and partial agonist, and its relevance to the use of drugs such as opioids, β-blockers and catecholamines;

■ formulate a suitable regime for a drug based on pharmacokinetic data, e.g. aminophylline and lidocaine and be aware of pharmacokinetic and pharmacodynamic changes which might occur in the perioperative period;

■ understand the actions of the main drugs affecting the sympathetic and parasympathetic nervous systems both endogenous and exogenous;

■ understand the principles of perioperative circulatory control.

Pharmacology

Introduction

Clinicians are now faced with an ever-increasing number of drugs that are being used by patients in the perioperative period. In addition, the likelihood of drug interaction increases with increasing numbers of drugs. It is very important that a clear understanding of basic pharmacology is needed to be able to use these drugs rationally. This chapter sets out some of these basic principles and provides a stimulus for further study. Information about the use of drugs is usually presented under the following three main headings.

Pharmaceutical

■ How the drugs are presented and administered, e.g. tablet, capsule, slow release and by what route. This is not of great relevance in the perioperative period. However, changes in the formulation of drugs (e.g. digoxin and phenytoin) have had profound effects on the absorption (and toxicity) of these drugs when given orally.

■ Speed and extent of drug dispersal in the gastro-intestinal tract (GIT).

■ Effects of other co-administered drugs and substances, e.g. L-dopa and carbidopa, tetracycline and milk.

■ Patient compliance problems, especially in the elderly with multiple drug regimes.

Other factors include the storage and cost of drugs. The latter is an extremely pertinent factor. It will not be considered further.

3

Pharmacokinetics

What the body does to the drug

This describes how the body handles the drug following its administration until it is eliminated. This concerns absorption (e.g. from the GIT, subcutaneous tissue, rectum), distribution, binding, metabolism and elimination. These factors can be quantified to give the pharmacokinetic parameters of half lives of absorption ($t_{1/2}$ abs), redistribution ($t_{1/2}\,\alpha$) and elimination ($t_{1/2}\,\beta$), loading dose (Ld), maintenance dose (Md), clearance (Cl) and volume of distribution (Vd). These are explained more fully in the sections that follow.

Pharmacodynamics

What the drug does to the body

This describes the effect of the drug and how it works. It concerns theory of drug action, usually in terms of receptor occupancy, description of effects in normal and diseased states, plasma concentration–response relationships (i.e. the concept of effective concentration, Ceff), interference with other drugs and effects of overdose, interactions and adverse effects. Present standards of practice demand extensive knowledge of pharmacological principles. The perioperative period provides excellent examples of the application of such principles.

Pharmacokinetic principles

Cell membranes

All drugs need to cross at least one cell membrane to produce their desired effects. This occurs by four main methods: passive diffusion, facilitated diffusion, active transport and pinocytosis.

Passive diffusion

This is the main method by which drugs move across a cell membrane from areas of higher to lower concentration. No energy is required and it is the unionised, lipid-soluble portion of the drug that diffuses most easily as it can cross the lipid bilayer of the cell membrane. However, cell membranes also contain protein molecules which float on this 'sea of lipid' and thus can also form hydrophilic ion channels to allow transport of different classes of *small* molecular weight (MW) < 100, water-soluble drugs alongside the bulk flow of water which occurs across all membranes.

Facilitated diffusion

This occurs when a molecule combines with a protein to cross the cell membrane at a faster rate than would be possible on its own. Examples include steroids, amino acids and glucose transport across the gut membrane.

Active transport

Active transport across the cell membrane is highly selective; i.e. it requires energy and can work against a concentration gradient. A good example is the Na/K-ATPase pump in the cell membrane and the maintenance of differential concentrations of Na^+ and K^+ inside and outside of the cell (Chapter 6).

Pinocytosis

This is where the membrane actually engulfs the drug (e.g. vitamin complex) and moves it into the cell.

Factors affecting these processes

Size and shape of drug molecules
The molecular size determines diffusion of drugs through pores in cell membranes, epithelia and endothelia by passive diffusion and is inversely proportional to the square root of molecular size (Graham's law), e.g. the relative confinement of high MW plasma expanders to the vascular compartment. Molecular configuration of drugs determines binding to specific cell surface proteins for active transport across the membrane.

Lipid solubility and ionisation
Lipid solubility is the most important determinant of passive diffusion across cell membranes because of the predominantly lipid nature of their constituents. The more

15

lipid soluble the drug, the faster is the rate of diffusion. However, most drugs are weak acids or bases, and therefore, dissociate into their unionised and ionised moieties in aqueous solution. Only the unionised fraction is lipophilic and easily diffusible across cell membranes. Acidic drugs are maximally unionised (lipophilic) at acid (low) pH, and basic drugs at alkaline (high) pH. The pKa of the drug indicates the pH at which the drug is 50% unionised. Most acidic drugs have a pKa in the acid range (<7.4) and vice versa for basic drugs. Thus, the proportion of a drug in the unionised, lipophilic form depends on the pKa of the drug, whether it is an acid or a base and the pH of the tissue or medium where it is present.

By rearranging the Henderson–Hasselbalch equation we get:

For acidic drugs:
pKa − pH = log(unionised/ionised)

For example, aspirin has a pKa of 3.5. Thus, if the pH of the stomach contents is 1.5, the log to the base 10 is 2. Thus, 100 times as much aspirin is present in the unionised compared with the ionised form in the stomach. Gastric absorption is thus enhanced. In the small intestine at a pH of 7.5, 10,000 times as much aspirin is present in the ionised form. Despite this, most of a dose of aspirin is actually absorbed in the alkaline medium of the small intestine, despite being mainly in the ionised form, due to the much larger surface area. Alkalisation of the urine can be used in aspirin overdose, rendering the aspirin ionised so that it is less easily reabsorbed by the kidney tubules.

For basic drugs:
pH − pKa = log(unionised/ionised)

For example, lidocaine has a pKa of 7.9, so at a pH of 7.4, pH − pK = −0.5. The log to the base 10 of −0.5 is 0.3, therefore, there is 0.3 times the amount in the unionised form or 75% is ionised and 25% unionised. Glycopyrrolate, being largely ionised at plasma pH, does not cross the blood–brain and placental barriers.

The degree of lipophilicity of the unionised fraction of a lipophilic drug is quantified by its ability to distribute *in vitro* between an octanol (oil) and water phase. The higher the octanol/water coefficient, the more lipid soluble the unionised moiety of the drug, and hence, the easier its passage across membranes. However, a highly lipid-soluble drug may be highly ionised at body pH, e.g. the opioid analgesic buprenorphine has a pKa of 8.4 which means that only 10% is unionised at pH 7.4. This will restrict its ability to cross the biophase to its site of action. The much less lipid-soluble opioid alfentanil has a pKa of about 6.4 which means that 90% is unionised and this means that there is more drug in the lipid-soluble form to cross cell membranes and accelerate its onset of action. This greatly offsets its inherent lower lipid solubility and the drug works much more quickly than buprenorphine as a result.

Absorption

Drugs may be given by a variety of routes. There is always some systemic absorption, even when drugs are applied topically.

Gastro-intestinal route

Lipid solubility and ionisation are important for absorption (see above). Drugs given orally are mainly absorbed in the small intestine and then via the portal system and liver before reaching the systemic circulation. For lipophilic drugs that undergo significant hepatic biotransformation, this '*first pass*' through the liver causes a large reduction in the amount of drug available (e.g. propranolol and most opioids). Sublingual (and to a much lesser effect, rectal) application bypasses this effect. *Bioavailability* is the fraction of an oral dose reaching the systemic circulation as compared with the same amount given i.v. and is affected by the combined effects of absorption *and* first pass metabolism (see later). Paradoxically, a highly lipophilic drug may be completely absorbed from the small intestine but then undergo extensive first-pass metabolism in the liver, thus reducing bioavailability. The opposite may be true for a hydrophilic drug.

It is important to know the bioavailability of the oral preparation of a drug that can

3

be given parenterally when switching routes in the perioperative period. Propranolol, e.g. is often given in a dose exceeding 100 mg orally in chronic use, but its equivalent i.v. dose is only 0.5–2 mg. This disparity is due both to its low oral bioavailability and the effect of chronic administration of the drug. For morphine, oral bioavailability is one-third to one-fifth of the parenteral version so a patient stabilised on a parenteral dose of 10 mg of morphine needs to be on 30–50 mg orally to get an equivalent effect.

Gastric emptying is greatly affected by transperitoneal surgery. It is important to make provision for continuation of drug therapy by an alternative route. If the patient is unable to swallow but has a nasogastric or duodenal tube in place, then the drug may be administered via that route. Some medications, such as anti-parkinsonian treatment, must be continued throughout the perioperative period. Here, an s.c. infusion of apomorphine may be appropriate as parenteral versions of the oral drugs are not easily available. Consultation with a specialist is often required in these cases.

Injection

Intravenous injection produces a peak plasma concentration within one circulation time (approximately 1 min). In terms of effect, it is the most predictable route and the one usually used in emergencies. Drugs given by intramuscular (i.m.) and subcutaneous injection are variably absorbed depending on local tissue perfusion. The latter is markedly reduced in shocked states and this greatly delays onset.

Mucous membranes and skin

These are used as a route for systemic absorption as well as for local effects limited to the site of application:

Systemic use
- *Sublingual:* Buprenorphine, nifedipine and glyceryl trinitrate (GTN), thus avoiding hepatic first-pass metabolism.

- *Rectum (as suppositories):* The NSAID diclofenac is often given by this route but

there is no evidence that bioavailability is any better than by the oral route.

- *Skin:* GTN, hyoscine, nicotine patches, buprenorphine and fentanyl can be given by this route. It provides the equivalent of long-term 'infusion' of drug, thus maintaining steady levels over many hours or days. It is only suitable for potent drugs as the amount of absorption through the skin is limited. In addition, absorption of active drug from skin depots continues for many hours following removal of the patch. This is obviously important with potent respiratory depressants such as fentanyl.

- *Nasal mucosa:* For example, arginine vasopressin (DDAVP for diabetes insipidus) and fentanyl.

- *Trachea and large bronchi:* This is a particularly useful route for administration of adrenaline during cardiac arrest prior to obtaining venous access. Roughly twice the equivalent i.v. dose must be given by this route, but the amount absorbed is often unpredictable.

- *Inhalation:* Inhalation of gases and vapours are of particular interest in this context, e.g. the administration of inhalational anaesthetics.

Local use
- *Skin:* A particularly good example in anaesthesia is the eutectic mixture of local anaesthetics (EMLA), prilocaine and lidocaine. A eutectic mixture is a mixture of two compounds in a certain proportion that has the lowest melting point. For prilocaine and lidocaine in a 50:50 mixture, the melting point is lowered to below room temperature (individually the melting points are 30–50°C), thus allowing the development of a very high concentration local anaesthetic cream which is capable of penetrating the skin.

Sometimes the systemic absorption of topically applied drugs (for local effects) can

3

3

inadvertently produce systemic toxicity. A few examples are:

- *Eye:* plasma pseudo-cholinesterase may be inhibited by ecothiopate eye drops thus prolonging the effects of suxamethonium.

- *Lung:* salbutamol and other bronchodilators may be given in sufficient doses to produce toxicity (e.g. tachycardia and dysrhythmias).

Distribution and binding

Drugs are not evenly distributed throughout all tissues of the body. Well-perfused organs such as the brain and heart in the 'central compartment' (see later) may initially be exposed to higher concentrations of drugs given parenterally before redistribution to other tissues. This is not so important for oral preparations.

A proportion may bind to plasma proteins; generally to albumin for acidic drugs and to α1-acid glycoprotein for basic drugs. Since only free, unbound drug is available for activity (or excretion by the kidney), the extent of protein binding influences the action of the drug. Some drugs compete for similar sites and can, therefore, displace each other leading to an enhanced effect of the displaced drug. The effect of this is slight in most instances as the free drug is then either rapidly redistributed or made available for metabolism and elimination.

Pharmacokinetic parameters

This is concerned with time-dependent changes in plasma concentration following administration of drugs (thus described as '*what the patient does to the drug*'). Knowledge of three pharmacokinetic parameters: volume of distribution (Vd), clearance (Cl) and elimination half-life ($t_{1/2}$ β) are used to calculate the loading dose (Ld), maintenance dose (Md) and interval and duration of action of drugs. These are most useful when dealing with drugs with a narrow toxic/therapeutic ratio.

Most studies of drug kinetics refer only to profiles of plasma concentration following i.v. injection. Fortunately, most drug effects are closely related to plasma concentrations, the Ceff (see above). After single injection, plasma levels decline according to well-defined patterns. Abstract models representing one or more 'compartments' are frequently used to help predict duration effects.

Single compartment model

Here, the plot of plasma concentration (following single bolus i.v. injection) against time is a simple exponential curve that appears as a single straight line if the logarithm of concentration is taken on the *y*-axis. This indicates that the drug is distributed into a single compartment from which it is being metabolised by *first-order kinetics,* i.e. a constant fraction (not amount) of drug present in plasma is eliminated per unit of time, the amount metabolised being proportional to the concentration of the drug in the compartment studied.

Two or more compartmental model (Fig. 3.1)

Most drugs do not behave as if they remain in a single compartment. After bolus i.v. injection they are rapidly redistributed to major visceral organs with a large blood supply such as the brain, heart, kidney and liver (central compartment) and then more slowly into less well-perfused tissues such as muscle and fat (peripheral compartment). As we shall see, each of these compartments has an apparent volume of distribution, e.g. the Vd of the central compartment (Vdcc) and the Vd steady state (i.e. the total combined Vdss). The concentration/time plot, therefore, shows a rapid initial decline in concentration with a consequently short *redistribution* half-life ($t_{1/2}$ α or alpha, usually measured in minutes). A slower decline in concentration (or series of declines) follows this due to the combined effects of elimination and continued redistribution with a consequently longer *elimination* half-life ($t_{1/2}$ β or beta, usually measured in hours). Drugs falling within this pattern of disposition are described as 'short acting' if the rapid initial fall in plasma concentration goes below Ceff during the redistribution phase, e.g. a bolus dose of

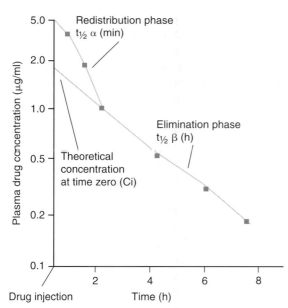

Fig. 3.1 Two compartment model following bolus i.v. injection.

thiopentone and fentanyl. They may, however, have 'cumulative' effects if administered repeatedly, due to a much slower elimination phase. Most drugs in current use show this pattern of distribution and elimination when given by i.v. injection. Obviously, the redistribution phase is much less prominent following other routes of administration.

Volume of distribution

If we take a beaker of unknown volume *V* and fill it with water we can calculate the volume by adding a known amount or 'dose' of dye (e.g. 10 mg), mixing it and then measuring the concentration in mg/l. If the final concentration is 1 mg/l then the volume of the beaker must be 10 l (i.e. volume = dose/concentration). The Vd of a drug in a human simply represents a theoretical 'volume' in which the drug distributes and which accounts for the concentration achieved in the plasma due to dilution after administration of a known dose of the drug. Thus, Vd in a single compartment model can be easily calculated by dividing the dose injected (D) by the estimated initial plasma concentration (Ci, obtained by extrapolating the straight line of the $t_{1/2}\beta$ back to time zero).

As many drugs bind to lipid and plasma proteins, this 'dilutional' volume, which is calculated by dividing dose administered by concentration achieved, as in the above example, may appear to greatly exceed total body water. In a similar way, we can surreptitiously place a sponge that absorbs the dye in the beaker in the example above. If we then measure the concentration, we find it is not 1 mg/l but perhaps 0.1 mg/l. Thus, the volume of the beaker would now appear to be 100 l, yet the external dimensions have not changed:

$$Vd = D/Ci \qquad (3.1)$$

Vd is more difficult to calculate in a two (or more) compartment model as the effects of continuing redistribution occur at the same time as metabolism and elimination. As mentioned earlier, it is convenient to divide the Vd into two parts in a two compartment model, Vdcc and Vdss. In this case, to calculate Vdcc we need the theoretical initial concentration Ci in the central compartment and this is obtained by extrapolating the redistribution curve back to time zero on the y-axis. Vdss can be obtained by similarly extrapolating the elimination curve back to time zero. In the case of opioids such as pethidine, Vdcc may be only 20–50 l while the Vdss is over 200 l (see Fig. 3.1).

Clearance

If, as stated above the amount of drug metabolised is proportional to concentration. Therefore

amount metabolised
    = a constant × concentration

The constant is known as clearance (Cl) and is the volume of plasma completely cleared of drug per unit time and represents the best measure of the elimination capacity of the body. It is only a constant if *first-order kinetics* apply to the metabolism of the drug because the body has excess capacity to metabolise the drug well beyond the clinical range. The units of clearance are volume per unit time and give no indication of the *amount* of drug metabolised. This will be dependent on

3

19

3

concentration of the drug at the particular time. If Ceff is the desired concentration of the drug (in mg/l) required to produce an effect and Cl is the clearance (in l/h), then the amount metabolised (in mg/h) is equal to

$$\text{amount metabolised} = \text{Cl} \times \text{Ceff} \qquad (3.2)$$

Note: Zero-order kinetics is seen for a few drugs that follow a quite different pattern of elimination (e.g. phenytoin, ethanol and thiopentone in high doses). Above a certain plasma level, saturation of metabolic processes occurs. At or beyond this level, a *constant amount* of drug is eliminated per unit time regardless of plasma concentration. If the dose is increased beyond this point, toxic concentrations can occur very rapidly.

Half-life ($t_{1/2}\,\beta$)

This indicates the time it takes for the concentration in the plasma to fall by half. It does not necessarily mean that the amount in the body falls by half or that half is eliminated. As seen above, in the two compartment model the rapid initial fall in blood concentration means that the $t_{1/2}\,\alpha$ is only a few minutes, while the shallower curve of metabolism and elimination means that the $t_{1/2}\,\beta$ is many hours. Indeed, for many drugs, further half-lives of increasing duration can be calculated reflecting slow return of the drug from peripheral-binding sites, often over many days. However, the plasma levels are usually well below Ceff so that no clinical effect persists.

Half-life is often utilised to predict 'wash-in' and 'wash-out' times, five half lives being taken to achieve wash-in or wash-out. This is particularly pertinent if the drug is commenced without a loading dose (see later). For a drug like digoxin with a $t_{1/2}\,\beta$ of 30 h, it will take 150 h to achieve steady-state concentrations if treatment is initiated as a daily maintenance dose. Manipulation of the dose to achieve a desired effect must take into account this long wash-in time if inadvertent toxicity is to be avoided. Trying to predict the duration of action of a drug by referring to its $t_{1/2}\,\beta$ is fraught with difficulties. For a start,

a drug may only achieve an effect at a specific concentration, thus even a slight fall will result in loss of effectiveness. On the other hand, receptor binding may be so avid that the half-life is irrelevant to the duration of action (see later).

Calculation of loading dose

In the perioperative period it is often important to bring drug plasma concentration to therapeutically effective levels immediately. Rearranging Equation (3.1), a loading dose (Ld) is administered which is sufficient to fill the Vd to a desired drug level, normally the effective concentration, Ceff:

$$\text{Ld} = \text{Ceff} \times \text{Vd} \qquad (3.3)$$

The level then falls unless it is followed by the administration of the maintenance dose. In the case of an induction agent like thiopentone no further maintenance dose is given and anaesthesia continued with an inhalational agent. In the case of a more rapidly metabolised drug such as propofol, a maintenance regime can be used to continue anaesthesia entirely by the i.v. route.

As stated above, for highly efficacious drugs given i.v., such as opioids, it may be necessary to give a small Ld rapidly to take account of the Vdcc and then a loading 'infusion' over an hour or so to take account of the Vdss. If only the Vdss was used to calculate the loading dose, toxic levels would occur initially. In anaesthesia, computerised infusion systems such as the 'Diprifusor®' target controlled infusion device for propofol take account of the three main phases. A small Ld is given to fill the Vdcc, then a fast but declining rate of infusion is given to maintain levels of propofol (and anaesthesia) during transit from the central compartment to the peripheral compartment. Finally, after about 20 min most of the Vdss has been filled with propofol, and thereafter, a near steady-state infusion level is given to compensate for the drug being metabolised and excreted. This is the maintenance dose and is discussed in the next section.

Calculation of maintenance dose

Ceff is often maintained by means of continuous i.v. infusions (e.g. propofol and lidocaine), where the rate of drug administration (Md) equals the rate of elimination (see Clearance):

$$Md = Ceff \times Cl \qquad (3.4)$$

Example of calculation of loading and maintenance doses for lidocaine:

- Desirable effective concentration (Ceff) in plasma is 2 mg/l (1.5–6)

- Volume of distribution (Vd) = 1100 ml/kg or 77 l (70 kg man)

- Clearance (Cl) = 9.2 ml/min/kg or 0.64 l/min (70 kg man)

Thus, from Equation (3.3):

$$Ld = Ceff \times Vd = 2 \times 77 = 154 \, mg$$

From Equation (3.4):

$$Md = Ceff \times Cl = 2 \times 0.64 = 1.3 \, mg/min$$

Thus, Vd determines the loading dose and Cl the maintenance dose. Cl is particularly important for drugs principally excreted via the kidney when administered to patients in renal failure. Loading dose will be the same or even higher than in patients with normal renal function, as Vd may be increased. Maintenance dose, however, will be markedly reduced (lower doses or longer dose intervals) in view of the much lower drug clearance. In congestive heart failure both Vd and Cl of lidocaine are reduced, necessitating lower loading and maintenance doses.

Note: In clinical practice, dose regimes are, normally, calculated on a mg/kg basis (e.g. lidocaine 2 mg/kg loading dose). The above calculations (Equations (3.3) and (3.4)) explain how these figures are derived. The above calculations apply to drugs eliminated by first-order processes, and the units used (e.g. mg, ml, min) must be consistent between equations.

It is important to realise that there is a fundamental relationship between Vd, Cl and $t_{1/2} \, \beta$, i.e.

$$t_{1/2} \, \beta = (Vd/Cl) \times 0.693 \qquad (3.5)$$

This relationship allows one to work out the third parameter when you know the other two, e.g. if you know the Vd and $t_{1/2} \, \beta$ you can calculate the clearance. It also shows that drugs with high volumes of distribution or low clearances (or a combination) tend to have long half-lives (and vice versa) (0.693 is the natural logarithm of 2, ln 2).

Drug metabolism and elimination

The pharmacokinetic patterns resulting from metabolism and elimination, described above, result from chemical alteration (metabolism) and/or excretion of the drug.

Chemical alteration (metabolism)

Having looked at the quantitative aspects of pharmacokinetics it is necessary to consider how drugs are metabolised. This is carried out mainly in the liver. In general terms the liver converts active, lipid-soluble drugs into inactive, water-soluble drugs which are able to undergo renal or biliary excretion (lipid-soluble drugs are filtered by the kidney but then immediately reabsorbed). Drugs already water soluble, such as digoxin and gentamicin, can be excreted directly. Obviously, there are many exceptions to this general statement (see below).

Although a few drugs are metabolised by a single process, hepatic biotransformation is usually carried out in two stages:

- *Phase I reactions* (non-synthetic) are carried out by hepatic intracellular microsomal systems requiring NADPH, oxygen and cytochrome p450. Examples are oxidation, reduction and hydrolysis. Drugs are usually prepared in this way for the second stage.

- *Phase II reactions* (synthetic) include conjugation with glucuronide, acetylation and methylation.

These reactions usually render lipid-soluble drugs water soluble, thus facilitating renal excretion. Some of the above reactions, particularly microsomal oxidation and reduction, can be significantly affected by patient genetic makeup and enhanced by previous exposure to similar drugs. This latter

3

is called enzyme induction. Classic examples are the chronic intake of phenobarbitone, rifampicin or alcohol that not only enhance their own metabolism but also metabolism of other drugs. Enzyme inhibition occurs with drugs such as metronidazole, cimetidine, erythromycin and sulphonamides.

The extent of hepatic biotransformation is dependent upon both hepatic enzyme activity (HEA) and hepatic blood flow (HBF). Hepatic clearance (HCl) can be calculated by multiplying hepatic blood flow by hepatic extraction ratio (HER). The latter is determined by looking at the ratio of amount of drug entering the liver (Di) via the portal system (e.g. following absorption from the gut) minus the amount leaving the liver and going into the systemic circulation (Do) divided by Di:

$$HER = (Di - Do)/Di \qquad (3.5)$$

$$HCl = HBF \times HER \qquad (3.6)$$

Thus, if the HBF is 1500 ml/min and the ratio (Di−Do)/Di is equal to 0.5 then HCl is 750 ml/min.

Clearly a drug which is not metabolised by the liver to a great extent has a high value for Do and thus the ratio of (Di−Do)/Di is low, e.g. 0.03 with aminophylline giving a clearance of 0.03 times 1500 or 50 ml/min. A drug which is almost completely extracted by the liver will have a very low Do and thus the ratio of (Di−Do)/Di will be very high, e.g. 0.9 with verapamil giving a clearance of 0.9 times 1500 or about 1350 ml/min. One can immediately see that if HBF falls by half, the clearance of aminophylline will fall by 25 ml/min. If the same occurs with verapamil, the clearance will fall by 675 ml/min. As HEA increases due to enzyme induction, HER increases along with clearance. This will have proportionately much more effect on low clearance drugs than high clearance drugs where the extraction ratio is already high, i.e. nearly 1 or 100%. Thus,

- The metabolism of *low clearance drugs* such as aminophylline is more dependent on the level of HEA than HBF. Thus, substances that induce HEA (such as nicotine in this case, phenobarbitone and rifampicin) increase HER and clearance and decrease the

effectiveness of the drug whereas those drugs that inhibit HEA (such as erythromycin, metronidazole and cimetidine) decrease HER and clearance and may lead to toxicity.

- The metabolism of *high clearance drugs* such as verapamil, opioids and β-blockers depend primarily on the level of HBF and have a clearance equivalent to HBF (1–1.5 l/m in the 60-kg patient). Clearance of these drugs are much more closely related to HBF than HEA as HER is already very high, a fall in HBF reducing clearance. When given orally, these drugs undergo substantial 'first-pass' metabolism, so blood levels are markedly increased if HBF is reduced. This, again, can cause toxicity.

- The metabolism of *medium clearance drugs*, such as alfentanil, lie in between these two extremes being affected both by HEA and HBF.

Drugs like suxamethonium and mivacurium are metabolised by plasma enzymes (pseudo-cholinesterase which is produced in the liver). More rarely, enzyme systems in other organs, e.g. kidney or lung, are involved.

As stated above, there are many exceptions to the general rule that the liver converts active compounds into inactive ones:

1. Active drugs are converted to compounds that are also active; e.g. diazepam is metabolised to desmethyldiazepam, which is equipotent to diazepam, but with a $t_{\frac{1}{2}}$ β of 53 h compared to 32 h for diazepam. This is of importance in long-term administration.

2. Inactive drugs (pro-drugs) are converted to active ones, e.g. enalapril into enalaprilat.

3. Active drugs are converted into toxic ones, e.g. pethidine to nor-pethidinic acid.

Excretion

Excretion of unaltered drug or its metabolites occurs mainly in the kidney for drugs with a MW of less than 300. There are three many processes, glomerular filtration (GF), tubular secretion and passive reabsorption. Renal clearance (RCl) *is equal* to fraction of drug unbound multiplied by the GF rate (GFR) for drugs which are filtered but not secreted or reabsorbed, e.g. gentamicin:

$$RCl = \text{fraction unbound} \times GFR \qquad (3.7)$$

As GFR falls so does clearance and maintenance dose must be reduced in renal impairment or failure (see above). For drugs that are reabsorbed, such as aspirin (see above) and amphetamine, RCl is less than GFR. RCl may be increased by alkalinisation of the urine, which reduces reabsorption (see above). For drugs, such as penicillin, which are actively secreted by the tubules, RCl is greater than GFR. To reduce RCl, this process of tubular reabsorption may be inhibited, e.g. by probenecid.

If the MW of the drug or its metabolites is over 300, then biliary excretion becomes more important (e.g. vecuronium and buprenorphine). Some antibiotics such as cefuroxime are excreted in the bile and this property is utilised in the treatment of cholecystitis. It is also important to be aware of enterohepatic recirculation of some drugs, e.g. oral contraceptives. These drugs are conjugated by the liver into a more water-soluble form and excreted in the bile. In the bowel, bacteria break down the conjugated form and the more lipid-soluble parent drug is reabsorbed and recycled. This recycling is an important component for the effectiveness of the drug. Administration of antibiotics destroys the gut bacteria and reduces enterohepatic re-circulation, which could lead to failure of contraception.

The lung is also an important route for drug elimination, e.g. inhalational anaesthetics.

Pharmacodynamics

Pharmacodynamics is the study of mechanisms of drug action or '*what the drug does to the body*'. Most drugs act upon receptors on the surface of cells in a highly specific fashion; very small modifications of the molecular structure of the drug may lead to a complete change of pharmacological activity. The study of this structure–activity relationship has led to the rational development of many new drugs in the past three decades.

Mechanisms of drug action

Drugs produce their effects via four main mechanisms: by direct action, by enzyme inhibition, by action on receptors and by direct effects on ion channels.

Direct action

These include drugs such as antacids that neutralise gastric acid, chelating agents such as desferrioxamine, which binds iron, volatile anaesthetic agents which may act non-specifically upon the lipid component of cell membranes and magnesium sulphate, which exerts its purgative action by an osmotic effect within the gut.

Enzyme inhibition

Many drugs come into this category such as anticholinesterases (e.g. neostigmine), monoamine oxidase inhibitors (MAOIs) (e.g. phenelzine), dopa decarboxylase inhibitors (e.g. benserazide), angiotensin converting enzyme (ACE) inhibitors (e.g. captopril) and phosphodiesterase inhibitors (e.g. aminophylline).

Receptors

This encompasses much the largest group of drugs and includes those that alter ionic permeability, alter intracellular metabolites especially calcium, enhance tyrosine kinase activity and those that modify gene transcription.

Ion channels

Ion channels may be affected such as nicotinic cholinergic for sodium ions and gamma amino butyric acid (GABA) for chloride ions as in the action of drugs such as thiopentone and benzodiazepines.

G-protein coupled processes

G-protein-coupled processes affecting receptors situated on the surface and interior of cells that mediate the action of natural chemical messengers upon intracellular

3

mechanisms. It allows the drug or chemical messenger to work rapidly as it does not have to penetrate the cell membrane and it often leads to amplification of the process. This is by far the commonest way that drugs work and include the actions of opioids, sympathomimetics, anticholinergics, dopamine and angiotensin effects. Activation of cell surface receptors associated with G-proteins may either activate (Gs) or inhibit (Gi) intracellular enzymes such as adenyl cyclase. The latter catalyses the conversion of ATP to cyclic AMP, which activates protein kinase C and instigates protein phosphorylation. This sets in motion intracellular events such as calcium mobilisation that leads to the inotropic effects of sympathomimetics. Other intermediates include cyclic GMP, nitric oxide, inositol triphosphate and diacylglycerol. An example is given in the section on anticholinergic drugs. It should be stated that the exact nature of transmitter–receptor interactions is not completely understood. The quantities of receptor molecules per gram of tissue is itself subject to complex regulation; e.g. thyroid hormone regulates the synthesis of β-receptors on heart cells.

Enhanced typosine kinase activity
Enhanced tyrosine kinase activity as with the effect of insulin on activation of tyrosine kinase and autophosphorylation of amino acids.

Gene transcription effects
Gene transcription effects such as the action of steroids and thyroid hormones which work by altering the expression of DNA and RNA.

Direct action on ion channels
This group includes the local anaesthetics-blocking sodium channels and calcium antagonists-blocking calcium channels.

Receptor-binding properties
To produce an effect, a drug must bind to a receptor.

Affinity
This relates to how well a drug binds to its receptor and conforms to the receptor-binding

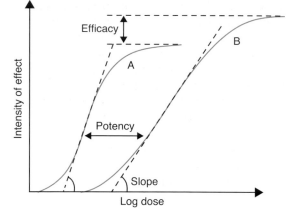

Fig. 3.2 Dose intensity effect showing potency (affinity) and efficacy (activity) differences.

site. For two opioids, the higher-affinity drug (e.g. fentanyl versus morphine) requires a lower dose to have a similar effect, i.e. fentanyl is more *potent* than morphine (0.1 mg being equivalent to 5–10 mg of morphine). In Fig. 3.2, drug A is more potent than drug B because it produces a similar effect at a lower concentration.

Activity
This relates to the magnitude of the effect of the drug once bound to the receptor and relates to how *efficacious* it is. Thus, looking again at Fig. 3.2 we can see that although A is more *potent* than drug B, at higher levels drug B is more *efficacious* than drug A because it produces a greater effect by having greater activity at the receptor.

Avidity
For the effect at a receptor to disappear the drug must dissociate again. Thus:

$$d + r \rightleftharpoons dr$$

In other words, as the drug concentration rises the receptor is occupied and an effect is produced, as it falls (due to distribution, metabolism and elimination) it becomes unoccupied and the effect diminishes.

For the majority of drugs this is true, the continuing effect being determined by the drug level as predicted by pharmacokinetic data.

Avidity is found with a number of drugs that do not act in this way and continue to occupy the receptor even though the level in the surrounding biophase is low. Buprenorphine and salmeterol (the long-acting β-2-agonist) are good examples of drugs with high receptor avidity. Although sharing almost identical pharmacokinetics with fentanyl, buprenorphine is only 50% dissociated from the opioid receptor at 1 h versus 90% at 10 min with fentanyl. Obviously, buprenorphine is much longer acting. With salmeterol the longevity is probably due to exo-receptor binding of the lipophilic tail of the drug, which allows it to repeatedly occupy the receptor.

Note: The term 'receptor' may also appear in a physiological context referring to 'sensory receptors'; these are complex structures such as muscle spindles or retinal rods.

Structure–activity relationship

The activity and other properties of many drugs are related to chemical structure. New drugs are 'tailored' to fit therapeutic requirements. For example, isoflurane and enflurane were designed to produce general anaesthesia based on the ether molecule, but with a lower solubility in blood, less irritant effects, and non-flammability.

Tolerance, tachyphylaxis and therapeutic index

- *Tolerance* is the decrease, over a period of time, in therapeutic effect produced by identical doses of the drug.

- *Tachyphylaxis* is the rapid development of tolerance.

- *Therapeutic index* or selectivity is the ratio between the dose producing undesired effects and the dose producing therapeutic effects. The median effective dose ED50 is that required to produce a certain intensity of effect in 50% of subjects. The median lethal dose LD50 is that which produces lethal effects in 50% of individuals (this evidently only applies to animal tests).

Drug–receptor interaction

Just because a drug binds to a receptor, it does not mean that it will produce an effect. Different types of interaction result in drugs being classified as agonists, antagonists and partial agonists.

- *Agonists* bind to receptors (affinity) and can initiate *maximal activity* (efficacy).

- *Antagonists* also bind to receptors (affinity) but have *no activity* (no efficacy). They may displace agonists and thus reverse their effects. This presumes that they actually have greater affinity for the receptor than the agonist. This is well demonstrated with naloxone that has higher affinity for opioid receptors than morphine, displacing the latter even at much lower concentrations.

- *Partial agonists* often bind with greater affinity but have less activity (efficacy) than full agonists. The circumstances in which a partial agonist may act as an antagonist or an agonist depends on both the efficacy of the drug and the pre-existing state of receptor occupation by agonist.

  - The *high-efficacy* partial agonist opioid buprenorphine only acts as an antagonist if there is excessive agonist already occupying the receptor. Thus, in fentanyl *overdose* buprenorphine acts like naloxone and reverses respiratory depression. However, in the presence of *small* amounts of agonist it acts in an additive way, e.g. a patient in pain following an inadequate dose of pethidine gains additional pain relief if buprenorphine is added (or vice versa). In normal clinical use buprenorphine is such a high-efficacy partial agonist that it is indistinguishable from other full agonist opioids such as morphine.

  - The *low-efficacy* partial agonist pindolol almost always acts as an antagonist (i.e. as a β-blocker). However, if there is zero underlying sympathetic activity (unlikely), the drug could act as an agonist (intrinsic sympathomimetic activity). Theoretically, there is a lessened risk of inducing

3

profound bradycardia in a patient with very low underlying sympathetic activity (unlike propranolol that slows the heart rate further still).

- The *medium-efficacy*, orally active, partial agonist xamoterol lies in between these two extremes and is used in the treatment of mild to moderate cardiac failure. It can act as an agonist (i.e. like adrenaline) if the underlying level of sympathetic activity is low to moderate thus improving cardiac function. In severe heart failure the underlying sympathetic activity is high so it acts like a β-blocker. This could lead to severe cardiac decompensation so the drug must be avoided in these patients.

Adverse effects of drugs
These can be divided into type A and type B. Type A occur as much more pronounced effect of the drug at normal dosage, e.g. excessive bradycardia with a small dose of propranolol. Type B (bizarre) reactions are not predictable and include immunological reactions such as penicillin allergy.

Plasma levels
Plasma levels may now be measured for a large number of drugs. It is an expensive complement to drug therapy and should be used only if there are clear advantages. Blood samples must be taken at specified times after drug administration to be of any value. The indications are as follows:

1. In some cases of treatment failure when there is a predictable relationship between plasma concentration and effects, e.g. anticonvulsants.

2. Use of drugs with a low therapeutic index or very serious side effects, e.g. lithium, gentamicin and theophylline.

3. In suicidal or accidental overdosage, e.g. paracetamol levels determine the management policy.

Drug interaction with anaesthetic agents
Caution about interaction of anaesthetic agents with other drugs is important. It may

occur by competition for binding sites in plasma proteins, saturation of metabolic pathways in liver or plasma, inhibition of inactivating enzymes, or by physiological potentiation. Some of the best-known examples are:

1. *Ecothiopate eye drops* used in glaucoma inhibit plasma cholinesterase prolonging the effect of suxamethonium.

2. *Aminoglycoside antibiotics* (e.g. gentamicin) have neuromuscular-blocking properties of their own, potentiating the effect of pancuronium and other relaxants.

3. *MAOIs* (e.g. iproniazid), by altering the metabolism of catecholamines and central analgesics, cause some patients to respond unpredictably to morphine or pethidine with hypotension, hypertension or coma. Response to inotropes and hypotensive agents is also unpredictable.

The physiology and pharmacology of the autonomic nervous system and circulatory control in the perioperative period

Introduction
The concept of the autonomic nervous system has resulted from anatomical and physiological studies carried out in the years since Langley first coined the term in 1898. The hypothalamus is the main site of integration of the autonomic nervous system, being a set of afferent and efferent nerve fibres and integrative neurones within the central nervous system (CNS). It represents the anatomical basis of regulatory reflexes which regulate visceral functions such as circulatory and temperature control, respiration, water balance, carbohydrate and fat metabolism. For this reason it has also been named the vegetative or involuntary nervous system. Studies in the past 20 years have shown that some regulatory functions can obey volitional control, suggesting cerebral cortical representation of some autonomic functions, e.g. BP control.

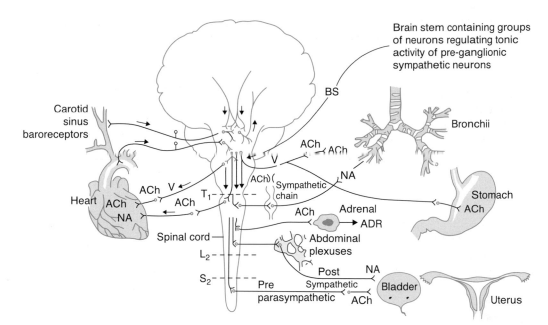

Fig. 3.3 Main components of the autonomic nervous system. NA: Noradrenaline; ADR: Adrenaline; ACH: Acetyl choline.

Anatomy and physiology

The first demonstration of the chemical nature of neurotransmission was made by Otto Loewi (1921) while studying the vagal innervation of the heart. The concept of a drug receptor (see above) has also emerged from experimental work in autonomic structures, on finding that different drugs may mimic or block different effects of the same natural neurotransmitter at different end organs. Traditionally, the autonomic nervous system has been divided into two anatomically and functionally distinct efferent divisions: the sympathetic and the parasympathetic (see Fig. 3.3).

Sympathetic system

Originating mainly in the hypothalamus, it emerges from cells in the intermediolateral columns of the thoracic and lumbar segments of the spinal cord (T1–L2) as the myelinated, white rami communicantes (B-fibres) that hitch a ride in the anterior nerve roots. They supply the pre-ganglionic innervation of the para-vertebral chain of sympathetic ganglia and abdominal plexuses. Synaptic transmission in the ganglia is mainly cholinergic with both nicotinic and muscarinic as well as

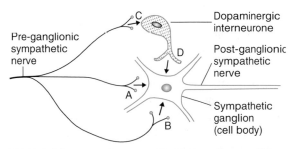

Fig. 3.4 Diagram of a sympathetic ganglion and the dopaminergic interneurone. For key to A, B, C and D please refer to Table 3.1.

dopaminergic receptors (Fig. 3.4). These involve both excitatory and inhibitory postsynaptic potentials (EPSP, IPSP). The unmyelinated, grey rami communicantes (C-fibres) leave the ganglia as post-ganglionic neurones to rejoin peripheral nerves and supply the end organs with noradrenergic nerve endings.

The pre-ganglionic neurones receive excitatory and inhibitory synaptic inputs from the spinal cord, brain stem and other higher centres. There is a constant background discharge in these neurones, which is referred to as underlying 'sympathetic tone'. This is responsible for maintenance of tone in the smooth muscle of capacitance and resistance

27

Table 3.1 **Transmitters and blockers in the sympathetic ganglion** (refer to Fig 3.4)

Site	Transmitter	Effect of transmitter	Receptor blocker	Effect of receptor blocker on ganglionic transmission
A	Acetylcholine (nicotinic)	Initial EPSP: facilitation of ganglionic transmission	Nicotine: pentolium, trimetaphan, d-tubocurarine	Inhibition
B	Acetylcholine (muscarinic)	Late EPSP: facilitation of ganglionic transmission	Atropine	Inhibition
C	Acetylcholine (muscarinic)	Stimulates the dopaminergic (inhibitory) interneurone	Atropine: pancuronium	Facilitation
D	Dopamine	IPSP: inhibits ganglionic transmission	α-blocking drugs	Facilitation

blood vessels, thereby maintaining BP. Since the B-fibres may synapse immediately in the sympathetic chain or go up/down the chain to a higher or lower level (including the adrenals, themselves modified sympathetic ganglia), the sympathetic system tends to respond to stimuli as an integral system. All nerve endings discharge noradrenaline, with two known exceptions: sweat glands and blood vessels in voluntary muscle, which are cholinergic.

Parasympathetic system

This has two main outflows from the CNS, one arising with cranial nerves and the other with sacral roots. Pre-ganglionic neurones are much longer than their equivalents in the sympathetic system but are also cholinergic. The ganglia are situated very close to or within the effector organs (e.g. Auerbach plexuses in the intestine). The post-ganglionic neurones are very short and release acetylcholine. The parasympathetic system tends to respond to stimuli in a more localised fashion. There is no evidence of parasympathetic tone regulating BP.

Innervation of effector organs

Most viscera are innervated by both sympathetic and parasympathetic systems; the effects of stimulation are usually antagonistic (e.g. sympathetic accelerates the heart, parasympathetic slows it, other examples being the pupil and bronchial smooth muscle). A few effectors receive innervation only from the sympathetic system such as sweat glands and 'resistance' blood vessels in the skin and gut.

Ganglia are far from being simple relay stations and are neuronal networks with more than one neurotransmitter involved. The diagram of a sympathetic ganglion, (Fig 3.4) displays the complexity of the system and the many transmitters involved.

The interaction between the sympathetic and parasympathetic nervous systems is best illustrated with reference to Fig. 3.5 and Table 3.2. Here, you can see that stimulation of the parasympathetic nervous system both slows the heart directly by release of acetylcholine but also presynaptically inhibits the release of noradrenaline.

In addition to the neural pathways and neurotransmitters described above, there are other fibres innervating the same end organs that release other chemicals. Some have a well-established role, but many of the newly described substances do not exhibit uniform effects in different species, and the relevance

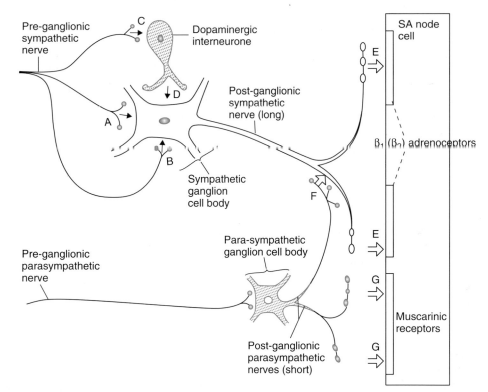

Fig. 3.5 Innervation of the SA node. Refer to Tables 3.1 and 3.2 for explanation of A–G.

Table 3.2 The autonomic innervation of the SA node. Nature and effects of the various transmitters and their respective blocking drugs (refer to Fig. 3.5)

Site	Transmitter	Effect of transmitter	Receptor blocker	Effect of receptor blocker
E	Noradrenaline	Stimulation of β-receptors leading to increased rate of SA node firing; heart rate increases	β-blockers, e.g. propranolol, labetalol	Heart rate decreases
F	Acetylcholine (muscarinic)	Presynaptic inhibition of noradrenaline from adrenergic neurone	Atropine: pancuronium	Increase in noradrenaline release; heart rate increases
G	Acetylcholine (muscarinic)	Stimulation of muscarinic receptors leading to decreased rate of SA node firing; heart rate decreases	Atropine: pancuronium	Heart rate increases

to human physiology is unclear. Examples are bradykinin, 5-hydroxytryptamine, enkephalin, substance P and vasoactive intestinal peptide (VIP).

Pharmacology

The natural transmitters adrenaline, dopamine and noradrenaline are often used therapeutically. A large number of synthetic drugs have been studied which mimic or block the effects of the natural transmitters at particular locations, depending upon the type of receptor present. Accordingly, they are designated agonists, partial agonists or competitive antagonists (see above).

The neurotransmitters described in the autonomic nervous system are also present in the CNS. Consequently, drugs prescribed for peripheral effects should always be considered to have central effects as well, their state of ionisation in plasma dictating whether they cross the blood–brain barrier (see above).

Cholinergic system

There are three types of peripheral cholinergic receptors, and there may be more within the CNS:

- *Nicotinic neuromuscular cholinergic receptors* occur at the neuromuscular synapse of voluntary muscle. It is named 'nicotinic' after nicotine was found to be the first drug having agonist effects. Stimulation of this receptor produces depolarisation and contraction of voluntary muscle.

- *Nicotinic ganglionic cholinergic receptors* are also present at the synapses of both sympathetic and parasympathetic ganglia (see Figs 3.4 and 3.5), and are also excitatory. The specific competitive antagonist drugs for this receptor are called ganglion-blockers and were the first drugs used to lower BP in the early 1950s (Table 3.1 A and Fig. 3.4 A). Their effect is to reduce traffic of sympathetic impulses that maintain tone in vascular smooth muscle. This class of drug is not used in ambulatory patients because of postural

hypotension, but pentolinium is still occasionally used during anaesthesia to lower BP. The neuromuscular blocker d-tubocurarine has marked ganglion-blocking properties. Vecuronium, rocuronium, cis-atracurium and atracurium are much more specific for neuromuscular nicotinic receptors.

- *Muscarinic receptors* occur at parasympathetic nerve endings (Fig. 3.5 G and Table 3.2 G); muscarine mimics the action of acetylcholine at this receptor (see below).

Anticholinergic drugs

Types and structure

Three anticholinergic drugs are in common usage. Atropine is a racemic mixture of d and l atropine of which the l form is much more active than the d form. Hyoscine exists in the l form and differs from atropine by the addition of an oxygen bridge. Glycopyrrolate is a synthetic anticholinergic and possesses a quaternary ammonium structure which means that it is a water-soluble, ionised drug at body pH, unlike atropine and scopolamine which are non-ionised and lipid soluble. Glycopyrrolate thus has limited membrane (e.g. gut, placenta and brain) penetrating potential. In comparison with atropine and hyoscine it is poorly absorbed orally, does not cause fetal tachycardia and does not interfere with CNS cholinergic function.

Mechanism of action

These drugs are competitive antagonists (almost exclusively) at the muscarinic receptor (e.g. Fig. 3.5 G) with little effect at nicotinic sites. Their broad range of actions throughout the CNS and autonomic nervous systems are mediated via three stages:

1. receptor binding,

2. activation of guanidine nucleotides (G-proteins),

3. transduction via G-proteins to produce intracellular effects including inhibition of adenyl cyclase (G_i) and activation of

phospholipase C, inositol triphosphate and diacylglycerol with ionic flux of calcium and potassium across cell membranes (G_q).

There are five well-defined subtypes of muscarinic cholinergic receptors in humans, denoted M1 to M5, each encoded by a unique gene and differing in their amino acid sequence. M1 receptors are mainly found in the CNS, M2 in the cardiovascular system (CVS), M3 in secretory glands (e.g. salivary), M4 in CNS and cardiac muscle and M5 in CNS. All three drugs are non-specific antagonists at these receptors, but atropine has a two-fold preference for M1 (CNS) receptors. M3-receptors (glandular secretion, blockade producing a reduction in salivation) are much more sensitive than M2-receptors (cardiac, blockade causing an increase in heart rate). Thus, for all three drugs, a greater dose is needed to prevent bradycardia when compared to reducing salivation.

Effects
In clinical practice, a 'normal' parenteral dose of hyoscine (0.4 mg/70 kg) does not cause tachycardia whereas an equivalent dose of atropine (0.6 mg) and glycopyrrolate (0.4 mg) does. Effects on reduction of secretions and intestinal motility are similar. Other major effects are summarised in Table 3.3.

Pharmacokinetics
Both atropine and scopolamine are well absorbed by the oral route whereas glycopyrrolate is not. Oral atropine has adequate M2 effects, thus preventing bradycardia, whereas oral glycopyrrolate is only effective in drying secretions (M3). Hyoscine is rarely used orally in anaesthesia but is available in a transdermal preparation that is useful for prevention of motion exacerbated vomiting in ambulant patients following day surgery. All three drugs are well absorbed by the i.m. route. After i.v. administration, the onset of atropine is much faster with a shorter duration of action when compared with glycopyrrolate. This is due to atropine's much higher Vd, presumably as a result of increased lipid solubility.

Uses
Atropine is used as a premedicant in those cases where excess salivation and bronchial secretion is problematical, e.g. babies and patients undergoing upper GIT or respiratory

3

Table 3.3 **Major effects of atropine, hyoscine and glycopyrrolate**

Heart rate	Increase (less with scopolamine)
Bronchi	Bronchodilation and reduction of secretions
Salivation	Reduced and dried secretions
Sweating	Reduced, may cause hyperpyrexia in children
GIT	Cardiac sphincter tone decreased
	Gastric secretion and acidity decreased Gut motility decreased: inhibits effects of metoclopramide on gastric emptying
Pupil size	Increased (mydriasis) with atropine and hysoscine, not glycopyrrolate
CNS	Atropine and scopolamine cause sedation and restlessness, even precipitating coma if the dose is high enough (central anticholinergic syndrome, the elderly are more susceptible) Glycopyrrolate has much less effect. Hyoscine may cause amnesia

3

endoscopy. During anaesthesia it is used to reverse or prevent bradycardia, particularly associated with anticholinesterases such as neostigmine, which are used for reversal of residual neuromuscular blockade (q.v.).

Hyoscine is still used for premedication in combination with papaveretum where it causes sedation, anti-emesis and reduction in salivation.

Glycopyrrolate is used exclusively by the parenteral route, due to poor absorption from the GIT. Uses are similar to atropine but lack of CNS side effects and better-matched onset and offset time with neostigmine make it the agent of choice in reversal of neuromuscular blockade, especially at extremes of age. It is also preferred in obstetrics for its lack of propensity to cause foetal tachycardia.

Adrenergic system

There are two main types of adrenergic receptors, α and β, which may co-exist in the same effector organ. Subtypes of these receptors, α-1 and -2 and β-1 and -2, have been identified with the advent of specific blockers and antagonists. They are distributed throughout the body, including the CNS, and both types are activated by noradrenaline and adrenaline. Activation of α- and β-receptors often has opposite physiological effects upon smooth muscle, such as in bronchi and in arterioles, a poorly understood phenomenon. Possibly regulation of synthesis of either type of receptor determines the relative effect of natural transmitters. A schematic diagram of a noradrenergic synapse is shown in Fig. 3.6.

With reference to Fig. 3.6, it is important to realise that the effects of *noradrenaline* are terminated at the adrenergic neurone by *reuptake* from the synaptic cleft (as shown by the arrow). Some noradrenaline is broken down in the synaptic cleft by COMT and in the adrenergic neurone by MAO. The effects of *acetylcholine* in the muscarinic nerve ending are terminated by *metabolism* by acetylcholinesterases.

Classic examples of location of β-receptors are the heart (excitatory), uterus (inhibitory), bronchi (dilation), platelets (aggregation) and

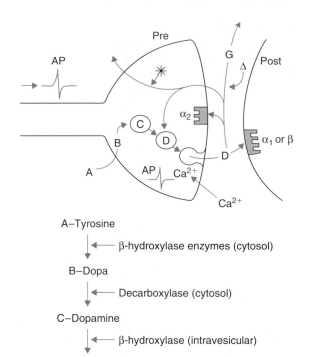

A–Tyrosine

$\downarrow$ ← β-hydroxylase enzymes (cytosol)

B–Dopa

$\downarrow$ ← Decarboxylase (cytosol)

C–Dopamine

$\downarrow$ ← β-hydroxylase (intravesicular)

D–Noradrenaline

Fig. 3.6 Noradrenergic synapse (adrenergic neurone ending) and the steps in synthesis of noradrenaline. AP is action potential; Pre, presynaptic terminal; Post, postsynaptic terminal; α, 1,2, α-receptors; β, β-receptors, O is storage vesicles for various stages of NAD synthesis, D is catechol-O-methyl transferase (COMT) and ✳ is monoamine oxidase (MAO). The letters A to Δ refer to the stages of NAD synthesis. G represents the breakdown products of norepinephrine.

brown adipose tissue (heat production). Examples of α-receptor location are the eye (mydriasis), skin and visceral arteries (constriction), veins (constriction) and bladder sphincter (contraction). α-receptors have been identified in many structures without a complete understanding of their physiological role; such as the spinal cord, associated with pain pathways, in the brain stem associated with the control of BP and temperature, and in human platelets.

The step between activation of α- and β-receptors on the cell surface and the intracellular response is mediated by G-proteins (see above), both stimulatory (Gs) and inhibitory (Gi).

Adrenergic drugs

α-blockers are no longer used on their own as hypotensive agents in ambulatory patients because of postural effects and reflex tachycardia; phentolamine is used in cardiac surgery to lower BP by a reduction in systemic vascular resistance (SVR):

- *α-1-agonists* such as phenylephrine are used to increase SVR and BP during cardio-pulmonary bypass and for maintenance of BP during carotid artery surgery. Large doses of dopamine may also produce α-1-effects (see below).

- *α-2-agonists* such as clonidine pre-synaptically inhibit the release of noradrenaline at adrenergic neurone endings. Interestingly, these agents have been found to produce anti-nociception when applied spinally and to augment the effect of general anaesthetics. A more specific α-2-agonist, dexmetotomidine, reduces anaesthetic requirements by up to 90% and is now licensed for sedation in ICU.

- *β-blocking drugs* have been extensively studied in recent years because of their application to long-term management of high BP, dysrhythmias and anginal pain. The specificity of drugs for β-1 and -2 receptors is far less marked than that seen between α- and β-receptors. Asthmatic patients should never be given β-blockers; even drugs claimed as β-1 specific may precipitate fatal bronchospasm.

- *β-agonists* are widely used as inotropic agents (e.g. isoprenaline), as bronchodilators in asthma (salbutamol) and to arrest premature labour in obstetrics (ritodrine). Dopamine and the synthetic inotrope, dobutamine, act on β-1-receptors and are used to increase cardiac output in myocardial infarction, cardiomypopathies and septic shock. Salbutamol, claimed to be β-2 specific, may cause severe tachycardia due to the presence of β-2-receptors in the atria. A newer inotrope, dopexamine, is also β-2 specific and used for inotropic support and as a vasodilator in chronic heart failure and in heart failure following cardiac surgery. It is claimed to have a preferential effect on maintaining gut and renal perfusion in septic shock but this is yet to be substantiated in a large clinical trial.

- *α- and β-effects:* some synthetic agonist drugs have both α- and β-effects like the natural transmitters. They may act indirectly by promoting the release of noradrenaline (e.g. ephedrine) or by direct action on the receptor (e.g. metaraminol). Labetalol has both α-1-, β-1- and -2-blocking activity.

Dopaminergic system

Dopamine is the immediate precursor of noradrenaline, the step being catalysed by dopamine-β-hydroxylase, an enzyme which is present within the microvesicles of noradrenergic nerve terminals (Fig. 3.6). Groups of central neurones lacking the enzyme secrete dopamine, such as those found in pathways controlling voluntary movement where depletion causes Parkinson's disease, and are also involved in vomiting reflexes (Chapter 18). Peripherally, dopamine receptors have been identified in the kidney (vasodilation) and in the carotid body chemoreceptor (inhibition).

Dopamine infused at rates of 1–3 mg/kg/min (renal dose) specifically increases renal blood flow; at higher doses it also has β, and finally α-effects. Examples of synthetic dopamine agonists are apomorphine and bromocriptine that are both used in Parkinson's disease. Dopamine blockers are used in psychiatric disorders (haloperidol) and as antiemetics (prochlorperazine, domperidone and metoclopramide). It is no longer accepted that dopamine has any renal protective effect.

Dopaminergic receptors

- DA 1 receptors mediate relaxation of renal blood vessels and gut smooth muscle

- DA 2 receptors mediate pre-synaptic inhibition of dopamine and noradrenaline

3

33

3

Other systems

There are other transmitter systems in the autonomic system, as stated earlier. A number of drugs related to these systems are finding a place in clinical practice, such as ketanserin (5-HT blocker), in the management of certain types of chronic limb pain and ondansetron and granisetron (5-HT3 blockers) in emetic chemotherapy regimes and post-operative nausea and vomiting.

Pharmacological effects unrelated to receptors

Many other drugs act upon autonomic functions without direct receptor interaction. They are mostly hypotensive agents:

- The action may be predominantly central, such as reserpine, which drops BP by reducing sympathetic 'tone' centrally.

- The action is at the pre-synaptic end of adrenergic terminals, by interfering with catecholamine synthesis (α-methyldopa), storage (reserpine), release (guanethidine) or re-uptake (desipramine).

The tricyclic antidepressants on the other hand block re-uptake of noradrenaline at the adrenergic neurone ending, thus enhancing its effect.

The enzymatic breakdown of neurotransmitter may be inhibited, enhancing the local concentration of transmitter. MAOIs slow down the breakdown of catecholamines, both peripherally and centrally; the latter effect may be beneficial in depression. Neostigmine acts by a similar mechanism on cholinergic terminals by inhibiting cholinesterase; it does not cross the blood–brain barrier. Another anticholinesterase, physostigmine, crosses easily into the brain; it is thus able to reverse central depressant effects of overdose with atropine, hyoscine or tricyclic antidepressants.

Finally, there is a group of drugs that act via nitric oxide and directly relax smooth muscle. Examples are sodium nitroprusside and nitro-glycerine whose hypotensive effects are initially mediated by relaxation of venous smooth muscle and at higher dosage by arteriolar dilation as well. Hydrallazine also acts in a similar way upon smooth muscle, with preference for the arteriolar side. Papaverine and theophylline are other examples of smooth muscle relaxants. The latter acts upon intracellular cyclic-AMP mediation of β-effects.

Circulatory control during the perioperative period

Introduction

Having discussed the physiology and pharmacology of the autonomic nervous system it is appropriate to look at how these systems work in collaboration with peripheral circulatory control during anaesthesia and surgery. It is obvious that safely conducted anaesthesia requires:

- sound knowledge of circulatory physiology and pharmacology;

- maintenance of adequate cardiac output and perfusion pressure;

- provision of normoxia and adequate oxygen delivery, normocapnea and adequate analgesia;

- minimisation of heat loss by maintenance of a warm operating environment (22–23°C), use of warming blankets, warmed fluids and humidification of the inspired gas.

Theoretical aspects of circulatory control

Pressure, flow and resistance

The Poiseuille–Hagen equation describes the factors that determine flow of a homogenous Newtonian fluid through a non-distensible cylindrical tube:

$$\text{blood flow} = \frac{\text{perfusion pressure} \times \text{radius}^4 \times \pi}{\text{length} \times \text{viscosity} \times 8}$$

The radius of the blood vessel and viscosity of the blood determine the resistive component above. Radius (being to the power of 4), therefore, has a dramatic effect on resistance.

Blood is a non-Newtonian fluid due to the presence of suspended cells (red blood cells, leucocytes and platelets). This results in non-linearity of viscosity (the Fahreus-Lindqvist effect) whereby it is effectively reduced as the radius of the vessel diminishes. This tends to counteract the effects of increased resistance as the vessel narrows.

Thus, in simpler terms:

■ *Blood flow* to a tissue is proportional to *pressure difference* divided by *resistance* (cf. Ohm's law of electrical resistance where V = IR or I = V/R).

Cardiac output (Q), BP and SVR: principles of peripheral circulatory control

Cardiac output is the product of stroke volume and heart rate. Stroke volume is determined by *preload* (mainly resulting from venous return), inherent *contractile* state (determined by sympathetic stimulation and endogenous (or exogenous) catecholamines and *afterload* (resistance of the circulation to ejection of blood). Again, rearranging the equation above, BP (V) is the product of Q (I) and SVR (R). Frequent measurement of BP is fundamental to good perioperative practice. However, it is clear from the above that a fall in BP may be due to, either a fall in Q, a fall in SVR or a combination of the two.

During surgery and anaesthesia, *a fall in Q* results from

■ *decreased preload* and thus stroke volume resulting from hypovolaemia (absolute, due to blood loss or relative or from vasodilation due to anaesthetic agents);

■ *decreased contractility* from the depressant effects of anaesthetic drugs or inadvertent hypoxaemia;

■ *increased afterload* due to peripheral vasoconstriction, often occurring in association with relative hypovolaemia and increased sympathetic tone.

Since maintenance of Q (and oxygen delivery) is of such crucial importance, it is surprising that methods to measure Q directly are not routinely used during anaesthesia. Newer techniques of non-invasive measurement will assume increasing relevance in the future, including oesophageal (Deltex Cardio Q®) and transtracheal Doppler ultrasound, pulse wave contour analysis (PiCCO and Lithium Dilution Measurement of Cardiac Output (LiDCO)), NICO and thoracic bioimpedance techniques (see Chapter 9). These methods have a good correlation with more invasive techniques such as thermal dilution. BP must be maintained by volume replacement to restore Q.

A *fall in SVR* usually results from the vasodilator effects of the agent (see below) either directly (as with isoflurane and propofol) or indirectly due to histamine release (such as morphine). It can also occur due to mesenteric traction during abdominal surgery.

Neural control of BP and vascular resistance

The reflex response to hypovolaemia and a falling *venous pressure* is mediated by the 'low pressure' cardiopulmonary baroreceptors situated in the vicinity of the superior vena cava and right atrial junction. This results in an increase in sympathetic tone and peripheral vascular resistance with arteriolar and venular constriction (Q is actually less than normal). The main site of increase in SVR is the arterioles and to some extent the small arteries and the pre-capillary sphincters. Although this may not be marked in some organ beds (e.g. cerebral), it is in skin and muscle.

The 'high pressure' baroreceptor reflexes are activated by sensors located in the arch of the aorta and the carotid sinus and respond to a falling *arterial* pressure (from any cause) by increased sympathetic activity. During anaesthesia, inhalational agents and i.v. induction agents effectively block this reflex increase in SVR (e.g. to hypovolaemia) and attenuate the central neural reflexes that stabilise BP. In addition, direct vasoconstricting effects on the peripheral circulation (e.g. to circulating catecholamines) are depressed. Nitrous oxide, benzodiazepines, ketamine, rocuronium, cis-atracurium and opioids such

3

35

as fentanyl (not morphine and pethidine) have much less effect.

The elderly, hypertensive and volume-depleted patients are much more sensitive to the haemodynamic depressant effects of anaesthesia and often respond with a precipitate fall in BP. It is thus crucial to adequately fluid resuscitate hypovolaemic patients prior to anaesthesia, avoiding where possible depressant agents. Conversely, high doses are needed to produce profound *hypotension* during anaesthesia in the young, normovolaemic patient who is surgically stressed.

Humoral control of BP and vascular resistance

Longer-term effects on BP and SVR are humorally mediated through release of agents with marked vasoactive properties such as adrenaline, noradrenaline, vasopressin, prostaglandins, kinins and angiotensin II. In general, the larger arterioles (first and second order) are under predominantly neural influence while the smaller arterioles (third and fourth order) respond mainly to humoral (and direct vasodilator) influences.

Local control of blood flow

Regulation of blood flow through capillary beds is mainly concerned with the supply of adequate oxygen and nutrients to cells requiring them. At any one time, only small sections of the capillary bed are perfused. As metabolism continues, hypoxia and hypercarbia supervene, together with the production of metabolic products such as adenine, hydrogen ions, potassium and lactic acid. These substances tend to cause relaxation of pre-capillary sphincters allowing blood flow to be re-established. Thus, given an adequate supply of blood to the tissue bed (dependent also on remote factors) it can then be appropriately distributed by local endothelial factors.

The role of the endothelium

The role of the intact endothelium in the production of vasodilator substances such as nitric oxide and prostacyclin (PGi2), is substantial. Nitric oxide (NO) is formed from l-arginine under the influence of the enzyme NO synthase. NO is a low MW volatile free radical (i.e. it has an unpaired reactive electron in the outer electron shell that can thus combine covalently with other molecules). It combines with and activates guanylate cyclase in vascular smooth muscle cells causing vasodilation, inhibition of platelet aggregation and adherence of neutrophils. NO synthase exists in two main forms. In basal conditions it is present as a calcium- and calmodulin-dependent enzyme which can be activated by vasodilators such as acetylcholine, adenosine, histamine and bradykinin. This form is controlled by cell-surface receptors. A calcium-independent form is produced by sepsis and cytokines, which once 'turned on' is no longer under control of cell surface receptors. Thus, excess NO synthase may cause the hypotension and myocardial depression of septic shock.

NO and PGi2 are produced in response to potentially vasoconstricting factors, such as thromboxane (TxA2) and adenosine diphosphate (ADP) produced from platelets following vascular damage and endothelial injury. These vasodilatory factors, together with fibrinolytic agents such as tissue plasminogen activator (TPA) limit stasis and thrombosis following endothelial damage. In their absence, coagulation and thrombosis occur, the endothelium and distal tissue become hypoxic and events are set in motion that can lead to irreversible cellular damage.

To complicate the issue still further intact endothelium also produces vasoconstrictor substances such as endothelium-derived contracting factors (EDCF) and endothelin. The latter is a 21 amino acid peptide that has greater vasoconstricting activity than any other hormone known. It is also responsible for the metabolism of renin and angiotensin I to produce angiotensin II, another potent vasoconstrictor. Additional factors of relevance during anaesthesia include the effect on the endothelium of smoking, ageing, arteriosclerosis and endothelial changes due to hypertension and hyperlipidaemia. It would appear that in

3

these circumstances the endothelium is much more sensitive to contracting substances as well as being less able to prevent the formation of thrombus due to tissue damage.

Conclusion

It is clear that circulatory control during anaesthesia, especially if compounded by the effects of surgery, hypovolaemia and sepsis, is extremely complex. The major points of note involve the provision of adequate anaesthesia and analgesia without compromising cardiac output and oxygen delivery, together with maintenance of normovolaemia.

3

4

Principles of preoperative assessment, optimisation and management

Aims

This chapter attempts to give an overall picture of the rationale of preoperative assessment and management. In particular, it outlines

- what we are trying to achieve and the rationale for preoperative preparation;

- the adverse effects of preoperative morbidity (e.g. diabetes, hypertension or obesity) on postoperative outcome and how can they be minimised;

- the favourable (and unfavourable) outcomes of doing preoperative tests, their significance and the concept of sensitivity and specificity;

- the resource implications of over (and under) investigation;

- the commonly prescribed drugs that have a relevance to perioperative management;

- the evidence that optimisation of patients' haemodynamic parameters improves outcome.

Objectives

After reading this chapter, you should

- have a clear appreciation of the rationale for preoperative assessment and its impact on patient morbidity and mortality;

- have a clear strategy for optimising the patient physically and mentally, and thereby reducing risk;

- appreciate that returning patients to a healthy state as soon as possible postoperatively is the overall aim of preoperative assessment and management;

- have a clear strategy for managing existing patient–drug administration in the perioperative period;

- appreciate that, above all, excellence in perioperative management requires a team approach between all parties involved, i.e. the patient, the patient's family (where appropriate), the general practitioner (GP), the surgical team, the anaesthesia team, other relevant medical and diagnostic specialties and the nursing and paramedical staff on the ward.

Introduction

Advances in anaesthetic and surgical technique coupled with an ageing population have led to an increasing number of 'high-risk' operative events; these events impose ever-increasing demands on patients' health and wellbeing.

The imperative of the preoperative visit is to assess the risks of surgery and anaesthesia, and to balance them against the benefits of the proposed operation. The surgeon and anaesthetist concerned must, therefore, jointly carry it out. Two elements combine to constitute a high-risk surgical event; firstly, the health of the patient, and secondly, the nature of the surgery.

The health of the patient, in turn, embraces two factors; firstly, the presence or absence of significant co-morbidities such as heart disease or respiratory disease and secondly, probably more subtly, the patients inherent physiological reserves.

The bulk of this chapter deals with identification and correction of reversible elements of any existing co-morbidities through well-established principles. However, recent studies are developing insights, which allow objective assessment not just of 'co-existing disease', but also more significantly of 'physiological reserve', and in turn ways of 'optimising' that reserve.

Managing the high-risk patient involves two essential stages:

- Identification of the 'high-risk' patient.

- Optimisation of the 'high-risk' patient.

Identification of the 'high-risk' patient

The scale of the problem
Although the overall role and recommendations of the National Confidential

Enquiry Into Perioperative Deaths (NCEPOD) have already been discussed in Chapter 2, it is worth re-emphasising some of the key points in the context of preoperative assessment. Annually, there are about 2.8 million operations in England, Wales and Northern Ireland. The risk of death within 30 days of operation is estimated between 0.7% and 1.7%. Thus, approximately 20,000 deaths within 30 days of an operation are reported to NCEPOD each year. A random sample from these deaths showed that

- one-third of deaths occurred on or before day 2 of the operation;

- the types of operation included are general surgery 46%, orthopaedics 22%, vascular surgery 11%, urology 7% and cardiac surgery 4%;

- the classification of operations was as follows: emergency 15%, urgent 52%, scheduled 24% and elective 7%;

- 87% of patients were aged over 60 years and 71% of patients were aged over 70 years;

- 84% of patients scored 3 or higher on the American Society of Anaesthesiologists (ASA) score (see below);

- 85% of patients had one or more co-existing diseases at the time of operation, 45% had cardiac disease, 30% had respiratory disease and 16% renal impairment;

- 23% had had their operation delayed to improve their condition;

- surgeons when questioned, indicated that in 58% of patients, a significant risk of death had been identified before operation, and that they knew that 8% of patients operated on were almost certain to die;

- 32% of patients were admitted to an ICU postoperatively, and 8% to an HDU;

- 5% of patients were denied ICU admission through lack of capacity;

- respiratory diseases were implicated in the death of 37% of patients, cardiac diseases in 36% and renal impairment in 22% of patients.

Other studies and data bases give an overall perioperative mortality of between 1% and 3%, however, in the age group of 65 years and above mortality associated with

- elective surgery is ~5–10%,

- emergency surgery is ~23–55%.

Thus, those patients who die after surgery are more likely to be elderly, to have co-existing medical disorders and require urgent or emergency surgery. The NCEPOD data suggests that in the majority of cases, these risks are identified before surgery both by surgeons and anaesthetists. Most deaths occur after abdominal, colorectal or major orthopaedic surgery.

Identification of the 'high-risk' patient: by clinical assessment

Various scoring systems are available as clinical tools to assess severity of perioperative risk, the two most commonly used are the ASA classification and the Goldman Index score for the presence of significant co-morbidities and are discussed below. However, Shoemaker in the course of his landmark studies, in the early eighties, identified a list of specific circumstances that are probably useful to include here:

- History of severe cardiorespiratory illness.

- Extensive ablative surgery for carcinoma.

- Severe multiple trauma (involving three or more organs and two or more cavities).

- Massive acute blood loss ~8 units.

- Age >70 years.

- Clinical shock, mean arterial pressure (MAP) ~60 mmHg.

- Septicaemia.

- Significant respiratory failure, $PaO_2 < 8\,kPa$ (60 mmHg) on room air.

4

- On mechanical ventilation for >48 h.

- Acute abdominal catastrophe with haemodynamic instability.

- Acute renal failure (ARF).

- End-stage vascular disease.

Identification of the 'high-risk' patient: by physiological assessment

Some patients have a level of cardiovascular reserve that is so low that they are unable to meet the physiological challenge of major surgery. Studies have shown that the ability to increase oxygen delivery in response to stimulation with filling and inotropes tested preoperatively, correlates directly with outcome postoperatively. Patients who readily elevate their oxygen delivery in response to stimulation do not die. Decreasing ability to increase oxygen delivery in response to stimulation is associated with increasing mortality.

Optimisation of the 'high-risk' surgical patient

Shoemaker, in a series of observational studies, demonstrated a group of patients whom he deemed high risk and who had a 28-day postoperative mortality of 30–40%. He used simple clinical criteria to identify these patients (see above). Shoemaker went on to establish which of the commonly measured variables predicted outcome within this patient group. He examined over 30 variables in several thousand patients and demonstrated that only variables related to blood volume and flow had prognostic value. Survivors of high-risk surgery demonstrated supra-normal values for cardiac index (CI), oxygen delivery (DO_2) and oxygen consumption (VO_2). Following on from this work, several studies have examined the hypothesis that these supra-normal values should be applied as therapeutic goals in prophylactically 'optimising' high-risk patients before surgery.

Survivors	Normal population
Cardiac index (l/min/m^2)	
4.5	2.8–3.5
Oxygen delivery (l/min/m^2)	
600	400–500
Oxygen consumption (l/min/m^2)	
170	120–140

Studies aimed at optimising high-risk patients towards supra-normal values either preoperatively or immediately postoperatively showed reduced mortality and morbidity in the treatment group. Interestingly, the same therapeutic goals applied to patients in established critical illness or sepsis lead to an increased mortality in the treatment group.

The preoperative visit

The preoperative visit should focus around two basic questions, namely:

- Is this patient as fit as he or she can be, to undergo this procedure? If not …

- What are the risks/benefits of delaying surgery while treatment is undertaken?

This approach may lead to the seemingly anomalous situation that an elderly man with optimally treated heart failure and stable, but severe respiratory failure may be accepted for surgery, whereas a young fit patient with a 'minor' chest infection is not. The former patient is 'as fit as he can be', the latter is not.

Adequate time must be allowed to assess the patients preoperatively, if delays and cancellations are to be prevented. For instance, many elderly patients benefit from treatment of preoperative cardiac failure, dysrhythmias and chest infections, but this may take several days. Pre-assessment clinics are ideal places to pick up such problems, but often difficult to organise at a time, which is close enough to the proposed operation date.

The house surgeon, nurse practitioner or medical student clerking the surgical patient is often the first person to detect and draw attention to the abnormalities likely to cause problems with anaesthesia.

General aspects

After introducing yourself, a general review of the patient is undertaken. Check the name, the proposed operation, the hospital number and the patient chart for indications of previous problems and pathology. Take time to answer any questions, the patient may still have about the operation and its effects, especially, the amount of pain that he or she may suffer, and how it can be alleviated in the postoperative period. In particular, make note of the following.

Complications (patient and blood relatives) with previous anaesthetics

These may range from nausea and vomiting to severe anaphylaxis with anaesthetic drugs. Pharmacogenetic problems, such as porphyria, absence of plasma cholinesterase and malignant hyperthermia (MH) (see later) may be detected from the history of the patient and require further investigation. If the patient has not had a previous anaesthetic or had only a minor one, then a history of specific anaesthetic problems in the immediate blood family should be sought.

Smoking

This is associated with increased cardiovascular and respiratory pathology in proportion to the 'pack-year' history (number of packs of 20/day multiplied by the number of years of smoking). Smokers have an increased incidence of postoperative pulmonary complications, especially, after upper abdominal surgery, where the incidence of clinically significant respiratory tract infection is about 70%, five times higher than non-smokers. Blood levels of carbon monoxide (COHb) in heavy smokers are increased three-fold up to 15% in some cases, resulting in a reduction in oxygen-carrying capacity equivalent to the loss of 2 g/dl of Hb. Should the patient be advised to stop smoking prior

to surgery? To significantly reduce the incidence of postoperative chest infection after upper abdominal surgery takes 3–6 months abstention. This would only be feasible in compliant patients with non-urgent surgery, but is nevertheless a worthwhile goal to achieve. Acute cessation of smoking (for 12 h or more) is also beneficial as it reduces COHb levels (half-life 60 min), and is equivalent, in terms of blood oxygen carriage, to a one or two unit blood transfusion!

Alcohol and drug abuse

High alcohol intake and long-standing sedative or analgesic therapy increases requirements of drugs used in anaesthesia, usually by hepatic enzyme induction. Studies have shown markedly increased opioid requirements for postoperative pain relief in opioid addicts. Knowledge of this preoperatively will allow a suitable dose strategy to be devised. Recent work has demonstrated very clearly the value of discontinuation of alcohol a month before major abdominal surgery in moderate to heavy drinkers (Chapter 18).

Obesity

This is a serious obstacle to anaesthesia and surgery for several reasons:

- *Practical procedures* such as venous access, airway control and intubation, local anaesthetic procedures and moving the patient are more difficult.

- *Increased demand upon the heart* with the possibility of hypertension (difficult to measure by cuff and auscultation) and left-ventricular failure being prominent associations.

- *Functional residual capacity (FRC)* is lowered by the weight of abdominal wall fat restricting diaphragmatic movement. There is increased risk of hypoxia and respiratory complications.

- *Sleep apnoea* is a common accompaniment together with an increased sensitivity to the respiratory depressant effects of opioids.

4

■ *Lowering of oesophageal cardiac sphincter tone*, together with the increased weight of abdominal contents, predisposes to regurgitation of abdominal contents. Antacid therapy (see later) should be prescribed, but endotracheal intubation (ETI), with a cuffed tube to prevent aspiration, is often required, even for minor procedures.

■ *Pressure areas* (see later) must be assiduously padded during surgery to prevent nerve trapping and pressure necrosis (Chapter 11).

■ *Associated conditions* may be present, such as diabetes, myxoedema and Cushing's syndrome.

Surgical problems are also common such as increased difficulty due to fat, poor wound healing and a higher incidence of deep vein thrombosis (DVT) and pulmonary embolus. Anti-thrombotic therapy (e.g. subcutaneous heparin and elastic stockings) should be carried out as a routine during the perioperative period.

Dehydration or hypovolaemia

These make induction and maintenance of anaesthesia very hazardous. They must always be corrected prior to anaesthesia with appropriate i.v. infusions.

Anaemia and bleeding disorders

Long-standing anaemia is remarkably well tolerated; in the days prior to erythropoetin, chronic renal failure patients often presented with Hb values as low as 6 g/dl. This chronic anaemia was 'tolerated' because of a compensatory increase in cardiac output and 2,3, diphospho-glycerate (2,3,DPG), which increase the ability of Hb to off load oxygen to the tissues (Chapter 16). However, in acute anaemia, compensation is usually inadequate; the Hb level should be brought up to 9 g/dl by specific therapy (such as iron, erythropoetin and folate) in elective cases, or by transfusion of packed red cells in urgent and emergency cases. Estimation of Hb concentration is only necessary if there are clinical indications of anaemia, such as the presence of significant pallor and shortness of breath on exertion, or if the operation is likely to be associated with significant (>15% of estimated blood volume) loss.

A sickle-screening test is performed prior to surgery in all patients of afro-Caribbean descent. A negative result indicates that no further assessment is needed. In routine cases, the test must be done early as a sickle-positive result can indicate a more serious problem, which can only be definitively diagnosed by Hb electrophoresis. The latter test may not be immediately available and takes several hours to perform, resulting in unnecessary delays in the operating schedule. Haemoglobinopathies, especially sickle-cell disease (SCD), should be diagnosed and treated in collaboration with a haematologist before anaesthesia. Traditionally, in preparation for major surgery, the patient underwent exchange blood transfusion until the level of HbS fell to <30% of total. However, recent work has suggested that restoration of the Hb level to around 9–10 g/dl (haematocrit 0.3) is all that is required. The haematocrit should certainly not be allowed to exceed 0.4 as this also increases the risk of sickling in the perioperative period. Following major surgery, the SCD patient is admitted to the HDU or ICU for close monitoring of cardiovascular and respiratory status. Sickle-cell trait does not require preoperative treatment, but throughout anaesthesia and recovery a higher fraction of inspired oxygen ($FIO_2 > 0.4$) should be used. Bleeding disorders are more a surgical than an anaesthetic problem, but should be noted if regional techniques are planned. Preoperative transfusion of concentrates of the missing factor may be indicated.

Drugs

A few drugs interact adversely with anaesthetic agents. Most regular medication should be given in the usual dosage right up to the last preoperative hour, with a few exceptions.

Stop before surgery:

■ *Long-acting oral anti-diabetic agents* should be stopped for up to 2 days preoperatively because of the risk of hypoglycaemia, e.g. chlorpropamide and tolbutamide. Most patients are now on the shorter-acting drugs, such as glicazide and metformin. These may be omitted on the morning of surgery. In patients undergoing anything but the most minor surgery, a change to insulin is made for the perioperative period to improve glycaemic control (see later).

- *Antidepressants* of the monoamine oxidase inhibitor (MAOI) group, now less commonly used, should be stopped 2 weeks preoperatively, because of their adverse interaction with pethidine and other opioid analgesics and anaesthetic agents (Chapter 19). Careful discussion with the patient's GP and psychiatrist is mandatory to assess the risks to the patient of stopping therapy for this period (e.g. suicidal depression). The anaesthetist often has to deal with patients in whom MAOI therapy must be maintained. For major surgery, *lithium* salts should be stopped for 3 days preoperatively, because they may unpredictably potentiate competitive neuromuscular blockers (NMB). If possible, a lithium level should also be obtained (therapeutic 0.4–1.2 mmol/l and toxic >1.5).

- *Anticoagulants* such as *warfarin* should be stopped at least 24 h preoperatively, and prothrombin time (International Normalised Ratio, INR) checked. It should be in the region of 1.6–2:1 with reference to control. If it exceeds 2:1, the operation should be postponed until this level is reached, but in an emergency a concentrate of vitamin-K-dependent factors (PPSB, obtainable from the haematology department) is administered preceded by a small dose (1 mg) of vitamin K. If necessary, change over to a heparin infusion to maintain anticoagulation. The effects of warfarin may be enhanced or reduced by many of the anaesthetic and analgesic agents, by alteration of plasma protein binding and liver inactivation. Non-steroidal anti-inflammatory drugs (NSAIDS) decrease platelet adhesion by inhibition of thromboxane synthesis and may increase bleeding in susceptible patients. *Aspirin* should be stopped for 2 weeks prior to major cardiovascular, urological or plastic/ reconstructive surgery. Other agents have a less marked and prolonged effect on platelet function, but can still cause serious bleeding in the occasional patient.

- *Oestrogen-containing contraceptives* (the pill) have been implicated in causing an increased incidence of deep vein thrombosis (DVT), particularly in smokers. Current recommendations for major surgery suggest stopping 'the pill' for a month prior to surgery and utilising other means of contraception during the time up to surgery. If they are continued to the time of surgery, or in an emergency, anti-thrombosis prophylaxis must be instituted.

The anaesthetist must also be aware of all other medication taken by the patient, which may affect the course of surgery and anaesthesia. In general, these should still be continued right up until the time of surgery.

Continue with treatment, but be aware of the most important points relating to:

- *Corticosteroids*, if given for more than 6 weeks, can cause adreno-cortical (and hence cardiovascular) depression. Supplementation with i.v. hydrocortisone (100 mg, 4 hourly) is necessary in the perioperative period.

- *Anti-hypertensive agents*, including β-blockers, because the regulation of pulse and BP is altered, particularly in response to blood loss.

- *Central analgesic and sedative drugs*, because their chronic use stimulates liver metabolism with consequent shorter duration and effect of anaesthetic agents.

Pharmacogenetic factors

As mentioned earlier, drugs used in anaesthesia may precipitate certain hereditary diseases associated with abnormal drug metabolism. Individual variation in response to drugs is a substantial clinical problem. Such variation ranges from failure to respond to a drug to adverse drug reactions and drug–drug interactions when several drugs are taken concomitantly. The clinical consequences range from patient discomfort through serious clinical illness to the occasional fatality. One UK study has suggested that about one in 15 hospital admissions are due to adverse drug reactions and a recent US study estimated that 106,000 patients die and 2.2 million are injured each year by adverse reactions to prescribed drugs.

Cytochrome P450s

The cytochrome P450s are a multigene family of enzymes found predominantly in the liver that are responsible for the metabolic elimination of most of the drugs currently used in medicine. Genetically determined variability in the level of expression or function of these enzymes has a profound effect on drug efficacy. In 'poor metabolisers' the genes encoding specific cytochrome P450s often contain inactivating mutations, which result in a complete lack of active enzyme and a severely compromised ability to metabolise drugs. Thus, mutations in the gene encoding cytochrome P450 CYP2C9, which metabolises warfarin, affects patients' response to the drug and their dose requirements. Polymorphism not only affects drug disposition but can also be important in the conversion of pro-drugs to their active form. For example, codeine is metabolised to the analgesic morphine by CYP2D6, and the desired analgesic effect is not achieved in CYP2D6 poor metabolisers.

Acute intermittent porphyria

Acute intermittent porphyria may be precipitated by anaesthetic agents such as barbiturates, so that these should be studiously avoided, as an attack may be irreversible.

Plasma pseudo-cholinesterase

A hereditary *plasma pseudo-cholinesterase* deficiency or inactivity of it is present in about one in 2000 people. Metabolism of suxamethonium is greatly prolonged leading to a requirement for postoperative sedation and ventilation for many hours.

Malignant hyperthermia (MH)

MH is a hereditary disease that is only manifested if the subject is exposed to an initiating stimulus such as anaesthesia with suxamethonium, halothane or other precipitating drug. In MH, there is failure of the sarcoplasmic reticulum in skeletal muscle to store Ca^{++} as a result of certain triggering agents. The resulting rise in Ca^{++} in the cell triggers excessive excitation/contraction coupling, which leads to muscle rigidity together with a massive increase in energy expenditure. The patient becomes tachycardic, tachypnoeic (if not paralysed), hypoxic and hypercarbic (easily detectable by pulse oximetry and capnography). Hyperthermia occurs relatively late. Unless MH is suspected, the triggering agent removed immediately and urgent measures taken, a metabolic acidosis supervenes together with hypotension and the possible demise of the patient. Although it is an uncommon syndrome, it can often be picked up from the history of unexplained pyrexia following previous surgery or a family member unexpectedly succumbing to minor surgery. Dantrolene sodium is a specific drug used both for prevention and treatment. It uncouples excitation/contraction coupling by interfering with the release of Ca^{++} from the sarcoplasmic reticulum. It must be readily available in the operating room. It is given in a dose of 1 mg/kg i.v. slowly and repeated up to a maximum of 10 mg/kg together with general supportive measures.

Cardiovascular system

History

Preoperative interrogation of the patient determines whether there are any indicators of cardiac disease such as chest pain and dyspnoea on exertion, presence of palpitations, orthopnea and paroxysmal nocturnal dyspnoea. This will indicate the need for more detailed systematic enquiry and examination, and special tests.

Detection by history and examination of patients with congenital or acquired heart defects (such as ventriculo-septal defect) and prosthetic heart valves is extremely important. In these patients, certain procedures such as dental extractions, genitourinary (GU) surgery, gynaecological and obstetric procedures, upper GIT endoscopy and respiratory tract operations (including tonsillectomy, adenoidectomy and instrumentation) all require antibiotic prophylaxis for the prevention of infective endocarditis. Regimes are tailored individually, but include parenteral amoxicillin for those not allergic and vancomycin + gentamicin for those that are. The antibiotics are administered immediately prior to surgery with a top-up dose given 6 h later. It is wise to consult with the medical microbiologist if in doubt (Chapter 11).

Examination
The presence of dysrhythmias, hypertension, cardiac murmurs and enlargement, and cardiac failure should be looked for (see below).

Investigations
Although a 12-lead ECG is a useful preoperative screen, it is not routinely performed prior to minor surgery, unless there are specific symptoms and signs. An ECG should always be obtained prior to major surgery in all patients over the age of 40 or earlier, if there are signs of cardiac disease. In equivocal cases of myocardial ischaemia with a normal ECG, exercise testing and echocardiography may be necessary.

It is, particularly, important to note the following.

History of myocardial infarction
Occasionally, a routine ECG is the only indicator that there has been a previous infarction, in such cases, it should be presumed to be recent. Expert cardiological advice and investigation may be needed in some cases. If there is definite evidence of a myocardial infarction having occurred in the previous 6 months, the operation should be postponed as the risks of perioperative re-infarction are very high (around 30%) with a high mortality (around 50%). If surgery is absolutely necessary (or an emergency), specialised cardiac monitoring is undertaken (e.g. invasive arterial pressures and Swan–Ganz catheterisation of the pulmonary artery) to warn the anaesthetist of impending problems with myocardial oxygen supply/demand, so that early action can be taken (see Goldman index Table 4.1).

Evidence of heart failure
This includes dyspnoea, basal crepitations, ankle swelling, increased jugular venous pressure or gallop rhythm. Heart failure must be treated with digoxin, diuretics and angiotensin converting enzyme (ACE) inhibitors prior to elective surgery.

Dysrhythmias
Are there more than five-ventricular ectopic beats per minute (bpm)? In supra-ventricular dysrhythmias such as atrial fibrillation (AF), the ventricular rate should be controlled with digoxin or amiodarone prior to surgery. Ventricular dysrhythmias warn of underlying cardiac pathology and although they are often left untreated preoperatively, the anaesthetist has anti-dysrhythmics ready intra-operatively.

Hypertension
Untreated hypertension increases the likelihood of perioperative cardiovascular instability, but the risks have probably been exaggerated. Nevertheless, most authorities recommend preoperative treatment of a diastolic pressure >100–110 mmHg. Hypertensive patients are definitely more labile at induction (big drop in BP), ETI (big rise in BP) and maintenance (big swings in BP due to blood loss and surgical stimulation). The anaesthetic technique is designed to minimise these changes.

Angina pectoris
This is not a serious risk factor in the absence of previous myocardial infarction. Neither hypertension nor angina figures in the Goldman index.

4

Table 4.1 **The Goldman index: a score of 13 or more indicates major risk, over 25 the risk is very serious**

Risk factor	Score
Heart failure	+11
MI in the last 3 months	+10
Not in sinus rhythm	+7
More than five VEs per minute	+7
Age over 70 years	+5
Emergency operation	+4
Aortic stenosis	+3
Major intra-abdominal/thoracic surgery	+3
Respiratory, hepatic or renal disease	+3

It should be noted that there is no evidence that regional analgesic techniques are safer than general anaesthesia in patients with cardiovascular disease. These preoperative cardiovascular risk factors have been combined in composite cardiac risk indices, such as the Goldman index (Table 4.1).

Respiratory system

History
Acute and chronic respiratory disease is justifiably worrying for the anaesthetist, so a detailed history should be taken including presence of chronic cough productive of sputum, wheeze and shortness of breath on exertion. Asking how far the patient can walk without shortness of breath, or asking the patient to count numbers in a single expiration easily assesses the seriousness of the situation. If the maximum uninterrupted walk is <50 m, or the patient is unable to count up to 10 in a single breath, or there has been more than one hospital admission due to respiratory disease, then pulmonary function tests are performed. The number of previous hospital admissions related to the respiratory condition is important.

Examination
Clinical examination looks for central cyanosis, finger clubbing, use of accessory muscles of ventilation, the extent of chest expansion, presence of wheeze, areas of collapse/consolidation, pneumothorax and presence of secretions.

Investigations
These include Hb, urea and electrolytes, chest X-ray (CXR) and ECG. Simple respiratory function tests are now available, which can be performed at the bedside using small micro-electronically based instruments.

Spirometry
- *Peak expiratory flow rate (PEFR)* is a useful screening test; a value below 100 l/min suggests serious ventilatory impairment in an adult. Coughing and clearing of bronchial secretions is unlikely to be effective, if the PEFR is <100–150 l/min. A value over 300 l/min shows that ventilatory function is unlikely to be seriously compromised following surgery.

- *Forced expiratory volume in 1 s (FEV1)* is <50% of normal, if there is a significant bronchospastic component.

- *Forced vital capacity* is <50% of normal, if there is a significant loss of functional lung tissue (e.g. emphysema) or a restrictive condition such as fibrosing alveolitis.

If both FEV1 is <50% and FVC is <50% of predicted, arterial blood-gas (ABG) analysis must be performed. These two parameters are combined in a useful diagram, which can be used to classify basic respiratory pathologies (see Fig. 4.1 below).

Reversibility of significant bronchospasm is attempted preoperatively, using suitable bronchodilators and chest physiotherapy instituted to maximise the available respiratory reserve prior to surgery.

4

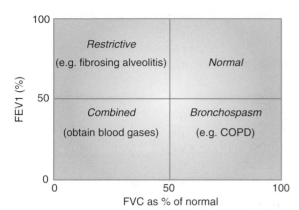

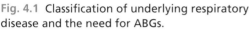

Fig. 4.1 Classification of underlying respiratory disease and the need for ABGs.

Arterial blood gases

The predicted postoperative course is best correlated with the resting PaO_2 and $PaCO_2$ values when breathing air (Chapters 8 and 17).

Three degrees of severity may present, with different postoperative prognoses:

1. $PaO_2 > 7.5\,kPa$ (55 mmHg) and normal $PaCO_2$: reasonable prognosis.

2. $PaO_2 < 7.5\,kPa$ and normal $PaCO_2$: requirement for short-term postoperative ventilation should be anticipated following major upper abdominal/thoracic surgery.

3. $PaO_2 < 7.5\,kPa$ and $PaCO_2 > 7.5\,kPa$ (55 mmHg): poor prognosis, with almost certain requirement for prolonged postoperative ventilation following major surgery.

Chronic respiratory patients benefit from regional analgesic techniques, if suitable for the operation. If general anaesthesia must be given, competitive neuromuscular blockers (NMBs) should be kept to a minimum, because the smallest interference with respiratory muscle function often leads to severe respiratory failure (Chapter 17).

Respiratory problems of particular importance for anaesthesia are as follows.

Acute respiratory tract infection

Paediatric patients, in particular, frequently present for surgery with clinically obvious upper respiratory tract infections and, as a result, have an increased risk of airway problems in the perioperative period. It is important to distinguish local rhinitis from laryngo-tracheo-bronchitis or pharyngitis/laryngitis, i.e. cough, sore throat, hoarseness accompanied by fever, malaise and vomiting indicating systemic infection. In such cases, the operation should be delayed while treatment is instituted.

Asthma

Intractable bronchospasm ranks high in the list of contributory causes of death under anaesthesia. Long-term bronchodilator therapy is continued right up to induction of anaesthesia. Antihistaminic agents, such as promethazine and oral theophylline, may be added to the premedication and salbutamol inhaled immediately prior to induction. The anaesthetic must be conducted with careful avoidance of all drugs and mechanical stimulation known to trigger bronchospasm. ETI is avoided, if possible, as it is a significant stimulus to bronchospasm, especially, if anaesthesia is too light. I.v. atropine (10–20 μg/kg) or glycopyrrolate (5–10 μg/kg) effectively prevents vagal reflexes; β-blockers, even if β-1 selective, must not be used.

Chronic obstructive pulmonary disease

Major surgery, particularly upper abdominal and intrathoracic, has profound effects on ventilatory function, even in the normal patient without respiratory disease. Patients with limited functional reserve are obviously at risk of serious postoperative respiratory complications. Preoperative physiotherapy, antibiotics and bronchodilators are necessary prior to major surgery to lessen the risk and severity of postoperative chest infection. This obviously necessitates careful screening in the clinic and timely admission to hospital to allow this to take place. Unlike asthma, most of the lung function impairment in COPD is fixed. However, there is often some degree of reversibility, and many patients will obtain symptom relief from using inhaled bronchodilators (Chapter 17).

Approaches to management include:

- Eradication of acute and chronic infection with appropriate antibiotics.

- Relief of bronchospasm with a bronchodilator.

- Chest physiotherapy to improve sputum clearance and bronchial drainage.

- Reversal of uncompensated or borderline cor pulmonale with diuretics, digitalis, improved oxygenation and correction of acidaemia by more efficient ventilation.

- Correction of dehydration and electrolyte imbalance.

- Cessation of smoking, if possible for 3 months, to improve mucociliary clearance and decrease sputum production.

- Abstinence from smoking for at least 12 h to reduce carboxy-Hb levels, resulting in improvement of blood oxygen content and increasing the release of oxygen from Hb.

- Consider steroid therapy in the week prior to elective surgery for patients with wheezing, despite optimal bronchodilator therapy. It has also been recommended that systemic steroid preparation should be used preoperatively in patients with moderate to severe asthma and a history of requiring steroids in the past.

Neuromuscular disease

Myopathies

Myotonic syndromes (such as dystrophia myotonica) cause a generalised contracture in response to suxamethonium. Responses to competitive NMBs may be either decreased or abnormally prolonged.

Myasthenia gravis

The use of competitive NMBs is usually contraindicated; a normal dose can cause incapacitating paralysis for more than 48 h. Postoperatively, the patient must be managed in the ITU.

Diabetes

Introduction

Diabetic patients fall into one of three classes: those managed on diet alone, those taking oral hypoglycaemic drugs and those taking insulin. They are all at an increased perioperative risk, because of the cardiovascular, renal and neurological changes associated with the disease.

History, examination and investigations

Assessment of the patient involves taking note of the quality of glucose control and the presence of associated cardiovascular, neurological and renal complications of diabetes. These include ischaemic heart disease (IHD), autonomic and peripheral neuropathy and renal failure. Minimum investigations include Hb, urea and electrolytes and glucose and ECG. Diabetics with autonomic neuropathy often complain of postural hypotension and are at increased risk of serious cardiac dysrhythmias during surgery under general anaesthesia.

Management

In minor (non-stressful) surgery, only patients on insulin or oral therapy require special management, mainly because of the fasting period surrounding the operation. Oral hypoglycaemics should be omitted prior to surgery to avoid the risk of hypoglycaemia.

All diabetic patients need special attention during major surgery because stress increases insulin requirements (partly due to release of catecholamines). A 5 to 10% glucose drip (with 20 mmol potassium chloride) should be instituted preoperatively and a constant infusion of soluble insulin started using a syringe pump (50 units insulin in 50 ml 0.9% sodium chloride). The hourly rate of insulin administration should initially be based on the patient's normal daily requirements (usually 1–6 units (ml) per hour), and adjusted at 2- or 4-h intervals depending upon blood glucose levels obtained from portable glucose monitors. This regime should be continued

4

during the operation and postoperatively, until the patient has recovered from operative stress and resumed a normal diet.

Renal disease

History, examination and special investigations

A full preoperative examination should concentrate on detection of complications of chronic renal disease such as hypertension and IHD. Patients may present with difficult anaesthetic problems, e.g. cardiovascular disease (ischaemia, left-ventricular failure and hypertension), diabetes, severe anaemia, high plasma potassium (avoid suxamethonium) and multiple drug therapy including immuno-suppression for transplantation. Minimum preoperative investigations include Hb, urea and electrolytes, ECG and chest radiograph (Chapter 18).

Management

Patients on regular haemodialysis should be dialysed in the 24 h preceding surgery, thus avoiding fluid overload. The activated coagulation time (ACT) should be checked and sufficient time should be allowed for the residual effects of heparin to wear off prior to surgery. Patients with pre-existing chronic renal impairment (raised urea and creatinine, but not requiring dialysis) usually tolerate badly the preoperative period of fluid restriction. They often exhibit an inability to conserve urinary sodium and can become fluid depleted in the perioperative period. This can even be severe enough to precipitate acute on chronic renal failure. An infusion of 0.9% sodium chloride should be commenced preoperatively to avoid this complication.

Anaesthetic drugs are available which do not rely on the renal route for their elimination. Inhalational agents such as desflurane or isoflurane, mostly eliminated through the lung, are good supplements. If competitive neuromuscular blockers must be used, atracurium, cis-atracurium or vecuronium are preferred.

Liver disease

History, examination and investigations

In assessing the patient with liver disease, it is important to determine what effects it is having on the functions of the liver and this is covered in detail in Chapter 18.

Anatomical difficulties

This is mainly directed towards spotting difficulties with the airway (e.g. ability to tightly apply a facemask and feasibility of ETI), prior to induction of anaesthesia. For example, consider the following.

Mouth opening

Is it sufficient to allow passage of a laryngoscope, airway or laryngeal mask? The Mallampati score is a useful system to classify and predict intubation difficulty as shown in Table 4.2.

Trismus due to infection, jaw fixation and temporo-mandibular pathology may limit mouth opening to such an extent as to make ETI impossible. Awake fibre-optic laryngoscopy via the nasal passages or tracheostomy under local anaesthesia may be the only safe option. If the uvula and posterior pharyngeal wall cannot be visualised, ETI may be very difficult.

Table 4.2 **Mallampati's modified classification**

Grade	Description
I	Faucal pillars, soft palate and uvula visible
II	As above, but uvula masked by the base of tongue
III	Only the soft palate visible
IV	Soft palate not visible

4

Neck movements

The extent of neck flexion and extension ('sniffing the morning air') should be established. Neck movements may be severely limited (and dangerous) in patients with rheumatoid arthritis (particularly young women with rheumatoid nodules). Radiological preoperative assessment is essential using lateral and antero-posterior neck X-rays. If necessary, the neck should be stabilised by a collar and the ETI performed on the awake patient using sedation and topical analgesia.

Spine

If epidural or spinal analgesia is anticipated, the lumbar spine should be examined for anatomical abnormalities and mobility. Severe spinal deformity, such as kyphoscoliosis can lead to severe respiratory embarrassment in the postoperative period.

Epilepsy

Most anti-epileptic agents, such as phenytoin and the barbiturates, induce hepatic enzymes, thus enhancing the ability of the liver to metabolise anaesthetic drugs. Higher doses of i.v. anaesthetics may be required for both induction *and* maintenance of anaesthesia. Anticonvulsant treatment is continued right up to the time of premedication and restarted as soon as it is practicable (i.m. or oral) postoperatively. Anaesthetic drugs that are liable to precipitate convulsions such as methohexitone and enflurane are avoided (Chapter 19).

Pregnancy

Only urgent surgery should take place, as there is an increased incidence of spontaneous abortion from the second trimester onwards, particularly if surgery is performed in the region of the uterus, e.g. appendicectomy. In the first trimester, drugs implicated in causing defects in organogenesis should be avoided. Thiopentone, suxamethonium, pancuronium, pethidine and halothane are examples of safe, well-tried agents that may be used in early pregnancy. After the 16–18th week, the risk of regurgitation of acid stomach contents at induction increases steeply.

Overall assessment of fitness for anaesthesia and surgery

The American Society of Anesthesiologists (ASA) has produced a classification of patients depending on their general condition before operation. This scale bears some correlation with morbidity and mortality due to operation or anaesthetic, and is useful as a means of recording and conveying to others the state of the patient. Thus, having examined the patient and noted the preoperative pathology, it should be possible to assign the patient to one of the following categories. For instance, patients attending a day surgery centre for surgery under general anaesthesia should usually be in ASA classes I or II.

- ASA I – Normal healthy patient.

- ASA II – Patient with mild systemic disease, which is adequately, treated, e.g. diabetes, chronic bronchitis and hypertension.

- ASA III – Severe systemic disease limiting normal activity, such as angina on exertion, chronic renal failure on dialysis and chronic obstructive pulmonary disease (COPD) with dyspnoea.

- ASA IV – Incapacitating systemic disease, which is a constant, threat to life, e.g. angina on minimal exertion, cardiac failure and COPD with dyspnoea at rest.

- ASA V – Moribund, not expected to survive 24 h with or without operation.

- E – Signifies that the operation is to be performed as an emergency. Generally speaking, this places the patient in the next highest-risk category.

4

Premedication

This is a traditional measure still thought by some to be essential for all patients undergoing surgery. It has its origin in the days of gaseous induction with di-ethyl ether, which was often 'stormy' and could cause intense salivation, coughing, breath holding and production of copious tracheal secretions. Combination of an opioid and anti-sialogogue decreased the likelihood of these problems on induction. Nowadays, with modern anaesthetic techniques, these drugs are rarely necessary, and the main purpose of premedication is to relieve anxiety.

Indications

The main indications for premedication all begin with 'A' and are outlined below. They can all be given either preoperatively on the ward (i.m., oral or p.r.) or by i.v. increments immediately prior to induction. Heavy premedication reduces requirements for anaesthetic drugs intra-operatively, but may also be responsible for delayed awakening at the end of the procedure. Premedication is used much less than formerly. Regimes usually include a benzodiazepine such as temazepam or an opioid and anti-emetic combination such as pethidine and promethazine.

Anxiolysis

The major requirement of premedication is usually achieved by a combination of preoperative assurance by the anaesthetist together with benzodiazepines as appropriate. A combination of an opioid and phenothiazine is equally effective, but must be given parenterally.

Analgesia

This is rarely necessary prior to surgery, unless the patient is already in pain, e.g. appendicitis and fractured neck of femur. Intra-operative analgesia is best achieved by i.v. administration of opioids. NSAIDS are increasingly utilised for postoperative analgesia, especially, in day surgery patients.

Although they can be given parenterally at or immediately after induction, a popular form of administration is by suppository. Ideally, this should be given an hour or so prior to anaesthesia.

Amnesia

Prior to major surgery, an amnesic component is useful in specific cases to reduce recall of unpleasant procedures carried out prior to induction of anaesthesia, e.g. insertion of major vascular catheters and awake intubation. This state is best achieved by a combination of lorazepam and hyoscine as premedication or as midazolam given in i.v. increments on arrival in the anaesthetic room.

Anti-sialogogue

It is usual to administer atropine, hyoscine or glycopyrrolate prior to anaesthesia for reduction of secretions in specific cases such as for infants and for patients having upper airway/GI tract endoscopy. An unpleasantly dry mouth is the commonest side-effect of these agents; hyoscine and to a lesser extent atropine cross the blood–brain barrier, exerting a depressant effect that can be excessive in the elderly and the very young.

Anti-vagal

Atropine and glycopyrrolate (less so hyoscine) are also anti-vagal drugs. They are useful to prevent bradycardia in infants (where cardiac output is mainly determined by rate, so bradycardia must be avoided at all costs) and patients receiving β-blockers. The incidence of bradycardia in patients undergoing certain procedures such as laparoscopy, especially, if non-vagolytic neuromuscular-blocking drugs are used has led to the routine use of these drugs in these cases.

Antacid

These include acid-buffering agents, such as sodium citrate, and H2 antagonists, such as ranitidine. They are administered as a routine in many centres to lower gastric acidity in order to reduce the risk of acid aspiration (see preoperative starvation below).

4

Autonomic blockade

The response to induction of anaesthesia on the CVS reflects the autonomic responses to anaesthetic drugs and to intubation of the trachea. Intubation causes the most dramatic changes, with hypertension and tachycardia occasionally requiring the use of blocking drugs; bradycardia with hypotension due to a vagal reflex is uncommon. Preoperative β-blockade may be indicated in patients with thyrotoxicosis, IHD or intracranial space occupying lesions.

Anti-emesis

An anti-emetic is usually included with opioid premedication to reduce the incidence of nausea associated with these drugs and with surgery.

Preoperative starvation

The dangers of pulmonary inhalation of acid gastric contents and particulate matter include severe bronchospasm, increased shunting of deoxygenated blood and acute respiratory distress syndrome (ARDS). To prevent this feared complication, the patient must abstain from food for 6 h preoperatively and clear fluids from 2 to 4 h preoperatively to ensure an empty stomach. Despite these recommendations, 30% of normal patients still have sufficient gastric volume and acidity to cause problems.

4

5

The process of the perioperative period: the patient's viewpoint and legal aspects of the perioperative period

Aims

- To present the process of anaesthesia and the perioperative period from a patient viewpoint.

- To present legal aspects of the perioperative period, particularly those relating to consent, confidentiality, patient death, do not resuscitate (DNR) orders and fitness to practise.

Objectives

After reading this chapter, you should be able to

- answer questions which the patient might have about what might happen to them in the perioperative period;

- appreciate that the process of anaesthesia and surgery in the perioperative period involves teamwork and the patient is the most important member of that team;

- appreciate how recent changes in the law are influencing the practice of medicine and the measures that practitioners must take to comply with the present legislation.

Introduction

There is usually a great difference between the views of doctors and patients about the overall process of anaesthesia and surgery. Many patients scheduled for surgery are clearly more worried about the anaesthetic than the operation, especially in minor surgery.

Most doctors without experience in the practice of anaesthesia admit to the lack of understanding of what happens during anaesthesia, its complications and risks. Thus, GPs often find it difficult to offer an informed, up to date, concise explanation of the process of anaesthesia to the patients whom they refer for surgery and who require more than the usual reassuring statement that 'everything will be all right'. Equally, surgical PRHOs and SHOs who were not exposed to an anaesthesia clerkship during undergraduate training will also find it difficult to reassure and inform their patients during clerking and when requesting a signed consent for operation.

This book provides the necessary material for doctors to be able to inform their patients of the general process of modern anaesthesia, the possible complications and the risk to life associated with anaesthesia alone. This written information, unfortunately, cannot replace the experience gained during a good anaesthetic clerkship. Although the anaesthetist is, normally, able to fully inform inpatients during the preoperative visit, for day cases the anaesthetist sees patients only in the morning of the operation. The proportion of day case surgery is increasing so more and more patients express their worries and request information about anaesthesia to their GP or to their surgeon. Day case surgery also tends to present the GP and nurse specialist with the postoperative complications occurring after the patient has returned home. We hope that this book provides some help in understanding the nature of and how to deal with such complications.

The patient's view of anaesthesia and the perioperative period is very varied. Some of the older generation tend to think that the practice of anaesthesia is either in the hands of non-medical technicians or in the hands of the youngest trainee surgeons, rather than medically qualified anaesthesia specialists. Those of the younger generation tend to think of anaesthesia as an automated 'high-tech' exercise under the control of a sophisticated computer and a technically minded specialist. Much of the general population is influenced by the occasional news and press reports of anaesthetic mishaps, including awareness during surgery, and by news of large monetary compensations to the unfortunate victims. Even the American film industry has somewhat contributed to the sources of anxiety in some patients with motion pictures featuring fictional criminal events in the operating room!

5

As a first step to address the natural worries of the patient the doctor should inform the patient that the anaesthetic will be administered by a specialised doctor who will be visiting before the operation. At that time he or she will be available to answer any questions related to anaesthesia, including the choice of type of anaesthetic (general or local). It gives great confidence to most patients to explain that the role of the anaesthetist is not only to give the anaesthetic but also to ensure good bodily function. This is not only during but also immediately after the operation, an important and most demanding task.

Patients should also be made aware that both the anaesthetist and the surgeon are responsible for pain relief during and after the operation. In some circumstances, e.g. in a GP's surgery, it may be helpful to provide patients with an information sheet designed to answer the most common questions and uncertainties about anaesthesia. The following set of questions that patients may ask and the 'jargon free' answers to those questions should provide sufficient information to allay most fears. It may also help patients define better the source of their anxiety.

Can I eat or drink before the operation?

You can normally eat until about 6 h and drink up to 4 h before your operation is due. This is because it is dangerous to be anaesthetised with food or liquid in your stomach; in most people, the stomach is almost empty 6 h after eating or 4 h after drinking. In the case of clear fluids, such as water or orange juice, the time to leave the stomach completely may be only an hour or so. In some people, however, food remains in the stomach for much longer times, especially if your disease involves your stomach or if you have been in pain after your meal. In these circumstances, having vomited is a positive advantage!

Do I need to tell anything (allergies, medicines I am taking, previous medical problems and operations) to the doctor beforehand?

Yes, this is very important. The anaesthetist must know of all medicines that you are taking regularly or occasionally even ordinary pain killers such as aspirin and paracetamol or the contraceptive pill. This is because many medicines interfere with the anaesthetic or with your blood clotting and you could suffer ill effects if your anaesthetist is not informed. Allergies are also important, especially to medicines such as penicillin or allergies to sticking plasters and iodine. Allergies to dust or food are not normally important. It is also important to tell the doctor of any medical conditions that you have or other operations you had in the past and also if any of your close blood relatives ever had an unexpected accident during an operation. This is because there are a few inherited tendencies to react in an unusual way to the anaesthetic medicines.

Should I wear anything special and should I have a bath and shave?

It is advisable to have a bath a few hours before surgery, if you have not been advised otherwise. For some types of surgery you may be asked to shave certain parts of the body. You do not have to wear anything special from home; the nursing staff will give you a gown to change into when you are admitted.

Will I have to remove jewellery, glasses, contact lenses and dentures?

It is advisable to leave at home all unnecessary jewellery and avoid using make up, lipstick or nail polish. All these have to be removed for

5

your safety; this is because they may cause damage when you are anaesthetised, and lipstick and nail polish may interfere with the monitoring of blood oxygenation. Devices such as hearing aids and spectacles may be worn up until the induction of anaesthesia as many patients feel terribly isolated without these aids. However, they will need to be safely stored during the procedure and returned to you as early as possible after awakening from anaesthesia.

Who gives the anaesthetic for the operation?

In the UK, a fully qualified doctor who has undergone many years of post-graduate training in the specialty always administers anaesthesia. In most cases, a fully qualified specialist or consultant gives anaesthesia; although the trainee may administer anaesthesia under supervision. Non-medical staff are not allowed to administer anaesthesia in the UK.

Do I have a choice of the type of anaesthetic?

In many cases, yes. Operations below the waist (such as hernia repair, transurethral resection of prostate) can often be performed by the use of regional local anaesthetic techniques without the need for you to be fully unconscious. This involves placing a needle close to the nerves of the spinal cord and 'freezing' them with local anaesthetic. In the case of an epidural, a very fine tube can be passed through the needle and alongside the main nerves serving the part of the body being operated upon. Local anaesthetic and other pain killing drugs are injected through this tube and can not only be used for the operation but continued into the postoperative period for pain relief. The anaesthetist will explain the 'pros and cons' of these techniques. Most operations are still performed under full general anaesthesia; in other words you will be unconscious and only

be awakened when the procedure is completed. General anaesthesia can be given entirely through a vein or by using an anaesthetic gas, although in the latter case an i.v. drug is given to induce sleep and anaesthesia continued with gas.

What will happen when I am under anaesthesia? Will I feel any pain or will I be aware of what is going on?

If you receive a regional block (see above) it is not necessary for you to be totally asleep and a light sedative may be all that is required. However, the regional block is designed to remove the pain of the operation. Many patients like to be awake and feel in control and aware of what is going on, others do not want to know what is going on and prefer to be asleep! In very rare cases it is possible for a patient to be conscious and aware of what is going on during the procedure. This is usually due to error on the part of the anaesthetist. However, modern anaesthetic machines monitor the concentration of anaesthetic gases and this ensures that a sufficient amount is given to virtually guarantee unconsciousness.

What are the risks of long-term effects or death during anaesthesia and surgery?

The risk to your life purely from the anaesthetic is exceedingly low. Estimates vary from 1:10,000 to 1:100,000. However, anaesthesia is never given on its own so the risks of surgery must also be considered.

Will I have to give consent for surgery and anaesthesia?

Surgery
It is important to realise that you must give consent for any procedure that a doctor

performs on you. This may just be for taking blood or examining your abdomen. Strictly speaking, doing a procedure without consent is a 'breach of civil law' or a tort, and a crime that could incur penalties. Thus, consent must be given. However, it is obviously not necessary in every case to give written consent, e.g. having blood taken. Indeed, although it is universal practice, it is not necessary in law to give written consent to surgery. However, on the other hand, simply signing a piece of paper also does not constitute true consent, as it is important that you receive enough information on which to base your decision. Consent is a process that occurs over time and ends up in your decision to sign on the dotted line. Consider a 55-year-old man who is discovered to have cancer of the prostate. There are many different treatment options and he naturally needs time and information before deciding whether to proceed to surgery, radiotherapy or drug treatment. Or maybe no treatment at all! This process may take many months and involve many specialists. Finally, having decided to proceed to surgery, he signs the consent form the day before the operation. The latter is the end stage of a long process rather than the single act of a signature.

Consent to a procedure such as major surgery obviously requires a decision on your part that must be taken in light of all the relevant information, such as complications and outcome. It is always up to the individual patient to decide how much information they want; you may feel that you wish to leave everything to the doctor. However, if there is a complication, you may feel that you would have liked to have known about it beforehand. Herein lies the dilemma, too much or too little information? Some doctors will hand the patient an information sheet that explains all the complications, sometimes in graphic detail, and leave the patient to make up their mind. This is an understandable approach but does not, in the author's opinion, substitute for a dialogue between patient and doctor. The need to give *informed consent* has meant that the doctor who asks you to sign will have a good knowledge of the operation and the

potential problems. Take the time to ask this doctor what you need to know.

Anaesthesia

At present, there is no legal requirement for there to be a separate consent form for anaesthesia. However, as explained above, this certainly does not mean that you would not get any information about the options available. Although many patients are worried about 'not waking up after the operation' or 'not being asleep during the operation' these complications are very rare. The other main concerns are postoperative pain and nausea and vomiting which are covered in the next sections.

Will I have pain after the operation?

This depends on the site of the operation. Minor operations on the face or a small lump removal will be remarkably pain free. However, major abdominal or chest surgery can be very painful after the operation and the effects of pain may make breathing and movement so difficult that it may produce complications of its own. For that reason, the anaesthetist will discuss with you what the degree of pain is likely to be and what means are available to alleviate it. In general, a combination of pain killing drugs such as local anaesthetics, non-steroidal anti-inflammatory drugs (NSAIDs) (such as are normally taken for headaches or arthritis) and strong pain killers such as morphine are the most appropriate. Very often, you will be offered a special device that allows you to administer a small dose of morphine when required. This is called a patient-controlled analgesia (PCA) device and allows you more control over the pain relief by not requiring you to call a nurse to get and administer the medication. As mentioned above, an epidural may be recommended in some circumstances and you will usually be able to make an informed decision about the pros and cons of any technique. For instance, although an epidural will provide very effective relief it does involve sticking

5

59

a needle in the back and placing a catheter close to the nerves in the spine (see above). Clearly this is more invasive and potentially dangerous than administering the analgesic through a vein or into the skin.

Will I have other side-effects from the anaesthetic?

Most side-effects from anaesthesia are very short lived as modern anaesthetics wear off very quickly. However, due to the increase in day case surgery you will be required to travel home on the afternoon or evening of surgery. Mobilisation tends to increase the propensity for postoperative nausea and vomiting (PONV). This can be so severe on occasions that patients who were intending to go home on the day of surgery have to be admitted to a hospital bed overnight. Patients more at risk from PONV include women, gynaecological procedures, squint surgery in children, previous episode(s) of PONV, tendency to be travel sick and so on. In cases where PONV has been a problem, a variety of anti-sickness medicines are available to reduce the intensity of PONV or abolish it altogether. It is important that you alert your doctor if you feel this might be a problem. Other symptoms such as dizziness and headache are usually mild and self-limiting (Chapter 19).

Conclusion

This section has been written from the viewpoint of the patient. It is very important that whoever is involved in the initial assessment of the patient, especially, if it is a non-anaesthetist, does not trivialise the role of anaesthesia. This limited perception of anaesthesia arises from lack of knowledge and experience often because there was no exposure to anaesthesia during the clinical training. In some European countries and the US, surgical trainees often undergo a period of anaesthetic training. Whether this improves awareness is open to debate!

Legal aspects of perioperative medicine

We live in an increasingly litigious society and the medical profession is not immune to the process of law. To counteract the threat of litigation, the Department of Health, the Royal colleges, the General Medical Council and the British Medical Association have all published guidelines concerning various legal aspects of medical practice. At the same time, it is hoped that the introduction and pursuit of clinical governance measures will allow for an improvement in service to consumers (patients), such that they will be less likely to sue doctors, and less successful when they do. Most hospitals now have a legal department which should be consulted at an early stage if legal problems occur or are foreseen.

Medical law is an extensive field; however, the most relevant issues, with reference to perioperative medicine, are those concerning consent, confidentiality, patient death and fitness to practise.

Consent

Obtaining informed consent is not the same as getting a patient to sign a consent form (see earlier). Consent is a state of mind that protects patient autonomy from intrusion by others. Legally, informed consent is an instrument that allows individuals to define their own interests and to protect their bodily privacy. Consent may be explicitly stated or implicit (e.g. holding out one's arm for a blood test). The form in which consent is given is irrelevant in law (i.e. written consent is unnecessary), although the courts do recognise that a written consent form may improve a doctor's legal defence against allegations of battery.

For consent to be valid, it must be

- voluntary (i.e. freely given);

- competent (i.e. the patient must be able to understand and retain the information presented, and use and weigh it in the balance when arriving at their decision);

5

informed (i.e. the patient must understand the nature and purpose of the treatment proposed – what is to be done and why – and the risks and consequences of the treatment).

No one over the age of 18 may be treated without their giving consent, unless:

- their consent is not valid,

- they are unable to give consent because they are unconscious.

In these cases, doctors may treat the patient in the patient's best interests, although 'best interests' do not necessarily equate to medical best interests, as they represent a summation of all those factors which a reasonable patient might consider important (e.g. a 90-year-old septic patient may require leg amputation for gangrene, although he previously expressed a wish never to become an amputee).

Competent, informed patients may consent to treatment OR refuse it, even if their refusal results in severe injury or death. However, persistent refusal that could be considered irrational may be a sign of a mental disorder, which might render the patient incompetent to consent. No one (e.g. relatives, care workers, legal representatives) may consent to treatment on behalf of an adult patient.

To treat someone without their consent is to commit a battery, which may be a common law or a criminal (i.e. imprisonable) offence. Battery may also be committed if the consent given was not valid because the doctor misled the patient as to what was to be done and why. The doctor may be liable in civil or criminal negligence if he misled the patient as to the risks and consequences of the treatment. Negligence occurs when the doctor breaches a duty to the patient, which causes harm.

In terms of consent, 16- and 17-year olds are treated as adults unless it can be shown that they are incompetent (in Scotland, they are always regarded as adults). The law requires a higher standard of competence in order for 16- and 17-year olds to refuse treatment, particularly, if refusal could result

in serious harm to the patient (e.g. refusal of food by anorexics).

Under 16s are considered incompetent to consent/refuse treatment, unless they can show that they are competent to make a decision (i.e. are *Gillick* competent, after *Gillick v West Norfolk and Wisbech Area Health Authority* (1986) 2 BMLR 11 (HL)). The more important and consequential the decision to be made, the greater the level of competence required. If under 16s are found not to be Gillick competent, a number of proxies may give consent for treatment:

- Parents – the usual repositories of proxy consent. Consent is only required from one parent, although that parent should inform the other, if possible. Parental refusals may be overruled by the courts, who are reluctant to martyr children to their parents' beliefs (e.g. the children of Jehovah's Witnesses).

- Local authorities – if the child is subject to a care order.

- Any adult who has parental responsibility for a child.

- Any adult who has temporary care for a child (e.g. teachers).

- The courts – who may issue wardship, prohibited steps or specific issue orders, or use its inherent jurisdiction.

Mentally disordered patients should not automatically be assumed to be incompetent to consent to medical treatment. The provisions of the Mental Health Act, 1983 only allow doctors to provide non-consensual treatment in order to improve the patient's mental condition. Thus, the patient's consent may still be required before surgical intervention.

Until recently the effects of drugs, illness and pain on patient competence was a grey area. However, it is now recognised that these influences must be acting to such a degree that the ability to decide is absent.

Confidentiality

The law concerning patient confidentiality is complex. Essentially, the doctor–patient

5

relationship is founded on trust, an important aspect of which is the doctor's duty of confidentiality concerning a patient's medical circumstances. Seven key legal aspects of confidentiality are recognised:

1. Doctors are generally obliged to maintain patient confidentiality.

2. This is not an absolute obligation – the law may either oblige or allow the doctor to breach their duty … although the breach must only be to the relevant authority, who in turn must maintain confidentiality.

3. Patient confidentiality is in the public interest of patients. Therefore, the question of whether or not to disclose depends on whether disclosure in the public interest outweighs the public interest duty of confidentiality.

4. Patient confidentiality may additionally be breached if the data disclosed is anonymous, if the patient consents to disclosure or if the information is shared with other health care professionals in order to optimise treatment.

5. Doctors should implement measures designed to prevent third parties from discovering information (e.g. firewalls on computer systems).

6. The courts require a compelling explanation if doctors transgress professional guidelines concerning confidentiality.

7. In law, confidential relationships between doctors, patients and hospitals are now regulated according to the provisions of the Data Protection Act, 1998.

Public interest concerns in which disclosure is allowed include information about human immunodeficiency virus (HIV) status to the at risk partner of an HIV positive patient, and informing the Driver and Vehicle Licensing Agency about a patient who is medically unfit to drive. Doctors are obliged to disclose information if the Court orders disclosure or if there is a statutory duty to disclose (e.g. Prevention of Terrorism Act, 1989, Notifiable Diseases (Public Health Control of Diseases) Act, 1984).

Since 1990 (Health Records Act), patients have had the general rights to see medical records, obtain copies of these and have the records explained, provided the records were made after 1991 and the patient (in the doctor's view) is unlikely to be physically or mentally harmed by viewing their notes. Doctors are expected to maintain the confidentiality of information about third parties who may be mentioned in patients' notes.

Patient death

Brain stem death is recognised as legally synonymous with actual death (and is not the same as persistent vegetative state (PVS), in which the brain stem remains intact). Medically it equates to the irreversible absence of brain stem function despite artificial maintenance of circulation and respiration. The criteria for diagnosing brain stem death are as follows:

- the patient is unconscious;

- a known, predisposing and irreversible cause has been identified;

- there is no CNS depression due to drugs, electrolyte imbalance, hypoxia, hypothermia, hypotension or endocrine disturbance;

- on testing (see Chapter 19), no cranial nerve reflexes are present;

- the patient makes no respiratory effort when disconnected for a period of time from the ventilator.

Testing should be performed independently by two doctors, preferably at least 6 h apart. One doctor should be an appropriately qualified consultant (e.g. neurologist, ITU consultant), the other an appropriately qualified doctor of at least 5 years post-graduate experience. Neither should work for a transplant team. Legally, the patient is considered dead after the first set of tests.

Advance directives

Advance directives are a legal mechanism whereby a patient can consent or refuse to treatment before an event that renders them incapable of consent (e.g. before the onset of dementia in Huntington's chorea). A recent court ruling has found that advanced directives are legally binding provided that, at the time the directive was made, the patient was competent and informed and consented/refused future treatment voluntarily, and that the directive was intended in broad terms to apply to the situation at hand.

Do not resuscitate orders

The BMA have recently reviewed the legal and ethical issues surrounding, 'do not resuscitate' (DNR) orders in light of the Human Rights Act, 1998 and in response to criticisms that doctors did not involve patients in such decisions. Legally, competent patients may refuse cardiopulmonary respiration, such that to attempt it would be considered an assault. However, neither patients nor their relatives may demand resuscitation attempts that are deemed inappropriate by doctors. Relatives may be involved in discussions about an incompetent patient's resuscitation status but can neither consent nor refuse cardiopulmonary resuscitation (CPR) on behalf of the patient. The BMA also suggest that, in the absence of an advance directive, CPR should be attempted unless the patient has refused CPR, the patient is clearly in the terminal phase of an illness, or the burden of CPR outweighs the benefit (i.e. CPR is, or is potentially, futile).

Fitness to practise

A doctor may be unfit to practise medicine on the basis of their conduct, their performance, their health or a combination of these. Medicine is a stressful occupation. Loneliness, tiredness, physical illness, overwork and interpersonal relationships can lead to, or be superimposed upon, other mental health issues or troubled circumstances outside medicine, resulting in depression, alcoholism and drug dependence, suicide, absenteeism and loss of temper. In turn, these may have deleterious effects on the doctor, his/her colleagues and on patients. There is an onus on doctors to self-diagnose and manage their problems themselves. However, it may be necessary for colleagues or friends and family to institute more professional assistance. In the first instance, confrontation is avoided, and ideally the case is referred to the head of department, who should act as the facilitator for access to a sick doctor scheme (run by all the Royal Colleges) and the GMCs Health Committee, although a number of less formal agencies can provide help. Return to work is only sanctioned after consultation between the doctor, his/her doctors and local medical directors ($\pm$the GMC), and may require that the doctor work through a period during which his/her work is constantly supervised by an appointed mentor. Further advice on fitness to practise can be found on the GMC website.

5

Perioperative fluid therapy

Aims

The aims of this chapter are to

- review the normal physiology of fluids and electrolytes and the role of the main fluid compartments of the body,

- show how the distinctive electrolyte composition of each compartment is maintained,

- define the terms osmolality and oncotic pressure and the differences between crystalloids and colloids,

- discuss the differences and importance of osmotic and oncotic pressure and the relevance of the Starling equation in health and disease,

- outline the normal maintenance fluid requirements and what types of fluids should be used to replace them,

- discuss the major changes in fluid and electrolyte homeostasis following trauma and major surgery and their management.

Objectives

After studying this chapter, you should be able to

- devise a suitable fluid and electrolyte regime for healthy patients needing maintenance fluids and for patients undergoing major surgery,

- use changes in electrolyte composition and osmolality of both urine and plasma to aid diagnosis and manage fluid changes in the perioperative period and in patients following trauma,

- optimise patient fluid management to help ensure adequate oxygen delivery to the tissues,

- rationally manage a postoperative patient who is hypovolaemic with hypotension and oliguria.

Introduction

Assessment of fluid requirements in the perioperative period can be complex. Fluid replacement must be primarily based on the clinical status of the patient. This is backed up and guided by measurement of plasma and urine electrolytes, while appreciating that they may be unrepresentative of changes in whole body electrolytes. For instance, in a 70 kg patient only about 15-mmol of K^+ is present in the plasma as compared to about 3000 mmol in the body as a whole. Na^+ forms the skeleton to which water is added to form the plasma volume (PV). Migration of Na^+ intracellularly (accompanied by water), as a result of cellular dysfunction, results in major changes in circulatory homeostasis, although the concentration in the plasma is unchanged. Hyponatraemia may occur with a normal extracellular fluid (ECF) volume, depletion or excess, the latter in the presence or absence of oedema. It is clear, then, that minor changes in serum electrolytes may mask major changes in cellular and total body concentrations that can result in or be the cause of significant cellular dysfunction. In addition, although we normally rely on sensors in the cardiovascular system (CVS), central nervous system (CNS) and kidneys for maintaining the *milieu interieur*, these control systems are disrupted and act unpredictably following surgical procedures, trauma or severe illness. Application of pharmacokinetic principles such as volume of distribution, concentration, redistribution and excretory processes are equally applicable to drugs and electrolytes and put changes in plasma electrolytes into context (Chapter 3).

Normal physiology

Water is the major component of mammalian structure. The percentage of total body water (TBW) to weight ranges from about 55% in the adult female, 60% in the adult male, to nearly 80% in the newborn. In the adult male of 70 kg, TBW is equal to about 40 l. There are three main compartments through which it is distributed, intracellular fluid (ICF), which contains about 27 l, interstitial fluid (ISF) 10 l and plasma volume (PV) of 3 l. The latter two, ISF and PV, constitute ECF. PV forms the medium in which red blood cells (RBCs) carrying oxygen can be transported to all cells of the body and together form the circulating volume (CV) of 5 l.

Transcellular fluid (TCF) is defined as fluid in transit between various compartments, usually in body cavities such as the gut lumen where it is continuously added to by ingested fluids, secreted and reabsorbed. The volume at any time is usually not large but may increase markedly in derangement of gut function such as paralytic ileus, diarrhoea and vomiting or is lost iatrogenically, as by nasogastric (NG) suction. TCF is extremely difficult to quantify but should always be considered when trying to quantify fluid losses and shifts in the surgical patient.

Control of volumes and constituents

In health, the volume and electrolyte distribution of these compartments of TBW are controlled by three major processes, the Na^+/K^+ pump, osmolality and the hydrostatic/oncotic pressure gradient in the capillaries.

The Na^+/K^+ pump
This is an active process, relying on ATP and a Na^+/K^+ exchange pump that controls the electrolyte composition of the ICF and ISF. The major intracellular cation is K^+ (140–160 mmol/l) with Na^+ of 10–40 mmol/l (depending on the type of cell), while in the ISF and PV the ratios are reversed with Na^+ being the predominant cation (132–145 mmol/l) with a K^+ of 3.5–5 mmol/l. Total body exchangeable Na^+ and K^+ are roughly equivalent to 40 mmol/kg body weight (BW). Derangement to this active process in disease results in K^+ leak from the cells and into the ECF with Na^+ (and water) going in the opposite direction.

Osmolality and tonicity
Maintenance of osmotic balance ensures that the total *concentration* of osmotically active particles is the same throughout all three compartments. The major osmotically active cation in ECF is Na^+ while in the ICF it is K^+. Osmolality is simply the number of osmotically active particles (osmols or mosmols) per kg of solvent (in this case per litre of water) (Table 6.1). A solution is hypotonic if it has fewer osmotically active particles than plasma, isotonic if it has the same number and hypertonic if it has more.

The osmolality or osmotic pressure of a solution depends on the number of osmotically active particles per kg of solvent (litre of water). This is normally equal to the number of mol or mmol, e.g. in 5% glucose there are 277 mmol of glucose and the osmolality is 277 mosmol/l. However, with an electrolyte such as NaCl, 1 mmol dissociates to 2 mosmol, i.e. Na^+ and Cl^-. However, with some solutions, dissociation may not be complete, so the calculated number of mmol may not equate with the total number of mosmol. For example, with 0.9% NaCl, the values are the same, i.e. it is almost completely dissociated and has a calculated and measured osmolality of 308. However, a balanced salt solution (BSS) such as Hartmann's or lactated

6

Table 6.1 **The major osmotic constituents of plasma**

Cation/anion	Concentration in m(os)mol/l
Na^+	135
K^+	5
Cl^-	110
HCO_3^-	24
Glucose	5
Urea	5
Total osmolality	284

Ringer's solution (see later) has a calculated osmolality of 277 mosmol/l but a measured osmolality (by freezing point depression) of 254 mosmol/kg due to incomplete dissociation. This may have implications for reduced osmotic pressure following large volumes of infusion (see later).

If two solutions of equal osmolality (i.e. the number of osmotically active particles are the same) are separated by a semi-permeable membrane and water is added to one side, then water will move across the membrane to equalise the osmotic pressure of the two solutions. Thus, with a fall in PV osmolality in comparison to that in the ISF, water will move initially from PV to ISF in an attempt to equalise the osmotic pressures (osmolality) in the two compartments. The resulting overall fall in ISF osmolality leads to further movement of water into the ICF. An opposite effect is seen with a rise in PV osmolality. In other words, a fall in PV osmolality always results in an increase in ICF and vice versa.

Example

This movement can be seen most clearly in the following example. A normal 2.5 kg infant has TBW roughly equal to 80% of BW with the ratio of ECF to ICF is 1:1. Thus, overall osmolality of both compartments is 280 with an ECF (and PV) Na^+ of 140 mmol/l. An infusion of 100 ml of 5% glucose in water is given over a sufficient period to allow the glucose to be metabolised. If no movement of water occurred, the overall osmolality of the ECF (PV and then ISF) would be reduced by dilution to 254 and the Na^+ would fall to 127. There is potential osmotic disequilibrium that cannot be sustained but it occurs gradually as the glucose is metabolised and the effective osmolality falls. Water moves from the ECF to ICF to re-establish osmotic equilibrium. This results in an expansion of the ICF by 50 ml and a final ECF (and PV) Na^+ of 133 (i.e. reduced from the original Na^+ of 140 but more than it would have been if the water had stayed in the ECF). The net result is that the 100 ml of water has distributed according to the relative volumes of the ECF and ICF (in this case

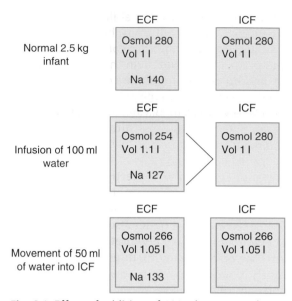

Fig. 6.1 Effect of addition of 100 ml water on the relative volumes of ECF and ICF and changes in osmolality (see text).

equally, but in an adult would be 1:2) and there is an expansion in ICF of 50 ml (see Fig. 6.1).

Hydrostatic and colloid osmotic (oncotic) balance

Obviously, the three compartments are not in a passive state. The dynamics of the circulation and the requirement to transport oxygen and nutrients around the body necessitates the generation of a pressurised flow of blood from left heart to right atrium (RA). The hydrostatic pressure generated by this column of blood in the capillaries would inevitably lead to a net loss of fluid from the PV into the ISF by filtration and eventual depletion of the CV. This hydrostatic pressure is balanced by the presence of *colloids* in the PV.

A semi-permeable membrane (the capillary endothelium) represents the barrier between the PV and the ISF as has been discussed above. High molecular protein constituents of plasma exert 'colloid osmotic' or 'oncotic' pressure. Colloids are molecules capable of exerting oncotic pressure and have limited (or zero) ability to cross a semi-permeable membrane due to their molecular size. At the same time, they have the ability to attract solvent (solvent drag) from the other side of the membrane into the compartment in which they are situated (in this case PV). The oncotic pressure of a plasma constituent is proportional to the amount (in g/l) divided by the MW. In man, plasma albumin (40 g/l) with a MW of 60,000 constitutes the most important component of plasma oncotic pressure (3 kPa or 20–25 mmHg). Albumin also exists in the ISF but its effective concentration is markedly reduced, due not only to the fact that it is bound to cells, but also that ISF albumin is mainly in a semi-solid gel form. The *oncotic pressure gradient* between the two compartments that is manifest as solvent drag from ISF to PV is around 1.5–2 kPa (10–15 mmHg).

Thus, the total *crystalloid osmotic* pressure of the PV is 680 kPa (6.8 atm or 5100 mmHg, see later) while the *colloid oncotic* component is only 3–3.5 kPa (20–25 mmHg). However, the former is equalised throughout the three main compartments (ICF, ISF and PV) while the latter is greater in the PV versus the ISF. This oncotic pressure gradient is responsible for maintaining the integrity of the PV.

The effects of the two opposing forces, hydrostatic pressure and oncotic pressure, have been summarised in Starling's equation, which states that

$$QF = K(HP_{pl} - HP_{in}) - \sigma(OP_{pl} - OP_{in})$$

where QF is the net outward flow of fluid from the capillaries into the ISF, K is a constant that expresses the flow of fluid outwards in ml per unit pressure gradient in kPa or mmHg, HP_{pl} is the hydrostatic pressure in the capillaries in kPa or mmHg, HP_{in} is the hydrostatic pressure in the ISF in kPa or mmHg, OP_{pl} is the oncotic pressure in the plasma in kPa or mmHg (almost entirely due to albumin), OP_{in} is the oncotic pressure in the ISF in kPa or mmHg (*Note*: over two-thirds of the body's albumin is in the ISF.), σ is the reflection coefficient of the capillary bed in question.

The reflection coefficient is a measure of the permeability of the capillary to albumin. If it is impermeable, then the full oncotic pressure gradient between plasma and ISF is

exerted, σ will be 1. If, on the other hand, the capillary is completely permeable to albumin, then no gradient exists, and fluid leaks out entirely as expressed by the hydrostatic pressure gradient. This would result in a σ of 0. In practice, depending on the capillary bed in question the range is about 0 (liver) to 0.7 (lung).

A fall in the oncotic pressure gradient, due to loss of albumin or a reduction in the reflection coefficient due to capillary endothelial damage (vide infra), causes a loss of PV and an increased propensity to the development of significant tissue and pulmonary oedema. This is seen experimentally in animals subjected to smoke inhalation injury where fluid leakage is greatest in those animals resuscitated with crystalloids compared to those resuscitated with colloids. The situation in human burn injury is still controversial.

Overall, plasma electrolytes represent a dynamic interchange between total body stores, input and output and passive and active movements between compartments as controlled by the processes alluded to above.

Figure 6.2 shows the effect of the Starling equation and the typical overall pressures in the capillaries and venules and the fluid shifts which occur. Please note that as fluid leaves the circulation at the arteriolar end, the hydrostatic pressure gradient gradually diminishes in the capillaries and the oncotic pressure gradient gradually increases. Thus, by the time we reach the venular end, the pressure gradients have been reversed and fluid re-enters the circulation again.

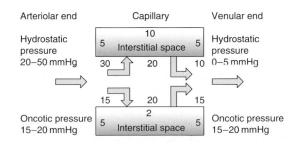

Fig. 6.2 Hydrostatic and colloid oncotic pressure gradients in the capillaries.

Conditions causing an increase in capillary endothelial permeability

Three common conditions cause an increase in *capillary endothelial permeability* (CEP):

- *Anaphylactic shock* (e.g. penicillin allergy) results in increased leakage of fluid leading to sudden hypovolaemia along with peripheral oedema and broncho-constriction. The initial treatment for a patient without venous access is i.m. adrenaline (0.5–1 mg, i.e. 0.5–1 ml of a 1:1000 solution) or in a patient with i.v. access, 1–2 ml boluses of i.v. adrenaline (1 mg in 10 ml or 1:10,000). Fluids and oxygen therapy should be used in addition.

- *Burn injury* causes a systemic 'capillary leak', which is proportional to the percentage of the burned area. The amount of fluid leakage is massive and is equivalent to 4 ml of Hartmann's or lactated Ringer's solution per kg per % area burn in 24 h (Parkland formula); e.g. in a 60-kg patient with a 40% burn this requires $4 \times 60 \times 40 = 9600$ ml, 50% given in the first 8 h, 25% in the next two 8-h periods) calculated *from the time of the burn injury*.

- *Septic shock* or systemic inflammatory response syndrome (SIRS) also leads to loss of CV and this fluid must be replaced in large quantities to maintain CV, despite the inevitable oedema that this causes (Chapter 13).

Regulation of blood volume

Day-to-day homeostasis

The factors mentioned above are all designed to maintain the integrity of the PV (and CV) so that it can form the medium to allow transport of oxygen and nutrients for cellular metabolism. This ensures optimal organ function, but in a dynamic process the volumes are not static. Adequate clearance of waste products of metabolism require the kidney to excrete about 1500 ml of urine per day containing about 400–800 mmol of urea,

50–100 mmol K^+ and 70–140 mmol Na^+, depending on intake (a volume of at least 500 ml of urine is needed to excrete the normal amount of urea per day due to a limit of about 1200 mosmol/l in the maximum concentrating ability of the kidney). Additional fluid losses are incurred from evaporation, the respiratory tract and faeces. The total loss of fluid is about 2500 ml of water plus about 70 mmol Na^+ and K^+ in a 70-kg adult per day. This has to be replaced to maintain TBW. The extent of maintenance fluid requirements is more closely related to body surface area (BSA) than weight. Since a newborn baby of 3.5 kg has about 2fi times the BSA/wt ratio of an adult (1/20 the weight and ⅛ the BSA) it consequently needs 2½ times the maintenance fluid per unit weight. A common formula used is shown in Table 6.2.

Normally, this fluid requirement is regulated both by changes in volume and osmolality in the PV being detected in the hypothalamus. An increase (due to fluid deprivation) stimulates anti-diuretic hormone (ADH) release from the supra optic nucleus which causes thirst and reduces urine output by increasing reabsorption of water from the collecting ducts in the kidney. A decrease in renal perfusion (due to fluid deprivation)

Table 6.2 **Maintenance fluid requirements**

Weight range	Fluids per 24 h
3–10 kg	100 ml/kg
10–20 kg	1000 ml for first 10 kg + 50 ml/kg for any additional weight over 10 kg
20 kg and above	1500 ml for first 20 kg + 20 ml/kg for weight over 20 kg

Thus, a 7-kg infant would require 700 ml/day, a 17 kg child would require $1000 + 350 = 1350$ ml/day, a 70 kg adult would require $1500 + 1000 = 2500$ ml/day.

increases renin output from the juxtaglomerular apparatus leads eventually to the formation of angiotensin II (AT II). This causes thirst, constricts the efferent glomerular artery to maintain glomerular arterial pressure and filtration and also causes release of aldosterone from the adrenal cortex. The latter increases renal Na^+ retention in exchange for K^+ in the distal tubule.

All these changes are increased by activation of the sympathetic nervous system (SNS). If fluid deprivation becomes greater or there are abnormal losses such as diarrhoea, vomiting, ileus or haemorrhage, these processes are amplified. It is important to note that volume is usually maintained at the expense of a reduction in osmolality due to hyponatraemia. This is due to the more powerful effect of ADH over aldosterone. As plasma Na^+ concentration falls, proximal tubular reabsorption of Na^+ (and water) becomes intense, limiting the ability of the kidney to produce dilute urine. Administration of hyponatraemic solutions in the postoperative period in the presence of a low serum Na^+ further compounds the problem. Five per cent glucose and 4% glucose 0.18% NaCl should never be given if the plasma Na^+ is low and 0.9% sodium chloride or Hartmann's solution (Lactated Ringer's) is more appropriate.

Acute changes in homeostasis

Acute surgical or traumatic hypovolaemia cannot be compensated for by the more chronic processes mentioned above. Additional mechanisms are brought into play. Acute reduction in CV reduces venous return and cardiac preload so cardiac output and BP fall. Reduction in BP reduces the afferent activity of the carotid sinus baroreceptors to the 'pressor' area in the dorsal hypothalamus, and results in increased SNS discharge. Reduction in venous return leads to a decrease in atrial natriuretic peptide (ANP) production (thus reducing urinary sodium loss) and a fall in output from the low-pressure baroreceptors in the atria and great veins to the 'depressor' centre. The resultant fall in parasympathetic

nervous system (PNS) discharge augments the action of the SNS (see also Chapter 3).

The effects of this are summarised as follows:

- *Direct neural effects* via α- and β-receptors.
- *Catecholamine release from the adrenal medulla.* In different shock states, and at different stages of shock, noradrenaline or adrenaline predominates.
- *Renin release* from the juxtaglomerular apparatus of the kidney (vide infra).
- *Increased Na^+ reabsorption* in the distal tubule.
- *Decreased Na^+ loss* due to a reduction in atrial natriuretic peptide (ANP).
- *Vascular redistribution of blood in the kidney* from cortex to medulla, the latter being the major site of Na^+ and water reabsorption.

The ISF compartment has an important role in maintaining CV. Sympathetic stimulation, particularly to the skin and splanchnic circulation, results in a reduction of flow to these non-essential areas, by α-adrenergically mediated arteriolar vasoconstriction. This results in a reduction of flow to the capillary beds by neuro-humorally mediated increase in the pre-capillary sphincter (PCS) tone. The hydrostatic pressure in the capillary beds falls, thus allowing fluid to enter the capillary circulation distal to the PCS as a result of the change in hydrostatic/oncotic pressure gradient (see Starling's equation and Fig. 6.2).

Intravenous perioperative fluid replacement therapy

Initially, it is pertinent to consider the types of fluids that are available and their uses. Fluids can be conveniently classified into crystalloids, colloids and blood (and blood products).

Crystalloids

These are solutions containing water and electrolytes and/or glucose made up in

Table 6.3 **Content of crystalloid solutions (amounts in mmol/l)**

Name	Known as	Na$^+$	Cl$^-$	K$^+$	Ca^{++}	Mg^{++}	HCO$_3^-$	Lactate	mosmol/l
NaCl 0.9%	Normal saline	154	154						308
Hartmann's (BP)		131	111	5	2			29	277[§]
Lactated Ringer's solution (USP)		130	112	5.4	1.8			27	276[§]
Glucose 5%	5% dextrose								252
Glucose 4% + NaCl 0.18%	Dextrose saline	30	30						286
Plasmalyte 148 + glucose	Plasmalyte	148	97	5		1		40*	552
Sodium bicarbonate 8.4%		1000					1000		2000

§ The measured osmolality is lower due to incomplete dissociation (see text).
* As gluconate/acetate.

a concentration that is usually isotonic with plasma. This means that they contain the same number of osmotically active particles as plasma, i.e. about 300 (normal physiological range is 280–310) mosmol/l of solute. Several solutions are available, 5% glucose, 4% glucose 0.18% NaCl, 'Normal' (0.9%) NaCl and Hartmann's (lactated Ringer's) solution (Table 6.3).

How do we make an isotonic solution? From first principles, if 1 g MW of solute is placed in a flask containing 1 kg of solvent (i.e. 1 l of water) it will form a molar solution. Thus, 180 g of glucose (180 = the m.w. of glucose) in a kg of water will have 1 mol or 1000 mmol/kg. By definition, if 1 mol of glucose is dissolved in 22.4 l of solution at NTP (i.e. 0°C) it will exert an osmotic pressure of one atmosphere (100 kPa or 760 mmHg). Thus, a molar solution will exert an osmotic pressure of 22.4 atm (2200 kPa or 15,200 mmHg) at NTP or 25.4 atm (2540 kPa or 19,340 mmHg) at 37°C. This amount is referred to as 1 osmol

or 1000 mosmol. One mosmol at 37°C thus generates an osmotic pressure of 2.5 kPa (19 mmHg). The total osmotic pressure of plasma is thus equal to 300 × 2.5 (19) = 750 kPa (5700 mmHg). However, a molar solution of 18% glucose (180 g/l or 18 g/100 ml) is hypertonic (1000 versus 300 mosmol/l). Each g per l therefore gives about 5.5 mosmol/l, so 50 g (5% solution of glucose) will produce an isotonic solution of 50 times 5.5 or 275 mosmol/l.

With an electrolyte such as sodium chloride, the molar solution (58.5 g of sodium chloride in 1 l of water) will contain nearly 2000 mosmol/l as in solution it is almost completely dissociated into sodium and chloride ions (1 mmol of NaCl giving 2 mosmol of Na$^+$ and Cl$^-$ ions). Thus, roughly 1/6 of 58.5 g/kg is required, i.e. 9 g/l (0.9 g/100 ml or 0.9% NaCl) with 154 mmol of Na$^+$ and 154 mmol of Cl$^-$. In a similar manner, 4% glucose and 0.18% NaCl will give 30 mosmol of both Na$^+$ and Cl$^-$ per l plus 220 mosmol/l from

6

glucose making 280 in all. It can be seen that normal (0.9%) NaCl is hardly *physiological* as it contains excess Na^+ (154 versus the normal 135) and excess Cl^- (154 versus the normal 105). Excess Cl^- administration can result in retention of H^+ and urinary loss of HCO_3^- and a dilutional hyperchloraemic acidosis if administered in excess. Thus, ideally, a BSS should be used for crystalloid volume replacement during surgery, trauma or burns. Such a solution is Hartmann's (BP) or lactated Ringer's solution (USP). This contains in mmol/kg, Na^+:131, K^+:5, Cl^-:111, Ca:2, lactate: 29 (the ionic concentrations of the two solutions are slightly different, see Table 6.3). The latter is a H^+ acceptor and is metabolised by the liver with net formation of 1 mol of HCO_3^- and 1 mol of pyruvate, which can be utilised as an energy source in the Krebs cycle. It does not cause a dilutional or lactic acidosis provided that liver perfusion is adequate.

Clinical relevance

The TURP syndrome

It is worth noting that a fall in serum Na^+ of 5 mmol/l (accompanied by a change in Cl^- of the same amount) will result in a pressure dysequilibrium between the PV, ISF and ICF of 1/30 (10/300) of total plasma osmotic pressure or about 25 kPa or 190 mmHg (1/30 of 750 kPa or 5900 mmHg, see above). This large pressure difference, should it occur rapidly, results in water leaving the PV into the ISF and then into the ICF in an attempt to restore osmotic balance between the fluid compartments. If this occurs acutely, as in excess absorption of non-sodium-containing irrigation fluid during transurethral resection of prostate (TURP), cerebral oedema and raised intracranial pressure may occur. The latter occurs in the *TURP syndrome*. However, it should be noted that glycine 1.5%, the irrigation fluid traditionally used during TURP, is hypotonic. The MW of glycine is 75, so 75 g dissolved in a kg of solvent (i.e. a litre of water) would be a molar solution and would contain 1000 mosmol/l. Thus, 1.5% glycine (or 15 g/l) has an osmolality of 200 mosmol/l. To aid detection of excess absorption of fluid,

ethanol (1%) is usually added as a marker. If a significant amount of irrigation fluid is absorbed, the ethanol component will be detectable in the breath (cf. a 'Breathalyzer'®). The concentration of ethanol thus reflects the extent of absorption. The addition of ethanol 1% to the 1.5% glycine affects its osmolality. The MW of ethanol is 46, thus 10 g/l (i.e. a 1% solution) will increase osmolality by 217 thus making the total osmolality of the irrigating solution 417, i.e. hypertonic! Since this combined solution is now commonly used it may account for the diminished incidence of TURP syndrome.

Thus, absorption of irrigation solution will increase overall osmotic pressure in the PV but still result in a fall in plasma Na^+. In fact, the TURP syndrome is more likely due to fluid overload and the possible cerebral effects of glycine than the effect of the drop in plasma Na^+.

In the same way, infusion of 5% glucose will cause a fall in plasma Na^+ due to a dilutional effect but osmotic pressure will remain constant, as the solution is isotonic. As the glucose is metabolised (the glucose concentration in 5% glucose is about 275 mmol/kg while in plasma it is 5), the osmotic pressure in the plasma will fall and water will go into the cells. The effect on cellular overhydration will depend on the rate of administration and metabolism of 5% glucose. Thus although non-sodium-containing isotonic solutions will eventually result in increased cellular water they do not do so rapidly enough in most circumstances to cause problems of dysequilibrium between the body compartments.

Chronic hyponatraemia

This may occur in patients on diuretic therapy, but since it occurs slowly, there is time to restore osmotic equilibrium without major pressure differences occurring between compartments. However, use of hypertonic NaCl may result in too rapid correction of Na^+ in the plasma and will cause rapid reversal of the above process and cerebral dehydration which can be equally dangerous. Thus, it is much easier to raise

6

Na^+ concentrations rapidly than to cause a fall. The commonest cause of excess hypertonic Na^+ administration is the use of $Na^+HCO_3^-$ solutions (see Table 6.3).

Electrolyte concentrations of commonly used crystalloid solutions are shown in Table 6.3.

Crystalloid solutions containing isotonic concentrations of Na^+ do not remain in the PV following i.v. administration. The volume of distribution (Vd) of these fluids is the total ECF volume and thus they only provide a short-term expansion of the CV. Approximately three times the volume of estimated blood loss must be given to maintain CV. In severe blood loss, massive doses of crystalloid for resuscitation (together with blood) have been implicated in the formation of pulmonary and generalised tissue oedema due to the large volumes required for resuscitation. Although this has not been substantiated in clinical trials, many anaesthetists employ colloid-containing solutions for resuscitation as lower volumes are required.

Colloids

Also known as 'plasma expanders', these solutions contain high MW substances such as dextrans, gelatins and hydroxyethylstarch, which exert oncotic pressure and thus retain fluid in the CV as stated above. In addition, naturally occurring colloid solutions such as 5% albumin and plasma protein fraction (PPF) can be used but they are expensive and have no advantages over the other synthetic colloid solutions (Table 6.4).

Intra-operative fluids

Introduction
Not all patients undergoing surgery need i.v. fluid therapy. Indeed, i.v. fluid administration is not devoid of risks (air embolism, deep vein thrombosis (DVT), overloading, discomfort to the patient, infection risk and considerable cost), so it should not be undertaken lightly. There are three components to fluid therapy in the surgical patient. Firstly, as it is customary to deprive patients of fluids for at least 4 h prior to a surgical procedure under general anaesthesia, there is an element of maintenance fluid deficit. Secondly, depending on the site and severity of the operative procedure, there will be an element of compartmental fluid shift due to tissue trauma (the so-called 'third space loss'). Thirdly, there will be the additional losses of other fluids

6

Table 6.4 **Commonly used colloid solutions**

Trade name	Source	Average MW	MW range	tfi in PV (h)	Effect on coagulation	Cost (2000) (£)
Albumin	Human	69,000	69,000	24	None	40
Dextran 70	Bacterial conversion of sucrose	38,000	10–250,000	12	Decreased platelet aggregation, reduced Factor VIII	4
Haemaccel	Gelatin	24,500	5–50,000	2.5	None	4
Gelofusin*	Gelatin	22,600	10–150,000	4	None	3.50
Voluven	Maize starch	130,000	15,000–380,000	3	No, if <33 ml/kg/day	10

*Contains no K^+ or Ca^{++}.

such as excessive urine output, ascites and fluid collections in the peritoneal or pleural cavities. Finally, blood loss must be considered.

Maintenance fluid
The average daily requirements stated above (Table 6.2) correspond to the normal physiological losses (70-kg patient) through the urine (1.5 l), faeces (100–200 ml), perspiration (300–500 ml) and respiration (500 ml). It is not necessary to replace this loss i.v. for many minor procedures where the preoperative period of fluid deprivation has been short and it is expected that oral fluids can be commenced within hours of the procedure's termination. If maintenance fluids are required then the aim should be to replace the preoperative deficit and then provide the requirements on an hourly basis until oral fluids are tolerated. On a 24-h basis, 4% glucose, 0.18% NaCl provides a suitable solution as 2500 ml (for a 70-kg patient) provides 75-mmol Na^+. On an hourly basis this equates to 100 ml, so 400 ml will compensate for the preoperative deficit and then 100 ml thereafter (see formula above). Addition of K^+ is not required for short-term (<48 h) therapy.

Third space losses
This only becomes relevant during major surgery (or trauma) where there is extensive tissue damage, e.g. major abdominal and thoracic surgery. Cellular damage at the site of injury results in an inability to maintain the Na^+/K^+ pump, so Na^+ and water leak into the cells, which become swollen and oedematous. The major loss of fluid, however, is from the PV into a non-exchangeable compartment of the ISF (the so-called 'third space'). This is due to alterations in the oncotic/osmotic balance between the PV and ISF, again as a result of tissue damage. In extensive surgery these losses can be considerable, although estimates that have been made of 15 ml/kg/h are now thought too high. A more reasonable figure is 5–10 ml/kg/h, nevertheless, this may represent a five-fold increase over basic maintenance requirements. This loss of functional ECF volume (FECFV), if not replaced in adequate quantities, leads to further activation of ADH

and aldosterone secretion as well as inhibition of ANP. It is not surprising that there is marked water and sodium retention with oliguria in the postoperative period. This fluid should be replaced with adequate quantities of a BSS such as Hartmann's (lactated Ringer's) solution.

Unphysiological losses
These may arise from surgical drains, NG tubes or vomiting, diarrhoea, excessive body temperature and excessive urinary output due to diuretic drugs. Losses arising from NG tubes, drains and urine output can be accurately measured while losses due to high body or ambient temperatures can only be roughly estimated.

The measurable losses must always be replaced as accurately as possible in volume, Na^+ and K^+ content: note that diarrhoea has a high K^+ content (20–50/mmol) and vomit has a high chloride content (80–100/mmol). Patients on thiazide diuretics or frusemide may lose 50–70 mmol of K^+ per litre of urine.

Elevation of body temperature is reasonably compensated for by an increase in the normal water, Na^+ and K^+ intake of 15% for each °C above the normal 37.

Blood loss
Maintenance of adequate oxygen delivery (DO_2) should be the primary aim rather than simply considering blood replacement.

$$DO_2 = \text{cardiac output (l/min)} \times \text{arterial oxygen content}$$

Arterial oxygen content = $SaO_2/100 \times$ Hb (g/l) $\times$ 1.34, ignoring the small amount dissolved in the plasma. Although the latter is not numerically important, it does form the all important interface between oxygen bound to Hb and cells which require it.

Thus, at a normal cardiac output of 5 lpm, oxygen saturation of 99% and Hb of 145 g/l:

$$DO_2 = 5 \times (0.99 \times 145 \times 1.34)$$
$$= 1000 \text{ ml/min}$$

In considering when blood loss should be replaced, it is pertinent to consider that a 50% fall in Hb can be compensated by a doubling

6

of cardiac output, provided CV is maintained. In addition, although similar big swings in SaO_2 are rarely observed, a 15% reduction to 85% is not uncommon in the postoperative period and would have the same effect as the loss of 1–2 units blood. It is therefore important to maintain (or increase) cardiac output and oxygenation, as a priority, in patients experiencing blood loss. Only when blood loss is likely to result in a fall in Hb to below 80 g/l, or when there are limitations on the ability of the patient to increase cardiac output should it be replaced. Although blood may not be required until 20% or more of the blood volume is lost (in a healthy patient) it is obviously necessary to replace the fluid component so that preload and thus cardiac output can be maintained (Chapter 7).

Also, please note that 1000 ml/min of oxygen can only be delivered to the tissues if a similar amount is being delivered to the alveoli. This is normally achieved by an alveolar ventilation of 5 l/min and an oxygen concentration of 21%. If oxygen demand is increased then more oxygen will have to be delivered to the alveoli. This can be achieved by increased ventilation, increased oxygen concentration (O_2 supplementation) or a combination of the two.

Three special problems in the perioperative period

Hypovolaemia associated with mild to moderate hypotension, oliguria and hyponatraemia

This is a common situation indicating depletion of isotonic fluid almost always accompanied by Na^+ depletion. Clinically, the symptoms and signs are:

- a low to low normal BP, e.g. mean BP less than 60 mmHg and a tachycardia;
- the signs of hypovolaemia, e.g. dry mucosae, cold extremities (as above);
- a low urine output of <0.5 ml/kg/h in the adult ;
- low plasma Na^+ (e.g. 125–130 mmol/l);
- high urine osmolality (>600 or at least 2:1 urine/plasma osmolality ratio);

- low urinary Na^+ (<20 mmol/l) due to Na^+ retention as a result of continuing 'third space' loss,
- a low central venous pressure (CVP);
- the Hb concentration may be relatively normal due to haemoconcentration or low if third space loss is exacerbated by blood loss.

Not all the above may be present and urine Na^+ may be higher, even in the presence of hypovolaemia, due to the injudicious use of diuretics to increase urine output.

Hyponatraemia is usually due to water excess rather than sodium depletion. In this situation it is usually due to low Na^+ (e.g. 30 mmol/l or less) containing fluids (e.g. 5% glucose or 4% glucose 0.18% NaCl) being given to compensate for continuing isotonic Na^+ (e.g. 135–150 mmol/l) 'third space' losses. Depending on the volumes given, signs of ECF deficit may not be obvious and the patient may even become oedematous with a high CVP. If the latter is associated with hyponatraemia then water restriction may be needed (see Water intoxication). Correction of low serum Na^+ should be done slowly with frequent measurements of serum Na^+. Aim to correct to a level of about 130 mmol/l. Chronic hyponatraemia (e.g. due to diuretics) should not be corrected quickly (see above).

Hypotension

As seen above, hypotension is a common accompaniment of relative fluid deprivation in the perioperative period. However, in making management decisions, it is very important to look at the physiological background (see also Chapter 2 and Chapter 15 for a more detailed discussion of cardiac function).

BP is equal to the product of cardiac output (Q) and SVR:

$$BP = Q \times SVR$$

Q is equal to the product of SV and HR.

$$Q = SV \times HR$$

SV is determined by the Frank–Starling mechanism that states that the force of

6

contraction of the ventricle is determined by the end-diastolic fibre length of the ventricular muscle. The greater the length (i.e. stretch or filling) the greater the force of contraction and (usually) the greater the SV. The three main factors at play here are:

1. *Preload*, i.e. the amount of blood returning to the heart and therefore filling the ventricle and is usually determined by the volume status of the patient and the compliance of the capacitance vessels, i.e. the venules and veins.

2. *Afterload*, i.e. the impedance to ejection of blood usually determined by the SVR, i.e. compliance of the peripheral arterial circulation. High SVR means low SV.

3. *Contractility*, i.e. the contractile state of the heart which determines the force of contraction for any given degree of filling pressure (i.e. the Frank–Starling mechanism, *vide infra*).

In the context of the perioperative hypotensive patient we can see that:

1. *Preload* may be diminished due to hypovolaemia or excess depressant drugs increasing venous capacitance (e.g. relative epidural or opioid excess).

2. *Afterload* may be increased in a shocked patient due to sympathetic overactivity and increased SVR as a compensatory mechanism to maintain BP.

3. *Contractility* may be decreased due to depressant drugs or increased in response to hypovolaemia and sympathetic stimulation.

In most cases, restoration of blood volume (with or without CVP monitoring) will restore preload, diminish sympathetic response and restore SV and thus Q.

If the patient is hypotensive and this is accompanied by bradycardia then the initial intervention should be to increase HR and then look at the state of the circulation.

These steps are summarised in the *Hypotension algorithm* (Fig. 6.3). Please note that it is important to exclude other causes of hypotension (as indicated in the boxes).

Oliguria

Oliguria is common in the postoperative patient following major surgery. It can be classified as pre-renal (e.g. hypovolaemia), renal (e.g. ARF) or post-renal (e.g. obstruction). The commonest cause is pre-renal due to insufficient fluid and sodium replacement in the perioperative period. Third space loss (see above) does not stop with the end of surgery and excess loss may persist for many hours. However, renal and post-renal causes of oliguria must always be sought, such as ARF and blocked catheter. Examination of the urine for casts, protein and glucose may indicate renal pathology. Measurement of urinary electrolytes and osmolality will distinguish between the two. As opposed to the values in hypovolaemia, in ARF the urine to plasma osmolality ratio will be about 1:1 and the urinary Na^+ >20 mmol/kg.

Do not give diuretics in this situation (unless the patient is on regular diuretic therapy) as they will only exacerbate the hypovolaemia. Although, a crystalloid such as 0.9% NaCl or Hartmann's (lactated Ringer's) solution may be used, a colloid such as Gelofusin® is preferred initially. Begin with a 5 ml/kg bolus over 10 min and follow the *Hypotension Algorithm*. Reduce to maintenance levels of 2–3 ml/kg/h of crystalloid once the above signs of hypovolaemia are reversed. 4% glucose and 0.18% NaCl should only be used if the blood Na^+ concentration is higher than 140 mmol/l.

The *Oliguria algorithm* (Fig. 6.4) gives a suggested course of action.

Potassium depletion

Chronic depletion is commonly seen in the ageing hospital population who have been chronically treated with diuretics for hypertension or cardiac failure. Plasma K^+ starts to fall below the normal minimum of 3.5 mmol/l only after 10% of total body K^+ has been lost (400 mmol). A good additional indicator of depletion is a high plasma

6

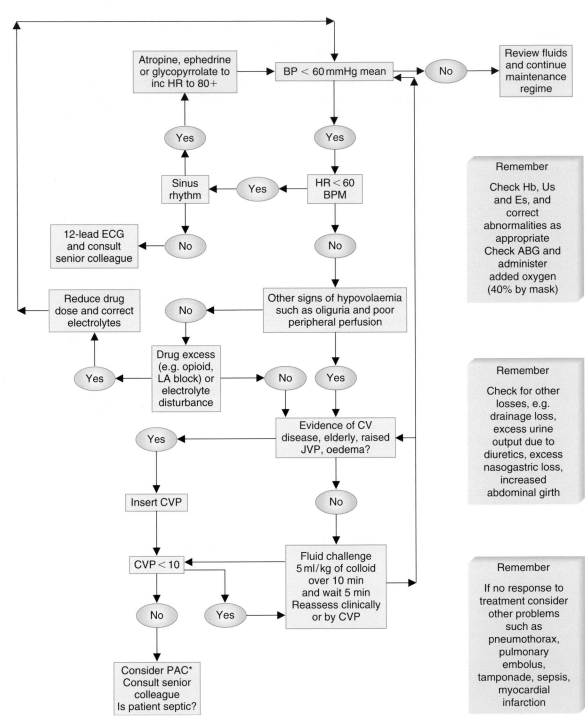

Fig. 6.3 Hypotension algorithm. *PAC: Pulmonary artery or Swan–Ganz catheter.

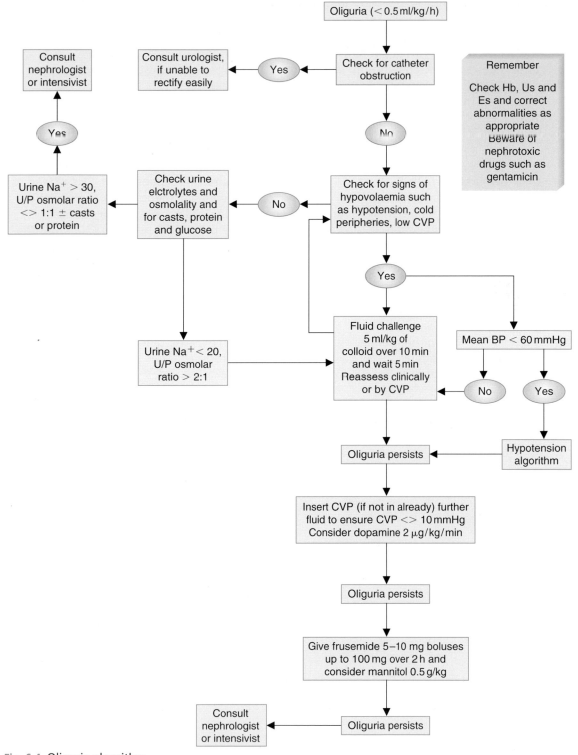

Fig. 6.4 Oliguria algorithm.

bicarbonate value (>28 mmol/l), associated with acid urine.

Depletion of 400–600 mmol K^+ causes intracellular acidosis as hydrogen ions enter the cells to maintain ionic equilibrium. Losses should be replaced over several days with oral supplements, and the underlying cause corrected.

If the patient is unable to take oral supplements K^+ must be given i.v. It is administered as KCl, and concentrations of more than 20 mmol/l in 0.9% NaCl or 5% glucose cause pain and thrombosis in peripheral veins. Rapid replacement is rarely advisable. If absolutely necessary, it is given through a CVP line (preferably in the HDU or ICU), with continuous ECG monitoring and frequent plasma K^+ measurements.

Water intoxication

This rarely occurs, but has dramatic consequences due to hyponatraemia. The cause is usually iatrogenic. Other causes include compulsive water drinking, transurethral resection of the prostate with excessive absorption of glycine irrigation fluid (see above), inappropriate secretion of ADH and a few rare medical disorders.

Excessive administration of i.v. 5% glucose and 4% glucose 0.18% NaCl solutions is the main iatrogenic cause. This was a not infrequent problem in labour wards. A fall in plasma Na^+, as stated above, leads to a movement of water from the hypotonic PV into the ISF and ICF to maintain osmotic equilibrium. This expansion of ICF can lead to cerebral oedema, mental disturbances and convulsions if plasma Na^+ falls rapidly. It should be noted that as plasma Na^+ falls the ability to excrete a water load falls also, thus exacerbating the water intoxication.

Frusemide (0.5 mg/kg) together with water restriction followed by 0.9% or 1.8% NaCl i.v. is an effective treatment of this emergency; a urinary catheter is needed. The speed of correction must be tailored to the speed on onset, chronic changes being corrected slowly.

6

7

Transfusion medicine in perioperative care

This chapter aims to review:

- the concept of oxygen delivery;

- the concept of optimum Hb concentration;

- the recent developments in the understanding of the physiology of haemostasis.

Objectives

After reading this chapter you should be able to

- manage patients with anaemia and formulate appropriate transfusion strategies;

- diagnose and manage haemoglobinopathies;

- diagnose and manage coagulopathies;

- formulate a suitable regimen for the prophylaxis of deep vein thrombosis (DVT) in the perioperative period;

- anticipate the potential problems in massive transfusion;

- appreciate the objective risks to the patient of blood transfusion.

Introduction

7

During the perioperative period, intravascular volume and Hb concentration may fluctuate significantly. Anaesthetists and surgeons should be prepared to respond to these changes in the most appropriate way. Frequent assessment of changes in intravascular volume, oxygen delivery and patient physiology are required.

Transfusion of blood products exposes the patient to significant risk and is also costly in resource, both in time and money. At the time of writing, it costs about £72 in the UK to produce a single unit of packed cells. This is mainly because all blood for transfusion in the UK undergoes the costly process of white cell depletion to reduce the (albeit negligible) risk of transmission of new variant Creutzfeld–Jacob disease (CJD).

Estimates for the frequency of inappropriate transfusion vary from 4% to 66% of all units transfused. The two prime reasons for transfusing blood products are firstly the restoration of oxygen-carrying capacity and secondly the maintenance of haemostatic competence. However, it is worthwhile remembering that

- blood loss up to 30% of circulating volume (CV) (estimated at 70 ml/kg) can be safely treated with colloid or crystalloid alone;

- when there is no pre-existing haemostatic problem, replacement of up to one blood volume (8–10 units of blood in the adult) with red cells and non-plasma fluids is unlikely to cause haemostatic problems due to dilution;

- wound healing is not affected until oxygen tension decreases below 6.5 kPa or haematocrit falls below 18%.

Transfusion of red cells to maintain oxygen delivery

Physiology of oxygen delivery

Within the context of red cell transfusion two aspects of Hb physiology must be borne in mind, namely, *oxygen content* and *oxygen affinity*.

Oxygen content: At atmospheric pressure, 1 g of Hb can combine with 1.34 ml of oxygen when fully saturated. Thus, 1 l of whole arterial blood which contains 150 g of Hb will carry 200 ml of oxygen fully saturated at 100%. Venous blood saturated at 75% carries 150 ml of oxygen per l. This means that from every l of arterial blood leaving the left heart, 50 ml of oxygen is extracted, giving an extraction ratio of 25% (normal range 22–30%). Since cardiac output is about 5 l/min this gives an overall oxygen consumption around 250 ml/min (Chapter 16).

Oxygen affinity: Hb is a two-quaternary compound, and may exist in one of two conformations, the 'Tense' or T-state with reduced oxygen affinity, or the 'Relaxed' or R-state with increased oxygen affinity. The prevailing combination of oxygen tension and pH at the alveolus cause the molecule to assume the R-state and thus bind oxygen. Conversely, the prevailing combination of oxygen tension and pH deep in metabolising tissue cause the molecule to assume the T-state and offload oxygen. Another factor affecting the conformation of Hb is the ambient levels of 2,3,diphospho-glycerate (2,3,DPG). Functional erythrocytes metabolise glucose via the Embden–Meyerhof pathway and the end product of that metabolic process is 2,3,DPG, which behaves as an allosteric effector in that it binds to deoxygenated Hb maintaining the T-state. In stored erythrocytes, maintained at 4°C, little metabolism occurs and levels of 2,3,DPG fall, thus oxygen affinity increases in available Hb, with reduced offloading to metabolising tissues. It can take up to 24 h for 2,3,DPG levels to normalise in freshly transfused erythrocytes.

Optimum Hb levels

It has been suggested that an Hb concentration of 8 g/dl is sufficient even in patients with significant cardiorespiratory disease. It is only in the most seriously ill patients that oxygen demands may occasionally exceed supply. Studies in healthy volunteers have shown that oxygen delivery is not compromised even when the Hb concentration is as low as 5 g/dl.

Reasons for transfusing red cells in stable patients

- Augmenting oxygen delivery may improve outcome.
- To decrease the risk of ischaemia in coronary artery disease.
- Age, disease severity and drugs may interfere with normal adaptive responses to anaemia.

- To improve the 'safety margin' in the event of further blood loss.

Reasons for not transfusing red cells in stable patients

- Red cell transfusions may not affect oxygen delivery.
- Pathological supply dependency is rare
- No evidence that higher Hb concentrations are advantageous in coronary artery disease.
- Transfusion may impair microcirculation – by increasing blood viscosity, by accumulation of platelet aggregates – because old red cells are rigid and non-deformable.
- Transfusion may cause immuno-suppression.
- The risks of transfusion may outweigh the benefits.

Guidelines for transfusion of red cells

- Normally patients should not be transfused, if the Hb concentration is above 10 g/dl.
- A strong indication for transfusion is an Hb concentration below 7 g/dl.
- Transfusion will become essential when Hb concentration falls below 5 g/dl.
- An Hb concentration between 8 and 10 g/dl is safe even for those patients with significant cardiorespiratory disease.
- Symptomatic patients should be transfused.

Ordering blood for planned procedures

For procedures that do not routinely require blood transfusion, only 'group and save' is necessary. For procedures that routinely require blood transfusion, the number of units ordered should be based on the number of units usually used.

For the purposes of ordering blood, 10 ml of the patient's blood should be returned to the laboratory, correctly labelled in a tube containing no coagulant.

7

Group and save

The process of group and save involves establishing the patients ABO and Rhesus antigen D type. The patient's plasma is also screened for immunoglobulin G (IgG) antibodies that can damage RBCs at 37°C. The sample is usually held in the laboratory for 7 days. If red cells are required within this period, they can be provided safely for the patient after a further rapid test to exclude ABO incompatibility. Thus, most hospital laboratories should be able to issue blood within 15 min of a request being made.

Cross-matching

In addition to the group and save, the patient's serum sample is further tested for compatibility with the units of red cells to be transfused. Compatible units of blood are then labelled specifically for the patient and are held in the laboratory for 48 h from the time of the request. If the patient needs further red cell transfusions, a fresh sample should be sent for cross-matching, particularly if more than 72 h have elapsed since the previous cross-match, or 24 h since the previous transfusion. This is because the patient may generate antibodies to red cells very quickly as a result of stimulation by the previous transfusion.

Emergency blood request

In an absolute emergency, when the patient is suffering catastrophic blood loss and no properly crossed-matched blood can be found, ABO-type specific or even O-negative blood may be administered. The risk here is that the patient may already possess antibodies to the red cells in these units.

Blood administration

Once the decision to transfuse has been made, the following procedures should be followed to minimise the incorrect administration of red cells to the patient:

- The identification of the patient must be confirmed.
- The blood compatibility label must be checked to ensure the blood is correct for the patient.
- The expiry date should be checked.
- The bag should be checked to ensure the integrity of the plastic casing.
- Blood left out of the fridge for more than 30 min should be transfused within 4 h or discarded.
- The blood must be infused through a blood-giving set. Stored blood contains micro-aggregates of approximately 200-μm diameter, thus no blood should be given through a giving set that does not include a 170-μm filter.
- Use of a blood warmer is advised as a routine for adults receiving infusion of blood in the operating theatre or emergency room and if rates of transfusion are greater than 50 ml/kg/h for adults or 15 ml/kg/h for children. A blood warmer is also indicated when transfusing a patient who has clinically significant cold agglutinins.
- No other infusion solutions or drugs should be added to any blood component.
- The details of the unit transfused should be recorded on the anaesthetic chart or as an entry in the clinical notes.
- The volume of blood transfused should be recorded.

Notes on red cell products

All red cell products are stored at a range of 2–6°C, and have a maximum shelf life of 35 days. They should all be compatible with the patient's ABO and Rhesus antigen D type and any clinically significant antibodies present in the patient's plasma. The maximum time between being removed from storage and transfusion should be no more than 5 h. Haematocrit ranges from 0.35–0.45 in whole blood to 0.50–0.75 in re-suspended red cell preparations. A dose of 4 ml/kg raises venous Hb by about 1 g/dl. Special types include:

- *Buffy-coat depleted:* Indicated in patients who have a previous history to reaction to blood transfusion.

7

- *CMV-negative blood:* Indicated in
  - all cases of haematological malignancy until their CMV status is known;
  - all CMV-negative patients receiving autograft or allograft bone marrow;
  - all HIV patients who are CMV negative, or whose CMV status is unknown;
  - patients receiving organ allografts who are CMV negative.
- *Irradiated blood products:* Engraftment of viable lymphocytes transfused with whole blood, red cells or platelets can cause fatal graft versus host disease (GvHD) in patients with severely depressed T-cell immunity, e.g. in HIV infection associated with a low CD4 count. This must be prevented by irradiation of all cellular blood components (25–30 Gy). Leucocyte depletion does not protect against GvHD.

Jehovah's Witnesses

It has been calculated that there are 5.9 million active Jehovah's Witnesses in over 230 countries worldwide. The prohibition of blood transfusion is a deeply held core value within this belief.

Most Jehovah's Witnesses will not accept a transfusion of whole blood or its major derivatives. This includes fresh-frozen plasma (FFP), packed cells, white blood cells (WBCs) and platelets. It should be noted that some Jehovah's Witnesses might also refuse gelatin-based colloids as these contain bovine products. *Absolute* rules regarding blood products, however, do not exist and some Jehovah's Witnesses may accept the use of plasma protein fraction (PPF) or components such as albumin, immuno-globulins or haemophilic preparations. Organ transplantation is not expressly forbidden for Jehovah's Witnesses and each individual is expected to come to their own decision.

Cardiac bypass may be accepted provided the pump is primed with non-blood fluids and blood is not stored in the process. Auto-transfusion is acceptable to many

Jehovah's Witnesses provided the equipment is arranged in a closed circuit that is constantly linked to the patient's circulation and there is no storage of the blood. Jehovah's Witnesses will not accept preoperative collection, storage and later re-infusion of blood.

To administer blood to a patient who has steadfastly refused to accept it either by the provision of an advance directive or by its exclusion in a consent form is unlawful, ethically unacceptable and may lead to criminal and/or civil proceedings. The doctor, on the other hand, has the right to refuse treatment in an elective situation.

Children of Jehovah's Witnesses below the age of 16 may cause particular difficulty. Should the parents refuse to give permission for blood transfusion, it may be necessary to apply for a legal 'Specific Issue Order' via the High Court in order to legally administer the blood transfusion. The first step is that two consultants must make both a written and signed statement in the medical notes that transfusion is essential to survival.

In terms of clinical management, it goes without saying that any preoperative anaemia should be treated appropriately. This could include the use of erythropoetin in some cases. Major procedures may be able to be carried out in stages to minimise blood loss. Intra-operative blood loss may be reduced by careful positioning to avoid venous congestion and by the use of hypotensive anaesthesia and haemodilution. Cell-saver systems may be acceptable to some Jehovah's Witnesses. Drugs to reduce bleeding in the postoperative phase include tranexamic acid and aprotinin. Excessive blood loss associated with bleeding down to an Hb of <7 g/dl may be an indication for elective postoperative ventilation with high FiO_2 to maintain oxygen delivery. This may increase complications and also imposes additional workload on ICUs and HDUs.

Management of haemoglobinopathies

Defects in Hb synthesis and structure are one of the major congenital causes of haemolysis.

85

The major examples are the thalassaemias (HbF) and sickle-cell disease (SCD, HbS).

Patients with thalassaemia major or severe complications of SCD may need long-term red cell support. All these patients require *specialist* investigation and management. Given their possible previous exposure to multiple blood transfusions, special precautions should be taken to reduce the risk of developing antibodies to red cells and white cells and the patient should be vaccinated against hepatitis B and hepatitis A.

Any evidence of splenic dysfunction should be covered with penicillin V. Accumulation of iron should be minimised by using a chelating agent such as desferrioxamine. Similar precautions apply to patients with hereditary red cell metabolic or membrane defects (Chapter 4).

Complications of blood transfusion

These may be classified as:

1. Early immune reactions:
   - anti-red cell – acute haemolytic transfusion reaction,
   - anti-white cell – non-haemolytic febrile transfusion reaction (NHFTR),
   - anti-IgA – allergic reaction.

2. Delayed immune reactions:
   - delayed haemolytic transfusion reaction (DHTR),
   - GvHD,
   - post-transfusion purpura.

3. Transmission of infection.

4. Transfusion-related acute lung injury (TRALI).

Acute haemolytic transfusion reaction

When blood is randomly administered to a patient without any typing, the chances of ABO incompatibility are about one in three. The most severe reaction will occur when group A red cells are infused into group O patients. The reaction will occur within 1–2 min of commencing the transfusion; symptoms, signs and treatment will include:

- symptoms:
  - agitation,
  - flushing,
  - pain at infusion site,
  - chest and/or abdominal pain;

- signs:
  - fever,
  - hypotension,
  - generalised oozing from wounds and puncture sites,
  - haemoglobinuria;

- treatment:
  - stop transfusing,
  - keep the patient well hydrated,
  - promote diuresis,
  - treat hyperkalaemia with 50 ml 50% glucose + insulin 10 units,
  - if disseminated intravascular coagulation (DIC) supervenes monitor and support, if necessary.

Antibodies other than ABO can cause haemolytic reactions. Severe reactions associated with complement activation occur to Jk (Kidd), and Fy (Duffy) antigens. Reactions occurring to Rhesus antigens – D, E and C typically do not activate complement and as a consequence are clinically less severe.

Non-haemolytic febrile transfusion reaction

NHFTR results from the interaction between anti-leucocyte antibodies raised by the recipient against donor white cells, and is thus not associated with red cell destruction. Simply terminating the transfusion and giving paracetamol to reduce fever is appropriate management for most reactions. Recurrent severe reactions sometimes occur in patients who have been exposed to repeated transfusions. In this situation, leucocyte-depleted blood products are indicated, or alternatively 'in-line' leucocyte-depleting filters are used.

Allergic reaction

Rare but severe allergic reaction can occur when the recipient has high circulating levels of anti-IgA antibodies present in their plasma. These patients typically present with chronically low levels of circulating IgA. Treatment is with chorpheniramine 10 mg i.v., or if more severe with hydrocortisone 200 mg i.v. and 1 ml increments of 1:10,000 adrenaline i.v. until BP is restored.

Delayed haemolytic transfusion reaction

This reaction occurs in about 1% of parous women requiring transfusion and is due to sensitisation to red cell antigens occurring during pregnancy. First exposure leads to limited production of these antibodies, and circulating levels are undetectable on routine screening. Subsequent exposure to transfused red cells in later life leads to a slow but sustained increase in anti-red cell antibodies. Thus, the reaction typically occurs 5–10 days following transfusion. Clinically significant DHTR is very rare.

Graft versus host disease

This severe and invariably fatal reaction is caused by the activity of *donor* T-lymphocytes reacting against *host* tissues. It typically occurs in the immuno-compromised patient receiving a blood transfusion. The reaction becomes clinically significant 3–4 days following transfusion beginning with fever and an erythematous rash which progresses rapidly to erythroderma and desquamation, associated with gut dysfunction, liver failure and pancytopaenia. GvHD is prevented only by administering irradiated blood products to patients' known to be immuno-compromised.

Post-transfusion purpura

This reaction occurs typically 5–10 days following transfusion and is associated with the production of platelet-specific allo-antibodies. Clinical presentation includes fever, bleeding tendency, thrombocytopaenia and purpura. Treatment is with steroids and γ-globulin.

Transmission of infection

The major risks of blood-borne infection are listed in Table 7.1.

Transfusion-related acute lung injury

This is the result of interaction between *donor* antibodies, and *recipient* leucocytes occurring in about 0.2% of all transfused patients.

Table 7.1 **The major risks of blood-borne infection**

Blood-borne infection	Frequency per unit transfused	Deaths per million units
Acute haemolytic reaction	1:250,000–1:1,000,000	0.67
Hepatitis B	1:100,000–1:400,000	<0.50
Hepatitis C	1:200,000	<0.50
HIV	1:4,000,000	<0.50
Bacterial contamination	1:5,000,000	<0.25
New variant CJD	Unknown	Unknown

7

If severe, it may progress to adult respiratory distress syndrome (ARDS) and require admission to intensive care. The reaction begins within 4 h of transfusion presenting as pyrexia, rigours, non-productive cough and dyspnoea. Chest X-ray (CXR) demonstrates the typical appearance of basal infiltration with perihilar nodules. There is no specific treatment and management, which is supportive. The implicated donors are almost always multiparous women who are found to have high circulating levels of anti-leucocyte antibodies. The recipient should be screened for the presence of anti-leucocyte antibodies, as should any remaining donor products. If the test is positive, then all products from that particular donor should be withdrawn. Mortality from ARDS associated with TRALI is lower than ARDS associated with other causes.

Haemostatic failure

Haemostatic competence involves maintenance of the balance between thrombogenesis on the one hand and thrombolysis on the other. Thrombogenesis involves the generation of fibrin through a 'cascade' of clotting factors, and its subsequent interaction with platelets. Thrombolysis involves cleavage of fibrin by plasmin again generated through a 'cascade' mechanism. The traditional view held that the initial clotting cascade resolved into the 'extrinsic' and 'intrinsic' pathways, and that these pathways functioned separately and at different times. The current modified view proposes that in fact, these pathways act in tandem, 'initiation' occurring via the *extrinsic* pathway, and subsequent 'propagation and amplification' occurring via the *intrinsic* pathway (Fig. 7.1).

Tests of haemostatic competence
- Static test of extrinsic pathway function: prothrombin time expressed in International Normalised Ratio (INR).

- Static test of intrinsic pathway function: activated partial thromboplastin time (aPTT).

- Static test of intrinsic pathway function: activated clotting time (ACT).

- Dynamic test of fibrin generation, platelet aggregation and clot lysis: thrombo-elastography.

Prothrombin time (INR)
Prothrombin time expressed as INR tests the *extrinsic* pathway, i.e. the vitamin-K-dependent clotting factors II, VII and X. Plasma is activated by tissue thromboplastin and calcium. This test is used to monitor the activity of the drug warfarin. The normal value for the prothrombin time is 12–14 s and the normal INR is 0.8–1.2.

Activated partial thromboplastin time
aPTT tests the *intrinsic* pathway, i.e. factors VIII, IX, X, XI and XII. Plasma is activated by kaolin. The test is used to monitor the activity of the drug heparin. The normal value is 39–42 s.

Activated clotting time
The ACT again tests the *intrinsic* pathway, as above. Again this test can be used to monitor activity of the drug heparin. The plasma is activated by diatomaceous earth, and the normal activated clotting time is 90–130 s.

Thrombo-elastography
Clotting is in reality a dynamic process with a balance between clot formation and clot lysis.

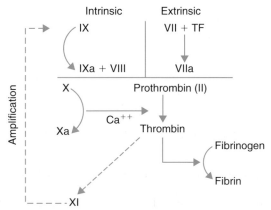

Fig. 7.1 Intrinsic and extrinsic pathway of coagulation.

7

Thus, an observed bleeding tendency could be due to either depressed clot formation or accelerated clot lysis. Further, platelet counts give only a quantitative, not qualitative, estimate of platelet function. In 1948, Hartert described a mechanical device that monitored the dynamic processes of clot formation, clot stability and clot lysis. A sample of fresh blood (0.35 ml) is placed in an oscillating cuvette heated to 37°C, a small probe connected through a system of levers to a recording pen is lowered into the sample.

As the clot forms and the viscosity of the blood increases, more of the oscillatory motion is transmitted to the probe which is recorded as increased excursions about a mid-point on the recording chart. Conversely, as the clot lyses and the viscosity decreases, the excursions transmitted to the recording pen decrease. Fig. 7.2 shows a schematic thrombo-elastograph trace and Table 7.2 indicates the parameters and activities measured, as well as the normal values obtained.

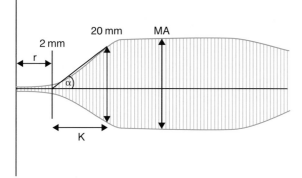

Fig. 7.2 A schematic diagram of a thrombo-elastograph trace.

Haemostatic defects encountered in the perioperative period

- Acquired haemostatic defects:

  - Patients prescribed warfarin.

  - Patients prescribed aspirin.

  - Heparin-induced thrombocytopaenia.

  - DIC.

  - Massive transfusion.

- Congenital haemostatic defects.

Table 7.2 Parameters measured, normal range and activity measured with the thrombo-elastograph

Parameter	Normal range	Activity measured
'r' reaction time (time to amplitude of 2 mm)	6–8 min	Clotting factors ↑ by heparin ↑ by clotting factor deficiency ↓ by hypercoagulable state
'K' clot time (time taken for amplitude to increase from 2 to 20 mm)	3–6 min	Combined activity of clotting factors, fibrin and platelets
α-angle (angle between 2- and 20-mm point)	50–60°	↓ In hypofibrinogenaemia ↓ In thrombocytopaenia
MA (maximum amplitude)	50–60 mm	Platelet function
Amplitude at 60 min	If this is 5 mm less than the maximum amplitude	Significant clot lysis

7

Patients prescribed warfarin

Several groups of patients at high risk of developing thrombosis are maintained on the coumarin derivative, warfarin. Warfarin interferes with the synthesis of the vitamin-K-dependent clotting factors II, VII, IX and X. The three major groups of patients routinely maintained on warfarin are as follows:

■ Patients with mechanical heart valves: INR maintained at ~3.5.

■ Patients with atrial fibrillation (AF): INR maintained at ~2.5.

■ Patients with mural thrombus detected on cardiac ECHO: INR maintained at ~2.5.

Unless contraindicated, warfarin is discontinued and prothrombin time (INR) is normalised prior to an elective surgical operation. Normalisation normally occurs within 48 h of the last dose but may require up to 5 days. In an emergency situation, PPSB together with parenteral vitamin K, 1 mg i.v. can restore coagulation within 6 h, alternatively, one dose of FFP will restore clotting function immediately. It should be noted that large doses of vitamin K will interfere with re-establishing good anticoagulation control for some days (p. 45).

In circumstances requiring continued maintenance of anticoagulation, the patient should be established on a heparin infusion preoperatively and warfarin discontinued. The heparin infusion should be continued until at least day 3 of warfarin reloading postoperatively.

Patients prescribed aspirin

Aspirin should be discontinued at least 14 days prior to major elective surgery, if it is safe to do so (Chapter 4). In an emergency situation, where aspirin is considered to contribute to a bleeding problem, a platelet transfusion is indicated.

Heparin-induced thrombocytopaenia

The overall incidence of heparin-induced thrombocytopaenia (HIT) in the UK is estimated at 3% of all patients prescribed unfractionated heparin. Two mechanisms of thrombocytopaenia are described:

■ Type 1: This is simply due to induced aggregation of platelets, typically presenting with a platelet count between 30,000 and 40,000/mm^3, qualitative platelet function however, is maintained.

■ Type 2: True autoimmune thrombocytopaenia, occurring between 4 and 14 days after commencement of heparin administration, presents typically with platelet counts of <10,000/mm^3. This type of HIT significantly impacts on qualitative platelet function. The basic mechanism involves antibody production to heparin–platelet–factor IV complexes, which then bind to specific FC receptors on the platelet membrane resulting in excessive platelet aggregation and significant thrombosis both venous and arterial. The condition, if unrecognised, carries a high morbidity and mortality. In suspected cases, an HIT screen should be carried out which detects heparin–platelet–factor IV complexes. Basic management involves removing all sources of fractionated heparin including the small doses used to flush arterial lines, and supportive therapy as indicated. The use of fractionated heparins is not associated with HIT.

Disseminated intravascular coagulation

DIC is a syndrome characterised by abnormal deposition of fibrin with associated consumption of plasma proteins and platelets. It is not a disease in itself but a response to various physiological stresses. The commonest causes of DIC accounting for 60–70% of treated cases are infection and disseminated malignancy. Common causes include:

■ *infection*: sepsis, viraemia, protozoal infestation;

■ *malignancy*: metastatic carcinoma, leukaemia;

■ *obstetric*: septic abortion, abruption, eclampsia, amniotic embolism, foetal death;

7

■ *shock*: multiple trauma, extensive burns;

■ *transplant rejection;*

■ *intravascular haemolysis.*

The mechanism driving the syndrome is an inappropriate and/or excessive activation of circulating platelets and/or coagulation cascade. Fibrin–platelet thrombosis occurs and can result in severe end-organ damage. The aggressive consumption of platelets and clotting factors leads to the clinical presentation of diffuse bleeding from wounds and puncture sites.

Laboratory profile
■ Prothrombin time >15 s (INR > 1.5 : 1).

■ Fibrinogen level <1.6 g/l.

■ Platelet count <150,000/m^3.

■ Fibrin-degradation products.

Treatment is firstly to treat the underlying cause, and secondly to provide supportive therapy in the form of FFP, and platelets as required. FFP is administered at a dose of 12–15 ml/kg to replace fibrinogen, factor VIII, and von Willebrand factor (vWF) to maintain INR <1.5 and fibrinogen at >1.0 g/l. Platelets are administered to maintain platelet count >80,000/m^3.

A potential adjunct to supportive therapy is the administration of protein C; the endogenous protein C has both anticoagulant and anti-inflammatory properties. Plasma levels of protein C have been noted to be depressed in DIC associated with sepsis, early augmentation of levels appears to be associated with an improved outcome.

Activated protein C exerts its anticoagulant effect via inhibition of factors Va and VIIIa, and its anti-inflammatory effect by inhibiting macrophage production of TNFα, IL-1 and IL-6. To date the major barrier to its use is its high cost.

Massive transfusion
Massive transfusion may be defined as the acute administration of more than 1.5 times estimated blood volume (normally 70 ml/kg).

For the reasons outlined below, routine monitoring of massive transfusion should include, core temperature, clotting function, urea and electrolytes, ECG and, of course, full blood count.

Complications of massive transfusion include:

■ dilution effect,

■ hypothermia,

■ hypocalcemia,

■ hyperkalaemia,

■ metabolic disturbance.

Dilution effect
In healthy individuals, replacement of up to 1 CV with red cells and colloid is unlikely to cause haemostatic defect due to dilution. There is no evidence that giving prophylactic platelets or plasma to a patient undergoing large transfusion reduces the risk of microvascular bleeding. Regular clotting studies should be carried out during the transfusion. A platelet count of <30,000/mm^3 alone or, <50,000/mm^3 with evidence of microvascular bleeding is an indication for platelet administration. Prolonged clotting times are an indication for FFP usually administered in increments of 15 ml/kg. Fibrinogen levels below 1 g/l require the administration of cryoprecipitate, equivalent to 3–4 g of fibrinogen (15 packs) (see Table 7.3).

Hypothermia
Infusion of cold blood at a rate exceeding 50 ml/kg/h risks exposing the patient to hypothermia. Core temperature should be monitored throughout the period of potentially massive transfusion, and blood administered via a blood warmer.

Hyperkalaemia
Some degree of red cell lysis occurs during blood storage and administration, releasing potassium into the plasma. ECG monitoring is also advised throughout the period of transfusion. The typical ECG changes consistent with hyperkalaemia are tall

7

91

Table 7.3 **Haemostatic blood components**

	Platelets	**FFP**	**Cryoprecipitate**
Single donation	40–60 ml plasma	200 ml plasma	10–20 ml
Dose	1 pool (4–6 donations)	15 ml/kg	15 packs
Concentration	240,000,000 platelets per pool	2–5 mg/ml fibrinogen	3–4 g fibrinogen in 15 packs
Storage	24°C	−30°C	−30°C
Shelf life	5 days	1 year	1 year

Note: Since sufficient donor plasma is present in platelet preparations to cause haemolysis, if the donor has potent red cell antibodies, platelet donations should be ABO compatible.

T-waves, wide P–R interval, and broad QRS complexes.

Hypocalcaemia
Citrate anticoagulant added to blood components, binds ionised calcium. Normally, the administered citrate is eliminated by rapid hepatic metabolism. The onset of ECG changes consistently with hypocalcaemia (prolonged Q–T interval and broad T-waves), occurring during massive transfusion, is treated with 5 ml of 10% calcium gluconate solution as required.

Acid–base disturbance
Large volumes of administered citrate have the potential to cause a metabolic alkalosis. However, as noted above, citrate is usually rapidly metabolised in the liver. Citrate effects on acid–base do not usually become apparent until the rate of blood infusion exceeds 1 unit in <5 min.

The council of perfection states that clotting factors should not be administered in the setting of massive blood transfusion unless guided by clotting studies. In situations, where such support is not available, a useful rule of thumb is that one dose of FFP should be administered for every 5 units of blood transfused, and one pool of platelets should be administered for every 10 units of blood

transfused together with 5 ml of 10% calcium gluconate.

Congenital haemostatic disorders

The three commonest congenital disorders of haemostasis occurring in the UK are the haemophilias A and B and von Willebrand's (vW) disease. They are summarised in Table 7.4.

All UK patients with haemophilia A, haemophilia B (Christmas disease) or vW disease, should be registered with a Regional Haemophilia Centre. The Local Regional Centre should be contacted for advice whenever such patients present for surgery.

Haemophilia A patients presenting for surgery may need supplementation with factor VIII concentrate, dose of 1 i.u./kg raising plasma levels by 2%.

Haemophilia B patients presenting for surgery may need supplementation with factor IX concentrate, a dose of 1 i.u./kg raising plasma levels by 1%.

If clotting factor concentrates are unavailable, cryoprecipitate is the appropriate treatment for haemophilia A, and FFP is the appropriate treatment for haemophilia B titrated against aPTT.

Table 7.4 **Congenital disorders of haemostasis**

	Haemophilia A	**Haemophilia B**	**vW disease**
Factor	Factor VIII	Factor IX	vW factor
Inheritance	Sex-linked recessive	Sex-linked recessive	Autosomal dominant
Diagnosis	Prolonged aPTT	Prolonged aPTT	Prolonged bleeding time
Presentation	Bleeding into joints	Bleeding into joints	Bleeding into mucous membranes

In patients with vW disease presenting for surgery, both the levels of factor VIII and vWF need to be established. Some patients can be managed with desmopressin alone without the need for blood products.

Desmopressin (DDAVP) may be used to reduce bleeding times in patients with mild forms of haemophilia A and vW disease. It promotes the release of vWF. It may also be useful in improving platelet function in uraemic patients. The dose of desmopressin for mild to moderate haemophilia A and vW disease is 0.4 µg/kg, it should be diluted in 50 ml of normal saline and given over 20 min immediately prior to surgery.

If clotting factor replacement is required in vW disease then the appropriate product is factor-VIII concentrate, which is also rich in vWF.

Pro-coagulant states in perioperative medicine

Pulmonary embolism in the postoperative period remains a significant cause of surgical mortality (7% of all surgical deaths). High-risk cases include, major orthopaedic surgery, surgery for abdominal or pelvic malignancy, amputation, a previous history of DVT, and patients with significant neurological motor deficit. The use of regional anaesthetic techniques is associated with a reduction in episodes of lower limb thrombosis in the postoperative period. Recent studies suggest that subcutaneous low-molecular-weight heparin is as effective as unfractionated heparin for the prophylaxis of thrombo-embolism. The basic advantage of the low-molecular-weight heparins is their once daily administration regimen and the fact that they do not seem to be associated with HIT. The theoretical disadvantage of their use is difficulty in monitoring their activity (via anti-factor Xa levels), and the fact that they are not reversed by protamine.

7

Practical procedures and arterial blood-gas analysis in perioperative care

Aims

The aims of this chapter are to

- describe what procedures may be employed by the perioperative physician,

- discuss the indications for carrying out those procedures,

- describe the practical aspects of each procedure,

- discuss the complications of the procedures,

- discuss changes in arterial blood gases (ABGs) and how they impact on patient management in the perioperative period.

Objectives

After reading this chapter, you should be able to

- understand which procedure is indicated for a clinical circumstance,

- be able to perform each procedure competently and confidently after gaining experience observing a skilled practitioner,

- recognise the complications associated with each procedure,

- understand common deviations from normality in an ABG sample and initiate appropriate management.

Introduction

Proficient perioperative management of patients combines rational diagnosis with appropriate treatment. Practical procedures may be performed either to assist diagnosis, or to enable therapy. Surgical patients are likely to have several practical interventions performed on them during each clinical episode. There is increasing awareness amongst medical educators that practical skills are poorly taught at medical school and during the PRHO year. 'Practising on patients'

is not appropriate – 'I got the i.v. line in on my sixth attempt' shows both a lack of respect for the patient and a lack of ability by the physician. It is also important to recognise your limitations and ask for help if you run into problems – every doctor, for example, has failed at least once to site an i.v. cannula. Although practical procedures are best taught on mannequins in a clinical skills laboratory, a certain level of understanding is required concerning equipment, anatomy and the risk/benefit ratios for each procedure. The procedures described are

- airway maintenance;

- i.v. line insertion and infusion of i.v. fluids;

- insertion of a central venous line;

- urinary catheterisation;

- insertion of a chest drain;

- arterial puncture, to obtain a blood-gas sample;

- passing a nasogastric (NG) tube.

Airway maintenance

Maintenance of a clear airway is of crucial importance during resuscitation, anaesthesia and intensive care. Respiratory obstruction, usually due to apposition of the tongue and the pharynx, is a major cause of perioperative morbidity and mortality, particularly in the recovery phase after emergence from anaesthesia. The principles employed to avoid airway obstruction in the perioperative period are applicable in other emergency situations, for instance following drug overdose, airway trauma and cardiac arrest. High flow oxygen (more than 10 l/min) should always be administered via face mask.

Recognition of airway obstruction

Airway obstruction in the conscious patient is easily recognised, as it leads to strenuous efforts on the part of the patient to overcome it. Inspiration may be impossible and expiration may be prolonged. However, the unconscious patient may not exhibit classical compensatory signs when obstructed. Paradoxical chest movement, where the upper abdomen and chest seesaw during attempted inspiration (the chest retracting and the abdomen sticking out) may be seen. Lack of air entry and exit means that air movement cannot be detected by listening at the mouth or by auscultation of the chest. The patient eventually becomes cyanosed.

Sites and treatment of airway obstruction

Nasopharynx

Although the nasal passages are the 'normal' portal for air from atmosphere to lungs, obstruction does not usually cause problems as air may equally well pass via the mouth. However, neonates are obligate 'nose breathers' and do not adopt mouth breathing easily, even when the nasal airway is totally obstructed (e.g. from choanal atresia). Insertion of an oral airway and placement of the infant in the prone position may allow temporary respite, but emergency surgical relief of the obstruction may be necessary.

Oropharynx

By far the commonest cause of obstruction in the mouth is relaxation of the jaw muscles due to anaesthesia or any CNS depressant (e.g. head injury, alcohol, benzodiazepines). The tongue falls back onto the posterior wall of the pharynx, which prevents air entry (Fig. 8.1).

Fortunately, treatment is straightforward. In the unconscious patient, the lower jaw is manually lifted anteriorly (jaw thrust), which disengages the tongue from the pharyngeal wall, clearing the airway. The efficacy of this manoeuvre may be improved by combination with 'chin lift' and insertion of an oral (Guedel) airway (that mechanically interposes itself between the pharynx and the tongue (Fig. 8.2)).

The patient who is unconscious from other causes, or who has a full stomach, should be turned on to their side (the 'recovery position') with a head-down tilt. This usually

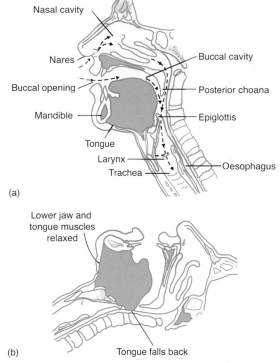

(a)

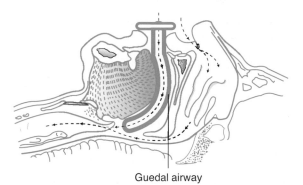

(b)

Fig. 8.1 Airway obstruction. (a) The normal upper airway: anatomical sites of obstruction. (b) Obstruction due to tongue falling back in the unconscious patient.

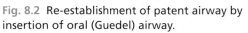

Guedal airway

Fig. 8.2 Re-establishment of patent airway by insertion of oral (Guedel) airway.

'automatically' clears the airway, by allowing the tongue to fall away from the pharynx. Should vomiting occur, this position protects against aspiration. All unconscious patients should be recovered on their sides where possible.

8

Other causes of oropharyngeal airway obstruction are far less common. In the neonate, maxillary hypoplasia, with a large tongue pushing back against the pharynx (e.g. Pierre Robin syndrome) causes obstruction that may need urgent treatment (the tongue is stitched and pulled forward, with the baby nursed prone). Trauma may lead to mechanical airway obstruction by teeth, dentures, blood, bone or oedema of the tongue and pharynx. Endotracheal intubation (ETI) may be required, if simple airway maintenance manoeuvres fail. Oropharyngeal infections (e.g. Ludwig's angina, retropharyngeal abscess) cause obstruction through swelling. Foreign bodies, especially vomit, should always be suspected and cleared manually, if necessary.

Laryngo-pharynx and trachea
Sudden obstruction is commonly due to infection (acute epiglottitis), trauma or foreign body aspiration, especially of vomit. If manual or instrumental clearance fails, cricothyrotomy or tracheostomy may be necessary to bypass the obstruction. Below the carina and main bronchi, blockage of air passages does not produce complete obstruction.

Special techniques

Endotracheal intubation
Relief of airway obstruction by the methods outlined above may only provide temporary relief prior to definitive ETI. To accomplish this skilfully and atraumatically requires considerable practical experience. The practice of some 200 ETIs is the minimum that most anaesthetists in training need to feel reasonably confident. This is usually accomplished in the first 6 months of training. There is great variability in the anatomy of the region, so unexpected difficulties arising in this manoeuvre are not uncommon.

As a life-saving measure, non-anaesthetists have a better chance of effectively providing respiratory support with a bag and mask (and airway if needed), than unsuccessfully attempting to place an endotracheal tube

(ETT). Turning the patient on the side and head-down, with careful observation and frequent suction of the oropharynx, is usually adequate to prevent gross inhalation of stomach contents. While preparations are made, it is important that the airway is maintained by other means as outlined above, and the patient fully oxygenated.

Equipment required (Fig. 8.3)
1. A pressurised source of oxygen and gas delivery system; a self-inflating bag is also suitable.

2. Mask and airway of suitable size (a mask size of 3 or 4 with a size 2 Guedel airway is suitable for female adults, with one size bigger for males).

3. A cuffed ETT for oral use (these are numbered according to their internal diameter in millimetres. A size 8 is suitable for females and 9 for males. In the emergency situation, smaller-sized tubes should be available).

4. A laryngoscope of appropriate size (a Macintosh size 3 or 4 for adults).

5. A syringe and clamp for cuff inflation, tube ties, etc.

6. Intubating forceps (Magill) for guiding the ETT and also for removing foreign bodies.

7. Drugs (such as i.v. anaesthetics and sedatives, neuromuscular blockers and atropine).

8. Good suction apparatus.

9. A bed with a 'head-down' facility.

10. A trained assistant.

Technique
The patient is turned onto the back and a pillow placed underneath the head. This flexes the neck so that the chin is directed towards the chest. Pulling back on the chin towards the operator then extends the head. This 'sniffing the morning air' position is

8

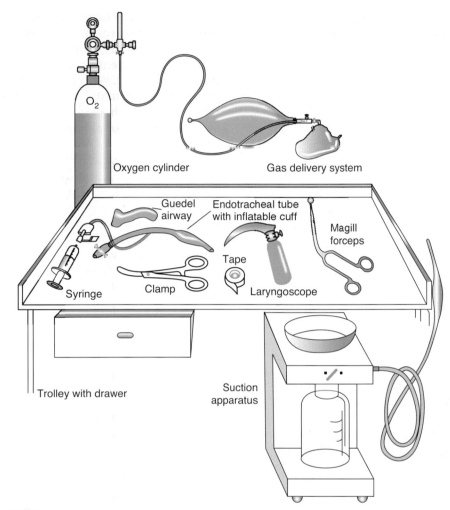

Fig. 8.3 ETI trolley.

designed to align the planes of the mouth with that of the larynx. Separating the lips and pulling on the upper jaw and lip with the index finger opens the mouth. The laryngoscope is held in the left hand, and enters the mouth with the blade directed towards the right tonsil. On reaching this level, the blade is swept to the midline, keeping the tongue on the left, and out of sight. At this point the epiglottis comes into view (Fig. 8.4).

The blade is gently advanced until it reaches the vallecula, i.e. the angle between the base of the tongue and epiglottis. It is important to get the earliest view of the epiglottis and not lose sight of it, so as to avoid going too far and misinterpreting the oesophagus for the larynx. At this stage the whole laryngoscope is lifted upwards and away from the operator so that the larynx comes into view. This may also require pressure on the trachea just below the cricoid ring to produce optimal alignment (Fig. 8.4).

The ETT is taken in the right hand with the inner curve of the tube facing the right side of the mouth so as to minimally impede the view of the larynx as the tube is inserted. If possible, observe the tube entering the larynx and push it in only until the cuffed portion disappears beyond the cords. This avoids inadvertent endobronchial intubation.

8

The cuff is inflated to provide an airtight seal and the bag squeezed to ascertain correct placement of the tube by listening to both sides of the chest with a stethoscope.

Laryngeal mask airway

The introduction of the laryngeal mask airway (LMA) markedly facilitated the management of the airway during anaesthesia. In the vast majority of adult patients, it provides a reliable airway (suitable for 'gentle' positive pressure ventilation) and limited protection against aspiration of regurgitated gastric contents. Insertion of an LMA is technically less difficult than an ETI because it does not require a laryngoscope and successful placement is less dependent on anatomical variations between patients. Educating non-anaesthetists to insert LMAs has produced encouraging results and the LMA is likely to be included in resuscitation kits in the future. The device is illustrated in Fig. 8.5. The external appearance of the airway, once inserted, is identical to that of an ETT. A large pear-shaped cuff is designed to fit in the oropharynx and once inflated with approximately 40 ml of air, it pushes the base of the tongue forwards. The masks are made of silicon rubber and can withstand many autoclave sterilisations. The device must be well lubricated before insertion and the patient's head positioned as if for ETI (head extended on neck, 'sniffing the morning air'). Insertion is facilitated by 'jaw thrust' and by the insertion of two gloved fingers into the mouth to push the tongue anteriorly and inferiorly, as shown in Fig. 8.5.

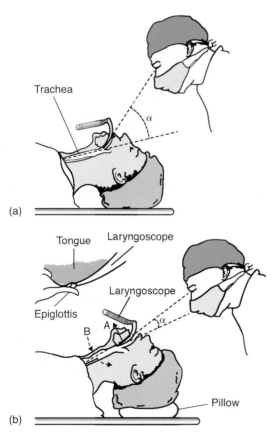

(a)

(b)

Fig. 8.4 Principles of visualisation of the larynx with laryngoscope prior to ETI: (a) Shows the patient in the incorrect position prior to attempted intubation. The greater the angle of 'α' the greater the difficulty in visualising the larynx. (b) Shows the position with the neck flexed on a pillow and the head extended (sniffing the morning air). Angle 'α' is now minimised, especially, if gentle traction is exerted on the laryngoscope in the direction shown in A (i.e. up towards the ceiling, NOT rotated) and gentle pressure applied just below the cricoid cartilage (B). It is easy to see that the visual and laryngeal planes are now more closely aligned.

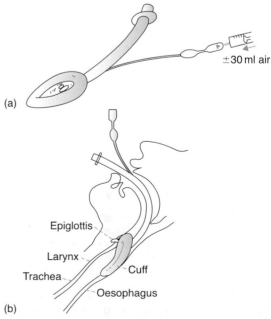

Fig. 8.5 Laryngeal mask: (a) the mask and (b) in correct position.

Care of unconscious patients: other aspects

Regardless of the cause, unconsciousness also means that the protective reactions to pain and discomfort are absent. Circumstances permitting, the patient should be placed in the recovery position with a slight head-down tilt. The cornea of the eye may dry and suffer irreversible damage, because tear flow and blinking are absent. Therefore, eyes should be carefully taped closed during unconsciousness.

Shoulder and hip joints should be protected from pulling and excessive passive movement, to prevent dislocation. Peripheral nerves may suffer prolonged compression or stretching. Particularly at risk are the lateral surface of the lower leg (superficial peroneal nerve), the medial surface of the elbow (ulnar nerve), the medial surface of the upper arm (radial nerve – particularly if the arms of a supine patient hang off the sides of a trolley) and the side of the face (facial nerve). Keeping the patient in the recovery position without additional support of the rib cage may damage the brachial plexus. Maintenance of body temperature is important. Body temperature should be monitored regularly. Wet garments should be removed, and the patient kept well covered with blankets if the room temperature is below 24°C. A warming blanket may be used. The position of unconscious patients should be altered at regular intervals (30 min) to avoid pressure necrosis of the skin (bed sores). Care must be exercised not to drop the unconscious patient on transferring to or from bed. Padded cot sides should be employed.

Intravenous line insertion and infusion of intravenous fluids

This process is best learnt by practise in a skills laboratory. Beginners should repetitively practise the sequence of assembling the giving set and bag of i.v. fluid, inserting the cannula, connecting the giving set to the cannula and checking for complications (Fig. 8.6).

The proper practise of connecting the three parts without contamination and presence of air bubbles can only be learnt by watching

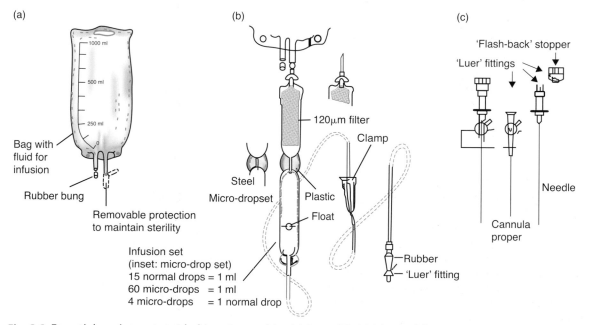

(a)

1000 ml
500 ml
250 ml
0

Bag with fluid for infusion

Rubber bung

Removable protection to maintain sterility

Infusion set
(inset: micro-drop set)
15 normal drops = 1 ml
60 micro-drops = 1 ml
4 micro-drops = 1 normal drop

(b)

120 μm filter

Clamp

Steel

Micro-dropset | Plastic

Float

Rubber
'Luer' fitting

(c)

'Flash-back' stopper

'Luer' fittings

Needle

Cannula proper

8

Fig. 8.6 Essential equipment needed to set up a drip. (a) Bag of fluid (checked for content and expiry date) for infusion. (b) Infusion set for giving blood (two chamber with ball float). Squeezing lower chamber causes the ball to rise up and prevent back flow during rapid infusion requirements. (c) i.v. cannula showing various components.

an experienced person first and then doing it oneself under supervision. Fifty cannulations is perhaps the minimum required to feel some confidence with the technique – the author reiterates that the time to gain experience in cannulation is not at 4 a.m. during the first few weeks of your time as a PRHO!

Any cannula bigger than 22 G (blue) should not be inserted without anaesthetising the skin to be punctured with a small amount of plain 1% lidocaine through a 25 G needle. In children and very nervous adults, a topical local anaesthetic such as amethocaine gel or eutectic mixture of local anaesthetic (EMLA) cream can be applied to the area for 30 min prior to cannulation.

Choice of vein

The choice of an appropriate vein is an important step. Except in very special circumstances, only the superficial veins of forearm and hand should be used. The wrist and antecubital fossa should be avoided, because splinting of the joint is required to avoid kinking of the cannula, and there is increased likelihood of cannula displacement and venous thrombosis at these sites. Veins forming an inverted 'Y' junction in the forearm are probably the best choice for beginners, because entry into the vein is more obvious. Do not despair if faced with a chubby individual, as veins have a characteristic feel when palpated, even if they cannot be seen. Try and use the non-dominant hand.

Choice of cannula

There is no evidence that the brand of cannula has any influence upon the success of peripheral vein cannulation. Of the presently available models, cost is the only consideration governing choice. To avoid needle stick injury, the needle should be carefully disposed of immediately after successful cannulation. New cannulae are being produced that incorporate a spring loaded stylet that protrudes through the bevel of the needle as soon as it is withdrawn, thus preventing needle stick injury. Such cannulae should be used in preference to the traditional models shown in Fig. 8.7.

Different sizes of cannula are required for different clinical applications.

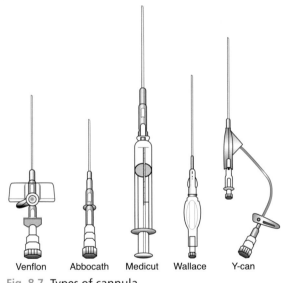

Venflon   Abbocath   Medicut   Wallace   Y-can

Fig. 8.7 Types of cannula.

Application	Internal gauge diameter (mm)	Standard wire gauge (SWG)	Maximum flow rate (ml/min)	Time taken to infuse 1 l (min)
Continuous infusion of drugs (pumped)	0.8–1.0	22–20	25–50	40–20
Normal daily fluid replacement	1.2	18	65	15
Slow blood transfusion or intra-operative fluids	1.7	16	150	7
Rapid blood transfusion	2.0–2.4	14–12	200–300	5–3

8

Preparation of insertion site

A tourniquet, BP cuff or a helper's hand must be placed proximal to the puncture site to distend the vein. The pressure applied round the arm must be such that blood flow in the arteries is not compromised (check for radial pulse if in doubt). If vein distension is insufficient, gently tapping it, rubbing it or applying a warm towel for 2–3 min, usually produces sufficient distension. Hanging the arm over the side of the bed and clenching/unclenching the fist may also be useful manoeuvres.

The operator must wash his hands and put on gloves before starting the procedure. However, the value and techniques of disinfecting the site of puncture are less certain. If a disinfectant is used (alcohol, chlorhexidene or iodine-based preparations), at least 1 min should be allowed for it to take effect prior to puncture.

Shaving of the skin produces small abrasions, which alter the skin flora, and should be done only to facilitate the application of adhesive tape. Scissors may be used to crop hair short, if visualisation of the vein is difficult in very hairy individuals.

Technique of insertion

The left hand of the operator holds the patient's arm (or hand) steady, the thumb pulling the skin taut, distally to the puncture site, without collapsing the vein. It is helpful to visualise the three-dimensional course of the vein prior to carrying on – think of roughly which direction you are going to advance the needle. With the bevel of the needle facing upwards, the cannula/needle assembly is advanced through the skin a few millimetre from the vein, using a quick jabbing action, at an angle of approximately 20° to the surface of the skin. This is the bit that hurts the patient, so warn them first. Note that the assembly must be held by the hub of the needle and not by the hub of the cannula. The cannula is then advanced until it enters the vein: a 'pop' is felt and a flashback of blood is seen in the hub. The cannula is then advanced some 3–5 mm inside the vein. The central needle is pulled back

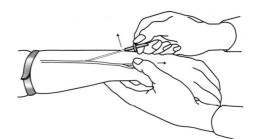

Fig. 8.8 Insertion of cannula into vein. Arrows indicate direction of pull.

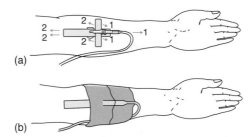

Fig. 8.9 Technique of securing cannula and drip set in the arm. (a) Arrows indicate direction of forces that may act to pull cannula out (1) and to keep cannula in place (2). Tape placed directly over the injection site should be sterile. When secured as in (a), a loop is made in the giving set and then the whole drip is secured with 3-inch tape as indicated. If the cannula has an integral injection port then this must be kept free of tape. Alternatively, a short extension with three-way tap can be used if injection of drugs is required.

through the cannula by about 1 cm. The whole assembly may then be advanced until the cannula is fully inserted (Fig. 8.8).

Fixation of the cannula and maintenance of flow

There are an infinite variety of methods of securing the cannula to the skin. Good common sense is the most important factor. Even the most perfect way of taping the cannula *in situ* can be defeated by greasy skin or a determined patient. If the drip is to be used in the awake patient over a few days, it is worth spending a bit more time in devising a firm way of securing the cannula in place, to avoid repeated re-cannulation (Fig. 8.9).

8

Important aspects that prevent accidental de-cannulation are

- the strength and adhesion of the tape,

- the area of adhesive surface in contact with dry skin and with the cannula,

- the direction of the tape applied on the skin with respect to the cannula,

- hair,

- shielding of the giving set from potential sources of pulling.

Preventing thrombosis and infection preserves drip patency. The longer the length of cannula inside the vein the higher the incidence of thrombosis; cannulae placed at the wrist or elbow tend to cause thrombosis more rapidly due to trauma to the vein wall. Injection of drugs through the drip increases the chances of thrombophlebitis; the irritant action of potassium, drugs and hypertonic or acidic solutions has the same effect.

Daily dressing of the puncture site and the use of local antiseptic agents are mandatory. In some hospitals in other European countries (but not the US) the routine practice of inserting a new cannula in a different site every 24 h (also changing the giving set and fluid container) has been found to be cost effective. At the first signs of local inflammation, the cannula *must* be removed and replaced elsewhere, preferably in the other arm.

Full recommendations on catheter-related infections can be obtained from the following URL: http://www.cdc.gov/ncidod/hip/IV/iv.htm

If all else fails...

- Central venous access may be attempted (see later).

- High volume resuscitation fluids may be given through an intraosseous needle in infants.

- Consider whether the patient really needs a drip – can those antibiotics be given orally, for example?

- Consider other routes for drug administration – i.m., rectal and s.c.

Insertion of a central venous catheter line (CVC)

This is a procedure that should only be attempted on a patient after lengthy practice in a clinical skills laboratory. It is a procedure with a high incidence of serious complications, for which the operator should be observant both during and after the procedure. Recent advice includes using an ultrasound device for catheter insertion rather than relying on the anatomical landmarks (see later). Apart from the methods mentioned below, central venous access can occasionally be obtained through the external jugular vein or a vein in the antecubital fossa using a long catheter. Neither of these routes has a high success rate of central venous placement of the catheter tip and is only used if the methods described below are unsuccessful.

Indications for CVC access

- Measurement of CVP (Chapter 15).

- Infusion of certain drugs that are highly irritant to peripheral veins (e.g. adrenaline, amiodarone and potassium).

- Total parenteral nutrition (TPN – Chapter 17), chemotherapy and long-term drug administration.

- Aspiration of air emboli.

- Inability to obtain peripheral venous access.

Contraindications/cautions

- *Coagulopathy:* These are not easy areas of the body in which to reduce haemorrhage by the application of pressure, and the consequences of haemorrhage can be severe.

- *Un-drained contralateral pneumothorax:* It is quite possible to cause a bilateral pneumothorax in this instance. One should always site a central line on the same side as a drained pneumothorax.

- Agitated, restless patient plus (or minus) agitated, restless, inexperienced operator!

- Take especial care in those with hyper expanded lungs, e.g. those patients with COPD.

8

Equipment required

There are many different brands of central venous catheter (CVC). They differ in length, lumen size, number of lumens, the material they are made of, the design of the J-wire holder and the presence or absence of a subcutaneous cuff.

The simplest resemble long peripheral cannulae. They have a single lumen and are usually available from 14G to 18G sizes. Their use is restricted to the rapid attainment of central venous access in an emergency situation, because they are somewhat tricky to insert and can cause big holes in vital structures. However, they are useful for infusing large volumes of fluid quickly and for administering 'cardiac' drugs. Double lumen lines are available, but rarely used except in infants.

The most common form of central venous access uses triple or quadruple lumen CVCs. These may be for short-term (up to 10 days) or long-term (up to 6 months) access. Long-term access uses a catheter with a subcutaneous cuff that is surgically tunnelled under the skin (Hickman line), to reduce the incidence of accidental de-cannulation and infection. In addition, the following items are required: a 16–18G 10 cm needle or cannula, a J-wire threaded on to a feeder, three-way taps (one per lumen), a blunt dilator, suture material (0/0 to 2/0 on a straight needle), a size 11 blade, cleaning equipment and drapes, 10 ml of NaCl, or heparinised NaCl, flush, a 22G (blue) locator needle and a 10-ml syringe. All these are present in the Triple lumen sets obtainable from many manufacturers.

Some anatomical considerations

Easy insertion, without causing complications, necessitates some knowledge of where the 'central' veins are and what other structures surround them. For our purposes, the central veins describe the large veins that drain the head, neck and arms, i.e. the internal jugular veins (IJVs), the brachiocephalic veins and the superior vena cava (SVC) (note that the femoral veins are also considered to be central veins – they may be cannulated, but this is less desirable due to an increased incidence of infection).

Three approaches to cannulation are commonly used.

The high internal jugular approach

The internal jugular vein (IJV) is a continuation of the sigmoid sinus. It collects branches from the face and neck, before joining the subclavian vein to become the brachiocephalic vein. With the patient supine, slightly head-down and head turned 10–20° to the left (for right IJV) or right (for left IJV), the locating needle (see below) is inserted at a point half-way between the sternal notch and the ipsilateral mastoid process, just anterior to the medial border of sternocleidomastoid. The carotid pulse should be felt medially, and the vessel avoided. The needle is advanced inferiorly and towards the ipsilateral big toe at an angle of 45° to the surface of the skin until the vein is punctured. Cannulation is then attempted using the method described below.

The low internal jugular approach

With the patient positioned as above, the locating needle (see below) is inserted at the point where the confluence of the two heads of sternocleidomastoid merge (i.e. at the apex of the triangle formed at the base by the clavicle, medially by the lateral edge of the sternal head and laterally by the medial edge of the clavicular head). The needle is advanced inferiorly and towards the ipsilateral nipple at an angle of 30° to the skin, until the vein is punctured. Cannulation is then attempted using the method described below.

Although traditionally these landmarks have been used, in the UK, the National Institute for Clinical Excellence (NICE) recommend that

1. the use of 2D imaging ultrasound guidance (USS) should be considered in most clinical circumstances, both elective and emergency, for insertion of CVCs into the IJV;

2. that use of USS should be considered the 'preferred' method for all elective cases and in children;

3. all involved should be given 'suitable training'.

8

105

Clearly, this has some significant implications for those of us inserting the 200,000 or so IJV catheters – not least the cost of the provision of enough USS machines and training.

The subclavian approach

The subclavian vein is a continuation of the axillary vein. It joins the IJV to become the brachiocephalic vein. With the patient supine and their head in the neutral position, the locating needle (see below) is inserted at a point a third of the distance along the clavicle from the suprasternal notch. The needle is inserted below the clavicle and advanced towards the suprasternal notch until the clavicle is encountered, at which point the needle is redirected more inferiorly and walked around the under surface of the bone, until the vein is punctured. Cannulation is then attempted using the method described below.

Technique of insertion (Seldinger method)

1. The indications and procedure are explained to the patient, and their consent is obtained, if possible.

2. The patient is placed supine, without a pillow, and covered with a blanket.

3. ECG electrodes are attached to the patient's chest.

4. The patient is placed in the Trendelenburg (head-down) position. This is wrongly assumed to be done to 'distend' the veins, but central veins do not collapse even when standing upright. The real reason for the head-down position is to prevent air entrainment through the catheter during insertion, leading to air embolisation; the position elevates the hydrostatic pressure of the blood at the point of insertion to above atmospheric pressure.

5. The operator dons gown, gloves and mask. This is a *sterile* procedure.

6. The patient's skin is sterilised using an alcohol-based cleaning solution, which should be applied for 3 min.

7. While waiting for skin sterilisation to be completed, the operator assembles and checks his equipment. Three-way taps are attached to each lumen port, except the distal port, which transmits the guide wire. All lumens are flushed to check their patency and remove air. The J-tipped guidewire is loaded appropriately on to its feeder. The patency of the guide wire needle and dilator should be checked.

8. The operator positions the patient's head, feels the appropriate landmarks and assesses the point of insertion.

9. Five millilitres of plain 1% lidocaine is inserted subcutaneously at the site of cannula insertion, and left for 1 min to take effect.

10. A locator needle is used to puncture the vein. This needle transmits the guide wire and is at least 18G and if used initially to locate the vein can cause significant trauma, making large holes in vessels and lungs. It is therefore more advisable to use a small 22G needle to locate the vessel.

11. Having gained an idea of the depth and direction of the vein, the guide wire needle, attached to a 10-ml syringe, is inserted through the skin and angled toward the vein. Gentle aspiration is applied using the syringe. Venous puncture is very obvious, as a rapid sudden flashback of blood is observed. (If the blood is pulsatile or bright red, an artery has been punctured; the whole assembly should be withdrawn, the patient tipped head-up and firm pressure applied for 10 min.)

12. The syringe is disconnected. Approximately 15–20 cm of guide wire is advanced along the guide wire needle. The ECG should be monitored at this point. Ectopics or other rhythm disturbances indicate cardiac irritation by the guide wire, which should be withdrawn by several cm. The guide wire needle is withdrawn over the guide wire.

13. The size 11 blade is used to incise the skin to a depth of 1/2 cm, adjacent to the guide wire.

8

14. The dilator is railroaded over the guide wire and inserted *for 2–3 cm only*, to dilate the tract around the guide wire. It is then withdrawn. Note: The dilator is very stiff and can do damage to valves and the vein wall if advanced too far. It is only necessary to form a tract through the skin and muscle to allow the soft tipped triple lumen catheter to be inserted.

15. The catheter is railroaded over the guide wire, to a depth of approximately 15 cm (three circumferential lines), depending on the size of the patient, their age and the site of insertion. The ECG should be monitored at this point. The guide wire is removed through the catheter.

16. The line is sutured into position. More sterile cleaning solution is applied to remove any excess blood. An occlusive dressing, or antiseptic spray, is placed over the catheter at the entry site. The patient is returned to a normal position.

17. Line position may be confirmed in three ways: one should be able to aspirate blood through all lumens, chest radiography should reveal the tip of the catheter to be sited at the junction of the SVC and the RA and transduction of the CVP should show a characteristic trace and be of a lower pressure than the systemic BP.

Complications of central venous catheterisation

The complications are divided into early complications (i.e. those associated with insertion), intermediate complications (within 24 h) and late complications (days to weeks), but are not mutually exclusive.

Early complications
- Allergic skin reactions to preparation fluid.

- Trauma to other structures: arteries (carotid, vertebral, aorta, thyroid, subclavian), oesophagus, trachea, thyroid gland, lung (pneumothorax, particularly with low internal jugular and subclavian approach), thoracic duct (left IJV lines), nerves

(phrenic, recurrent laryngeal, cervical plexus, brachial plexus).

- Haematoma and airway obstruction.

- Cerebral ischaemia (never attempt contralateral cannulation if the ipsilateral carotid artery has been punctured).

- Air embolism.

- Thrombo-embolism.

- Cardiac arrest or dysrhythmia, due to cardiac irritation by the guidewire or catheter.

Intermediate complications
- Allergic reactions to catheter components/coating.

- Infection – necessitates removal and contralateral reinsertion.

- De-cannulation.

- Pneumothorax, haemothorax, chylothorax, hydrothorax, parenteral feed thorax.

- Air embolism.

- Thrombo-embolism.

- Cardiac arrest or dysrhythmia.

Late complications
- Infection.

- Difficulty in removal.

- Mural perforation.

Note: it is very important to make sure that the catheter is not advanced too far. If it advances into the atrium then wall perforation can occur and this is uniformly fatal. It is not uncommon for a correctly placed catheter to perforate the SVC. This may occur without clinical signs and is only detected on post mortem where the patient has died from another cause. However, it can cause catastrophic haemorrhage into the thorax and requires urgent thoracotomy. If this is suspected in a patient who suddenly deteriorates with a triple lumen catheter *in situ*, attempts to aspirate blood through the

8

catheter should be made. It is imperative that NO attempt is made to drain the haemothorax, as this will precipitate more haemorrhage, which may well prove to be fatal.

- Catheter embolisation, i.e. a piece of the catheter detaches itself and embolises the RA or ventricle.

- Air embolism.

- Thrombo-embolism.

- Cardiac arrest or dysrhythmia.

Urinary catheterisation

Catheterisation of the bladder is an important aspect of surgical care. Catheterisation may be required to bypass obstruction to urinary flow (which can be painful and cause ureteric dilation and infection) or as a method of managing urinary incontinence (urine drenched bed sheets hasten the formation of bedsores and increase the likelihood of their infection, as well as being detrimental to the psychological status of the patient).

Specifically, urinary catheterisation is indicated for

- accurate perioperative monitoring of urine output;

- prolonged immobilisation, particularly of unconscious patients;

- urethral obstruction and urinary retention, due to stricture, clot, foreign body or prostatic hypertrophy;

- urinary incontinence;

- prolonged epidural anaesthesia.

Remember that males and females have different urethral anatomy. The indications and the process of the procedure should be explained to the patient, and their consent should be obtained when possible. Ideally, male doctors should catheterise male patients, and female doctors female patients. In practice, this arrangement is not always possible. Nevertheless, a chaperone should accompany the operator throughout the

procedure. Only the practice of transurethral catheterisation is described here, but it should be remembered that in instances of urethral blockage or failure of urethral catheterisation (e.g. due to urethral strictures, foreign objects, trauma or prostatic hypertrophy), trans abdominal, suprapubic catheterisation may be attempted.

Equipment

A general schematic representation of a urinary catheter (Foley) is presented in Fig. 8.10. (The irrigation channel is usually absent from a conventional Foley catheter used in the perioperative period.)

Urinary catheters are sized according to their French gauge, 12F (smaller) to 16F (larger) being the most commonly used. The French gauge is a unit of distance in mm used for measuring the external circumference of small tubes such as tracheostomy tubes, catheters and fibre-optic bundles. Thus, a 36FG tracheostomy tube has an *external* diameter of 11.5 mm (circumference = π × diameter), which is equivalent to an 8 mm (*internal* diameter) ETT.

The following items are also required: gloves, sterile dressing pack and disinfectant (chlorhexidine or similar), 1% lidocaine gel, 10-ml syringe and saline, and a urine collection bag.

Technique of insertion

The patient is asked to lay supine on a bed, with their genitals exposed. In men, the foreskin is retracted and the glans penis and genital area cleaned. Women are asked to bend their knees, with the soles of their feet together, which opens the legs – the genital area is cleaned and the labia lifted and retracted to expose the urethral meatus. Drapes are placed around the cleaned area.

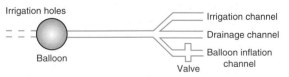

Fig. 8.10 Schematic representation of a urinary catheter.

8

Lidocaine gel is gently injected into the urethra, and a period of 3–4 min should be allowed for this to take effect (unless the patient is unconscious). The catheter is introduced gently. In women, the passage of the catheter is usually unobstructed. In men, the catheter is advanced with the penis held at 90° to the patient's body, until the external sphincter is encountered, at which point the penis is moved horizontally towards the lower body, before the catheter is advanced into the bladder. The catheter is advanced as far as possible, before the balloon is inflated with 10 ml saline. The catheter is then gently withdrawn until the resistance of the balloon at the internal urethra is felt. Urine should be seen to flow (gentle pressure to the suprapubic area may assist urinary flow, as may the injection of 10 ml of saline into the catheter to unblock any debris in the lumen), and the catheter is connected to the urine collection bag. In male patients, the foreskin, if present, should be un-retracted. Bloody insertion or failure to pass the catheter necessitates referral to a urologist.

Complications

- Early
  - Failure to insert.
  - Urethral trauma.
  - Creation of a false passage.
  - Haemorrhage.
  - Leakage around the catheter.
- Intermediate
  - Urinary infection.
  - Haemorrhage due to bladder irritation.
  - Clot retention/blockage.
  - Haemorrhage due to rapid deflation after chronic distension.
- Late
  - Urethral stricture.
  - Sphincter incompetence.

Insertion of a chest drain

Chest drains are trans-thoracic catheters that are sited in order to drain blood, fluid or air from the pleural cavity. Their placement is, therefore, indicated for the drainage of a pneumothorax, haemothorax, chylothorax (lymph, due to damage of the left-sided thoracic duct), pus or pleural effusion. Their use is often routine after cardiothoracic surgery or trauma, and they may be placed prophylactically when there are rib fractures or lung contusions in a patient requiring emergency general anaesthesia (positive pressure ventilation may rupture contused lung tissue, leading to an intra-operative tension pneumothorax).

Equipment required

Chest drains are sized according to their internal circumference, the most commonly used being 20–34 Ch (Ch is Charriere gauge, which is the same as the French gauge (F), see above). They are supplied with a central introducer (trocar) – all current guidelines for the insertion of chest drains recommend that the trocar is discarded before insertion is started because its use is associated with a high incidence of severe complications (e.g. liver, diaphragmatic, lung and cardiac laceration). The operator also requires a sterile gown and gloves, 10 ml 1% lidocaine and a green needle, a dressing pack containing antiseptic, scalpel, artery forceps and a size 0 silk or nylon suture, a chest drain bottle filled to the zero mark with sterile water, adhesives, dressings and a trained assistant.

Technique of insertion

The patient should give their consent if possible, and the operator should explain that the procedure might be uncomfortable. With the patient supine, the fifth or sixth intercostal space in the mid-axillary line is identified by palpation and the skin around the area sterilised. Lidocaine is injected into the skin and subcutaneous tissues as far as the parietal pleura and a period of 5 min should

8

109

be allowed for local anaesthesia to become established (unless the patient is unconscious). A 2-cm incision is made parallel to the direction of ribs and superior to the upper surface of the rib below (to avoid damage to the intercostal neurovascular bundle, (Fig. 8.11(b)), as deep as the intercostal muscle, and a purse string suture is placed around the incision. A blunt dissection method using first the artery forceps and then the index finger is used to make a hole through the intercostals muscles as far as the pleura, which should be incised under direct vision. The artery forceps are used to advance the chest drain into the pleural space, which may be accompanied by a sudden loss of air or blood through the drain, and the drain is connected to the underwater seal. The drain is directed anteriorly in the chest in order to drain air, and posteriorly to drain fluid, before being tied into place with the purse string suture, and dressed. A post-procedure CXR should confirm the position of the drain and re-inflation of the lung (after pneumothorax). Oral analgesia should be prescribed (Fig. 8.11(a)).

The water level of the underwater seal is initially seen to swing up·and down in time with the respiratory cycle, according to the intrapleural pressure (more negative on inspiration – meniscus moves up; less negative/positive on expiration – meniscus falls/bubbles escape if a pneumothorax is present). If the water level is not swinging, the drain has fallen out of the pleural space or is blocked.

Chest drains are removed when there is no further bubbling and the lung has re-inflated on CXR (pneumothorax has resolved), or when the fluid drainage is less than 100 ml/day. A CXR is mandatory after removal. Persistent bubbling indicates a broncho-pleural fistula, and necessitates application of gentle suction to the drain (approximately 5 cmH₂O pressure) and referral to a chest physician or thoracic surgeon (for possible pleurodesis).

Complications

■ Early

- Haemorrhage.

- Pain.

- Laceration of liver, spleen, diaphragm, inferior vena cava, aorta, lungs, heart.

- Pneumothorax, chylothorax.

■ Intermediate

- Blockage (especially due to clot).

- Haemorrhage.

- Displacement (air/fluid recollects).

- Subcutaneous emphysema (tube is mildly displaced – air tracks from pleural space to subcutaneous tissues).

- Infection.

- Pain (particularly when coughing, or due to diaphragmatic irritation).

■ Late

- Broncho-pleural fistula.

- Transthoracic fistula.

Arterial puncture and blood-gas sampling

ABG analysis forms an essential part of the perioperative management of seriously ill patients. In addition, routine analysis may be employed for patients with respiratory disease scheduled to undergo surgery, and during complex operations. The method for

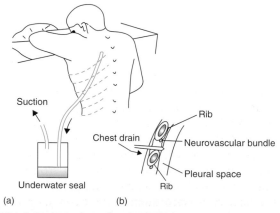

Suction

Chest drain

Underwater seal

Rib

Neurovascular bundle

Pleural space

Rib

(a)   (b)

Fig. 8.11 Insertion of a chest drain.

obtaining ABGs described below obtains a single sample. A necessity for repeated samples requires cannulation of an artery; a procedure that is beyond the scope of this book, but which also enables the physician to monitor invasive BP. Interpretation of ABG sample analysis is described later in this chapter.

Equipment

An alcohol swab, gloves, a 23G (blue) needle, a pre-heparinised syringe and gauze are required.

Procedure

One of three sites is commonly used from which to obtain a sample. The radial artery is located by the radial pulse on the lateral aspect of the ventral forearm at the level of the proximal wrist crease. Allen's test should be negative before the radial artery is punctured – that is, occlusion of both the ulna and radial arteries after clenching the fist, followed by release of the ulna artery should result in reddening (i.e. blood flow) of the palm. The femoral artery is located half-way along a line connecting the symphysis pubis and the anterior superior iliac spine, with the patient supine (Fig. 8.12). The dorsalis pedis artery is located just laterally to the tendon of flexor hallucis longus on the upper surface of the foot, more towards the ankle than the toes.

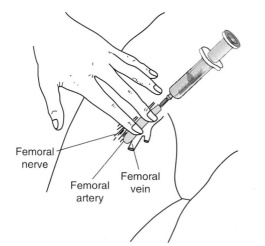

Femoral nerve

Femoral artery

Femoral vein

Fig. 8.12 Sampling arterial blood from the femoral artery.

In all cases, the patient should consent to the procedure, if possible. The skin overlying the artery should be swabbed. The artery is palpated with the index finger and the needle (connected to the syringe) advanced through the skin at an angle between 45° and the perpendicular. If using a low resistance syringe, arterial puncture will register as a flashback into the syringe, which will proceed to fill. Normal syringes require the operator to pull back gently on the plunger to fill the syringe. Two millilitres of blood is collected, before the needle is withdrawn. Firm pressure is placed over the puncture site. Air should be dispelled from the syringe (to avoid continued gas exchange). The sample should be placed on ice if analysis is to be delayed (which prevents further cellular metabolism). The patient's core temperature should be recorded (which alters the dynamics of gas binding).

Complications

The procedure is associated with minimal complications. Haemorrhage may occur through the puncture site, particularly if patients are coagulopathic, or pressure is not applied for long enough (5 min) after the needle is withdrawn. Occasionally, femoral nerve injury may occur. The main complication in ABG analysis concerns poor interpretation of the results, particularly the failure to recognise that the sample taken is venous (rather than arterial) in origin (see Interpretation of ABGs at end of this chapter).

Passing a nasogastric tube

An NG tube is a two-way conduit between the patient's stomach and the outside world. They are employed either to drain the stomach contents (e.g. acute obstruction, gastric dilation, ileus) or in order to administer drugs or food to a patient (e.g. postoperative enteral nutrition, or to bypass malfunctioning/absent oropharyngeal/oesophageal swallowing mechanisms). They may be passed when the patient is awake (described below), or intra-operatively.

8

Equipment

A chilled NG tube (10–12F), gloves, KY gel® and lidocaine throat spray and a bladder syringe.

Procedure

Consent is obtained for the procedure. The operator sprays four to five jets of throat spray to the back of the patient's throat under direct vision, and waits for a minute, to establish anaesthesia. The patient is placed in a semi-recumbent position. The tip of the NG tube is lubricated with KY gel and advanced along the infero-medial border of one nostril, as far as the pharynx. The patient is then asked to flex their neck and start swallowing, while the operator continues to advance the NG tube (up to 50 cm). Persistent coughing may indicate tracheal placement of the tube. A satisfactory tube position is confirmed by auscultation of borborygmi over the stomach area when 25 ml of air is flushed down the NG tube. In addition, stomach contents may be aspirated through the tube (these turn blue litmus paper red). The tube is capped off with a spigot or connected to a drainage bag, and taped to the nose. A CXR should be used to confirm the position of the tube before any fluids are administered down it.

Complications

Again this is not a procedure associated with many complications – failure to pass the tube being the most common problem (particularly, in cases of abnormal oesophageal anatomy or stricture). NG tubes have been cited as possible colonisation routes for gastrointestinal bacteria to enter the lungs, but this is of more concern in the ICU than on general surgical wards.

8   Arterial blood gases and interpretation

Introduction

The role of hydrogen ion (H^+ or proton) in living cells is as important as that of sodium or potassium. Its intracellular concentration has not been reliably measured in most mammalian tissues (except erythrocytes), but it is thought to be critically important. It is affected by such factors as its extracellular concentration and the transmembrane balance of potassium ions. Hydrogen ions are constantly produced (about 15 mol/day) by metabolism and additional amounts are ingested with food. There must be a balance between production and excretion. Some 80% (12 mol/day) is eliminated through the lung as carbon dioxide and water, and the rest through the kidney (3 mol/day). The human body has several built-in mechanisms to maintain the extracellular concentration of hydrogen ion within narrow limits, namely 35–45 nmol/l (pH 7.45–7.35). In blood, sustained concentrations above 100 nmol/l (pH < 7.0) or below 10 nmol/l (pH > 8.0) are incompatible with life.

Regulatory mechanisms

There are two major regulatory mechanisms which tend to keep the hydrogen ion concentration at the physiological 'set point' of 40 nmol/l (pH 7.4): a fast mechanism operated via the lung and a slow one operated via the kidney. Finally, the liver plays a major role in recycling lactate to bicarbonate to replace that lost in the periphery by buffering H^+.

Respiratory homeostatic mechanisms

The immediate determinant of hydrogen ion (H^+) concentration in blood is the partial pressure of carbon dioxide ($PaCO_2$), which is acutely dependent on pulmonary ventilation. In a mechanically ventilated subject, the relationship between minute ventilation and the $PaCO_2$ in arterial blood is a curve close to a hyperbola, varying its shape with the metabolic consumption. Note that the same increase in minute ventilation produces a much smaller fall in $PaCO_2$ as levels decrease below normal. An excess of H^+ in arterial blood stimulates both the peripheral chemoreceptors in the carotid bifurcation and the respiratory neurones in the brain stem. This causes an increase in ventilation that leads to a fall in $PaCO_2$ and H^+ in blood, closing the negative feedback loop of this regulation. It should be noted that chemoreceptors are also stimulated by an increase in $PaCO_2$. The arterial chemoreceptors are independently stimulated by (PaO_2) values below 8 kPa (60 mmHg); the three stimuli interact with each other in a multiplicative way.

Carbon dioxide and hydrogen ion are interrelated through the reaction of the former with water to form carbonic acid; the latter dissociates into hydrogen H^+ and bicarbonate HCO_3^- ions, a major buffer system in blood

$$CO_2 + H_2O = H_2CO_3$$

(catalysed by carbonic anhydrase)

$$H_2CO_3 = HCO_3^- + H^+$$

Traditionally, H^+ concentration has been measured in pH units, pH being the negative logarithm (base 10) of the H^+ concentration. Its quantitative relationship has proved more convenient.

$$pH = pKa + \log(HCO_3^-)/(a \times PaCO_2)$$

where pKa is 6.1, and 'a' the CO_2 solubility factor (0.2, if $PaCO_2$ is measured in kPa, 0.03 if in mmHg).

The latter is known as the Henderson–Hasselbalch equation. It has three variables, pH, HCO_3^- and PCO_2. So, it cannot be represented by a single curve, but rather by a family of curves forming a 'surface'.

Various authors have represented this relationship in different ways: Davenport chose to plot pH against (HCO_3^-) at different $PaCO_2$ values. Sigaard–Andersen plotted pH against $PaCO_2$ at various HCO_3^- values. These plots were of great practical value before the era of electronic calculators to estimate HCO_3^- and the amount of excess acid or base present in blood. Most blood-gas machines in clinical use now have a microcomputer incorporated that instantly calculates these derived variables.

The way each variable in the Henderson–Hasselbalch equation depends on each other is a predictable function of temperature, concentration of Hb (buffer) and Hb saturation. This is also taken into account by the computer in the blood-gas machine. Temperature is not measured but the blood sample is warmed (or cooled) to 37°C in the measuring cuvette.

The printout of most blood-gas machines shows eight or more results, four from direct measurement (pH, $PaCO_2$, PaO_2 and Hb), and the others derived by calculation. The latter include base excess, bicarbonate, standard bicarbonate and Hb saturation. Base excess is a calculation of the amount of acid (HCl), or base (NaOH), that would need to be added to a litre of blood (*in vitro*) to titrate the pH back to 7.40 at a normal $PaCO_2$ of 5.3 kPa (40 mmHg) and at 37°C. The base excess result is negative in acidosis (it is really a 'base deficit', since NaOH would be added) and positive in alkalosis (HCl added). The standard bicarbonate is a calculation of the bicarbonate value if the blood were to be equilibrated with a $PaCO_2$ of 5.3 kPa (40 mmHg).

Renal homeostatic mechanisms

One of the many functions of the kidney is to excrete hydrogen ions. The H^+ in urine may be as high as 30,000 nmol/l (pH 4.5), 800 times that of plasma. At such high H^+, the total quantity of H^+ that can be excreted in the urine depends on its buffering power.

Two main buffer systems exist in urine: the phosphate system and the ammonia/ammonium system:

$$H^+ + HPO_4^- \leftarrow \rightarrow H_2PO_4^- \quad (pK = 6.8)$$

$$NH_3 + H^+ \leftarrow \rightarrow NH_4^+ \quad (pK = 5)$$

Note that these only work as buffers in the region of their respective pKs. The renal synthesis of ammonia is subject to regulation. Normally, about 30 mmol of ammonium are excreted per day; after three days of severe acidosis as much as 200 mmol may be excreted per day. The excretion of each H^+ ion into the urine leads to reabsorption of a Na^+ ion, and it is dependent upon the local $PaCO_2$ and availability of carbonic anhydrase. The K^+ ion competes with H^+ in urinary excretion; K^+ depletion leads to urinary loss of H^+ and alkalosis, and acidosis leads to K^+ retention and hyperkalaemia. The kidney also compensates for alkalosis by excreting excess bicarbonate; it is more effective in metabolic

8

alkalosis because the respiratory compensation leads to an increased $PaCO_2$.

The role of the liver in acid–base balance

About 1300 mmol of lactate and associated H^+ (lactic acid) are produced in the tissues every day. H^+ ions are buffered locally by HCO_3^- and lactate is released into the general circulation. The liver is the main site of lactate uptake (70%) as well as the heart and kidneys. In the liver, lactate can be converted to glucose or oxidised, either reaction consuming H^+ and generating HCO_3^-, which is re-circulated to the periphery to replace that which was lost. (A similar reaction accounts for the generation of HCO_3^- from the lactate in Hartmann's or lactated Ringer's solution.) It is clear that failure of the liver to take up lactate in proportion to its production could lead to depletion of bicarbonate and a metabolic acidosis. This is particularly likely to happen during hypovolaemic shock where diminished oxygen delivery to the tissues generates *excess* lactic acid (anaerobic glycolysis). The H^+ are buffered by HCO_3^- as usual but results in excessive bicarbonate consumption and lactate formation. Although acidaemia increases the ability of the hepatocyte to take up lactate (and generate the necessary bicarbonate), reduced hepatic blood flow (due to hypovolaemia and cardiac depression from acidaemia) leads to a vicious cycle of lactic acidaemia and loss of bicarbonate.

Acid–base disturbances

Introduction

It is important to understand the time course of acid–base disturbances. If it is caused by an abrupt change such as acute respiratory failure, the renal homeostatic mechanisms only develop fully after 3–5 days. A sudden acid challenge, such as that following release of a tourniquet applied to the lower limb for 2 h (e.g. orthopaedic operation under epidural anaesthesia), causes alterations in the values of the blood acid–base status that change rapidly with time as respiratory compensation occurs. Following this rapid respiratory phase over the course of a few minutes, a slower hepatic and renal phase follows in the course of the next few hours.

The four clinical situations described below usually progress in two phases. The initial phase is well understood and could easily be mimicked *in vitro* by adding or removing CO_2 or acid to a sample of arterial blood in a test-tube and measuring the pH and $PaCO_2$.

What are the differences between -aemia and -osis?

The terms acidaemia and alkalaemia refer only to the status of the blood, acid or alkaline in pH or H^+ concentration. Acidosis and alkalosis refer to pathological situations resulting from a positive or negative balance of protons, where there is a change in $PaCO_2$ or HCO_3^- in an acid or alkaline direction. However, as these changes may be compensatory, they may not lead to acidaemia or alkalaemia.

Consider a patient that develops an increased H^+ of 60 (pH 7.2), i.e. they have an *acidaemia*. If the HCO_3^- concentration is also found to be low they have, by definition, a metabolic *acidosis*. The effect of the increase in H^+ leads to respiratory centre stimulation that increases ventilation to reduce CO_2 to develop a respiratory *alkalosis*. But, how do we know which change is primary and which is secondary? Did the patient develop the metabolic change first and then respiratory compensation or the other way round? The important point to remember is that compensation on its own will never be enough to bring H^+ or pH back into the normal range. So, it is easy to see in this example that the primary event must be the metabolic acidosis that has led to the acidaemia and a secondary or compensatory respiratory alkalosis.

Example

A diabetic with a metabolic acidosis and acidaemia with a low HCO_3^- and pH of <7.1 or H^+ >60 responds with hyperventilation that results in a low $PaCO_2$. The latter constitutes a respiratory alkalosis, but the patient is not alkalaemic as the change is secondary.

To decide the primary and secondary changes:

1. look at the H^+ (pH) to decide whether the patient is acidaemic or alkalaemic,

2. look at the HCO_3^- and CO_2 levels to see whether they have a metabolic or respiratory acidosis or alkalosis,

3. the -osis that agrees with the -aemia is the *primary* change.

So, if the patient is acidaemic with a high $PaCO_2$ then it is this primary respiratory acidosis that has led to the acidaemia. There will often be a higher than normal HCO_3^- (especially, if it is a chronic CO_2 increase) to match this change, in other words a secondary or compensatory respiratory alkalosis.

It is not possible to quantitate precisely metabolic acidosis and alkalosis in the whole body. Clinical observation is the only reliable indicator of the severity of the situation. In the blood sample, the degree of metabolic acidaemia or alkalaemia is easily seen by looking at the base excess value: values below -12 tend to be associated with severe acidosis, needing urgent therapy, and values above $+12$ are usually associated with severe alkalosis (see later).

Respiratory acidosis
This is the commonest situation and follows retention of CO_2 due to acute or chronic respiratory failure due to inadequate ventilation of the lungs.

In acute CO_2 retention, blood (H^+) rises by about 6 nmol/l for each 1 kPa (7 mm) rise in $PaCO_2$ (pH drops 0.1 unit per 10 mmHg CO_2 rise). For each 1.5 kPa (10 mmHg) acute rise in $PaCO_2$, HCO_3^- increases by 1 mmol/l due to reaction of CO_2 with H_2O.

Example
Acute $PaCO_2$ retention occurs postoperatively due to excess opioid in an otherwise fit patient. $PaCO_2$ rises acutely by 3–7.5 kPa (21–61 mmHg), pH will then drop by 0.2–7.2 (H^+ increases by 1858 nmol/l). HCO_3 will be 26 mmol/l.

In chronic CO_2 retention, renal mechanisms allow reabsorption of plasma (HCO_3^-), which increases by about 4 mmol/l for each 1.5 kPa (10 mmHg) CO_2 rise. This is often sufficient to restore pH to near normal values.

Example
An elderly patient with chronic CO_2 retention has a $PaCO_2$ of 8 kPa (60 mmHg). Renal retention of HCO_3^- has been sufficient to raise the HCO_3^- by 8–32 mmol/l. H^+ is 45 (pH is 7.3), i.e. nearly normal.

Metabolic acidosis
The second commonest situation may appear in a variety of disease states, such as:

- grossly uncompensated diabetes (ketoacidosis);

- lack of oxygen delivery to tissues, as in shock or severe hypoxia;

- loss of intestinal alkaline secretions, as in severe diarrhoea or fistulae;

- transplantation of the ureters into the ileum after total cystectomy;

- acetazolamide therapy, which impairs bicarbonate re absorption in the kidney;

- failure of normal homeostatic mechanisms, as in generalised renal or hepatic failure.

If a patient develops a metabolic acidosis and acidaemia they will develop a compensatory respiratory alkalosis, i.e. the $PaCO_2$ will fall. It is important to have some idea of what degree of compensation is likely. In an experiment where healthy subjects were made acidaemic by infusion of dilute solutions of HCl it was found that the resulting lowered $PaCO_2$ was related to the HCO_3^- concentration by the following formula:

$$PaCO_2 \text{ (in mmHg)} = 8.4 + (HCO_3^- \times 1.3)$$

For example, if HCO_3^- is 10, the normal subject should be able to reduce $PaCO_2$ to 21 mmHg (3 kPa). Anything much higher than this will mean that the patient is unable to compensate fully (e.g. has respiratory depression due to drugs or ventilatory

8

inadequacy). It is important to make this assessment since the efficacy of exogenous administration of $NaHCO_3$ in patients with metabolic acidosis and acidaemia relies on adequate ventilation to blow off the CO_2 generated by the reaction of H^+ and HCO_3^- (see later).

Respiratory alkalosis

This is a less common situation and may be due to spontaneous hyperventilation that occurs in certain patients for unknown reasons. Respiratory alkalosis occurs commonly in mechanically ventilated patients under anaesthesia or sedation in the ICU. Acutely, it causes a fall in H^+ of the same proportion as for respiratory acidosis (6 nmol/l H^+ change for 1 kPa $PaCO_2$ change).

Metabolic alkalosis

A rare situation, that sometimes presents clinically as tetany with normal plasma calcium levels. It is due to

- loss of acid secretions as in compulsive vomiting or in pyloric stenosis;

- excessive ingestion of alkali (over treatment of 'indigestion'), or i.v. administration of bicarbonate (frequently seen after successful resuscitation from cardiac arrest);

- potassium depletion (extracellular alkalosis and intracellular acidosis).

Interpretation of blood-gas values

Introduction

Blood gas results are nearly always obtained from arterial blood (see later). In very special circumstances mixed venous blood may also be analysed to compute oxygen consumption, cardiac output or other variables. The sample must always be heparinised by priming the dead space of the syringe (just the hub) with a 1:1000 solution of heparin. Failure to do this results in damage to the machine taking hours of expensive labour to repair, see above.

The interpretation of results includes examination of the acid–base status of the blood and its oxygen-carrying capacity. It must be remembered that examination of the clinical state of the patient is the most important factor in any therapeutic decision. Arterial blood measurements are only a narrow observation window of a very complex and poorly understood homeostatic system. However, following a logical routine in the examination of the results increases the chances of a correct diagnosis.

The use of integral microcomputers in blood-gas machines will soon be extended to provide interpretation of the results as well, following the same logical steps as the clinician. Although, SI units are now officially in use, it will be found that in the great majority of establishments blood gases are still reported in pH and mmHg.

Artefacts

The blood-gas result should match the clinical assessment of the patient; a PaO_2 of 5 kPa (38 mmHg) in a conscious, non-narcotised patient without evidence of dyspnoea or central cyanosis is almost certainly an artefact. The commonest artefact is the sampling of venous blood instead of arterial, due to faulty technique of arterial puncture (see above). Extreme values of pH or derived parameters are likely to result from mixing of the blood sample with some acidic or basic residue in the syringe. For example, if highly concentrated subcutaneous heparin solution is used to prevent sample clotting, a very acidic result may be obtained.

Samples taken from indwelling arterial catheters attached to long plastic tubes should be preceded by withdrawal of 6–8 ml of blood into another syringe to remove the priming heparinised saline. Mixing of blood with saline will give an unexpectedly low $PaCO_2$ and a low Hb (if measured). If the machine measures Hb, care should be taken to stir the sample well just prior to injection into the cuvette, to prevent the effect of sedimentation of red cells in the syringe. The Hb value measured enters many of the calculations.

The time elapsed between taking the sample and analysing it is of little importance in clinical practice. PaO_2 and $PaCO_2$ change only by about 2% of the original value, if kept in a 2-ml syringe for 1 h at room temperature.

8

If stored in ice samples may be kept for up to 12 h with little change in values; this precaution is only necessary for research purposes.

Diagnosis

The method used in interpretation is based on the above.

Firstly, look at the pH or hydrogen ion changes:

Normal arterial blood pH is 7.4 ± 0.05 (H^+ = 40 ± 5); it can be below that value or above it.

If the pH is below 7.35 ($H^+ <$ 45), there is acidaemia. If the HCO_3^- is <22 mmol/l, metabolic acidosis is the likely cause of the acidaemia. If the $PaCO_2$ will be <5 kPa or 40 mmHg, a reduction in HCO_3^- occurs due to excess H^+ production and a failure of HCO_3^- recycling by the liver. As HCO_3^- falls and H^+ rises, the chemoreceptor stimulation causes an increase in ventilation and a reduction in $PaCO_2$. This respiratory alkalosis tends to limit the resulting acidaemia.

If the $PaCO_2$ is >5 kPa or 40 mmHg, respiratory acidosis is the likely cause of the acidaemia. In a pure respiratory acidosis, the HCO_3^- is always raised above normal.

If the pH is above 7.45 ((H^+) <35), there is alkalaemia.

If the HCO_3^- is >26 mmol/l, metabolic alkalosis is present and is the likely cause of the alkalaemia. The $PaCO_2$ will be >5.5 kPa or 40 mmHg as a secondary change limiting the effect on pH or H^+ of the metabolic changes.

If the $PaCO_2$ is <4 kPa or 30 mmHg, respiratory alkalosis is present and is the likely cause of the alkalaemia. HCO_3^- will be lowered as the kidney attempts to excrete HCO_3^- to limit the alkalaemia, i.e. a compensatory metabolic acidosis is present.

Oxygen changes

The partial pressure of oxygen (PaO_2) in arterial blood falls with age. On average, it is approximately 13 kPa (100 mmHg) in the young adult, and declines steadily to about 10 kPa (75 mmHg) at the age of 80. There is hypoxia when PaO_2 values are 2 kPa (15 mmHg) below the expected value for the patient's age.

The peripheral arterial chemoreceptors in the aortic arch and in the bifurcation of the carotid arteries are the only known oxygen sensors in the body. They are progressively stimulated by PaO_2 values below 8 kPa (60 mmHg), causing a reflex increase in ventilation. Hypoxic drive to ventilation, such as in pulmonary oedema or at altitude, usually leads to a fall in $PaCO_2$. In acute respiratory failure, hypoxia may be accompanied by CO_2 retention (Chapter 16).

Treatment of acid–base disturbances

The cause of the acid–base disturbance must be treated and the normal respiratory and renal homeostatic mechanisms allowed to restore the balance of protons (H^+). Only rarely is it indicated to infuse i.v. an alkali or an acid. HCl infusions in severe alkalosis have been described in a few instances, but with doubtful benefit for the clinical status of the patient. On the other hand, sodium bicarbonate infusions have been widely employed in the past to treat severe metabolic acidosis; presently their indication has been much restricted as more deleterious side-effects have been found. Its precise role in diabetic acidosis and cardiac arrest is hotly debated.

Sodium bicarbonate (84 is the MW) of 8.4% (or molar) carries a considerable load of sodium (1 mmol Na^+ per mmol HCO_3^- per ml of solution). High CO_2 pressures are generated on mixing with acidic blood, which cause diffusion of CO_2 into cells and intracellular acidosis. This is more likely to occur in mechanically ventilated patients or those in respiratory failure who have inefficient pulmonary CO_2 elimination (see above).

When sodium bicarbonate is considered necessary to correct acidosis, it should be remembered that the figure for base excess refers to the deficit of bicarbonate in the ECF. Thus, it is necessary to calculate ECF in litres and multiply this value by the BE to arrive at a figure for sodium bicarbonate in mmol. In adults, about 1/3 to 1/5 of BW is ECF; while in babies it is about 2/5.

8

Usually, only half of the calculated amount is given initially, e.g.

weight = 60 kg

BE = −12

ECF = 0.2 × 60 = 12 l

Thus, the initial dose of $NaHCO_3$ needed equals 0.5 × 12 × 12 = 72 mmol.

Note: As stated above, sodium bicarbonate must never be given if $PaCO_2$ is raised or there is any evidence that the patient has respiratory impairment.

9

Cardiorespiratory and temperature monitoring in the perioperative period

Aims

The aims of this chapter are to

- describe the operating principles of monitors used in the perioperative period,
- discuss the indications and limitations of monitors.

Objectives

After reading this chapter, you should be able to

- appreciate and make informed choices about the role different monitors play in the provision of optimal perioperative care,
- use monitors rationally and safely realising that they do not replace sound clinical examination and judgement.

Introduction

As discussed elsewhere in this volume, the key to proper patient management through all phases of perioperative care is the maintenance of oxygen balance. The two key organs in relation to oxygen delivery are the heart and the lungs. For the purposes of monitoring oxygen balance they should be regarded as a single functioning unit – the cardiopulmonary system.

Oxygen delivery depends on two basic factors, blood flow and oxygen content. (Chapters 7 and 18). Thus, monitoring essentially provides information on the two basic functional aspects of the cardiopulmonary system namely, *mechanical efficiency* in relation to blood flow, and *metabolic efficiency* in relation to oxygen delivery, extraction and consumption.

It should be stressed from the outset that near-patient monitoring devices should be deployed simply as an *adjunct* to support the conclusions of thorough clinical examination. No clinical device is without inherent sources of functional and measurement error.

Many recently developed near-patient monitoring devices purport to provide a whole battery of clinically 'useful' parameters. In assessing their real utility it is important to distinguish between which parameters are directly (physically) *measured* and which parameters are (mathematically) *derived*. Failure to make this distinction will lead to erroneous identification of functional relationships between parameters which are in reality artefact, arising from the fact that displayed values for those parameters are actually calculated from a common set of measured variables – the problem of *mathematical linkage*.

The patient suffering a major surgical crisis presents a constantly changing dynamic of physiology. It is axiomatic that the key to proper assessment and appropriate management of these patients lies not in single measured events, but in examining *trends in physiological variables* – properly tabulated!

The monitoring of mechanical function: pressure, flow and work

The basic mechanical function of the cardiopulmonary system is to sustain blood flow, through maintenance of a pressure gradient across the circulation. A measure of the efficiency of the system is the work required to generate that flow. These concepts are linked by some very elementary physics.

Ohm's law states that the *potential difference* across an electrical circuit is proportional to the product of the *current* flowing through the circuit and the inherent *resistance* of the circuit.

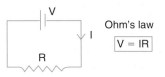

Ohm's law
$$V = IR$$

The same basic principles apply to the cardiovascular circuit, only here we have blood flowing around the circuit rather than a current of electrons. The potential difference driving the flow is equivalent to the pressure gradient across the system, for the systemic circulation this equates to the difference between the *mean arterial pressure* (MAP) at the aortic root, and the *central venous pressure* (CVP) at the great veins of the heart. The current in the electrical model is equivalent to the *cardiac output* (CO), and the resistance is equivalent to the *systemic vascular resistance* (SVR).

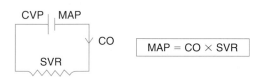

In practice, because the CVP is so small in relation to the MAP, we eliminate it from the equation leaving us with the expression:

MAP = CO × SVR
EMF = current × resistance

Both MAP and CO can be directly *measured* by feeding these values into the expression above – a value for SVR can be *derived*.
Further,

work done = force × distance moved

Since,

force = pressure × area

Then,

work done = (pressure × distance) × area
work done = pressure × volume

Thus, an estimate of mechanical work (and hence efficiency) can be derived from the product of measured pressure and volume.

Non-invasive measurement of BP
Techniques based upon inflation of an arm cuff are by far the commonest method of measurement, but these give only intermittent readings; automated devices based on this principle are now in common use and are able to measure pressure at intervals as short as 1 min, if necessary. The basis of sphygmomanometry (Fig. 9.1) is

that estimation of both systolic and diastolic pressures is possible, because of the sudden onset and offset of turbulent flow as the pressure in the cuff becomes less than systolic and then diastolic pressure, respectively.

In automated machines, an air pump initially inflates the cuff above systolic pressure, then allows slow deflation (Fig. 9.2). Turbulence is detected electronically as

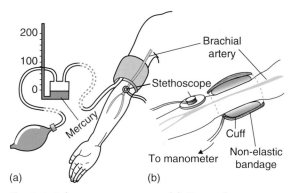

(a)   (b)

Fig. 9.1 Sphygmomanometer: (a) General arrangement of the mercury manometer and cuff. (b) Effect of inflating the cuff upon the artery.

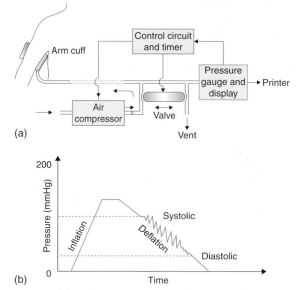

Fig. 9.2 (a) Schematic diagram of an automatic non-invasive BP monitor; (b) approximate profile of pressure detected by the gauge. Onset of oscillations during the downward slope indicate systolic pressure.

pressure oscillations in the cuff. The width of the cuff should be 20% greater than the diameter of the arm. Errors in non-invasive measurement of BP may be as much as ±30%, typically low pressures are overestimated and high pressures are underestimated.

Invasive measurement of BP

In certain circumstances, *continuous* direct measurement of BP may be required, e.g. in certain types of surgery – typically cardiothoracic surgery, neurosurgery or major vascular surgery, or if the patient is simply very haemodynamically labile for whatever reason.

This requires the insertion of a cannula into a peripheral artery, usually the radial, or occasionally the femoral. The cannula is then connected to a length of plastic tubing primed with heparinised saline, connected at the other end to a measuring device placed at the same level as the heart. If only MAP is required, a simple aneroid manometer may be used. If systolic and diastolic pressure values and information about the shape of the pressure waveform are needed, a pressure transducer must be used (Fig. 9.3).

The observed values for systolic and diastolic pressures obtained from direct measurement depend at which position in the arterial tree the pressures are measured. Moving from the great vessels to the periphery the precise waveform obtained changes becoming *narrower* and *increasing* in amplitude. This alteration in waveform is caused by the general reduction in both

vascular diameter and compliance as one moves from the aorta to the peripheral vessels. When comparing values from indirect and direct measurements of BP in the same patient, typically direct measurement gives a systolic value 5 mmHg higher, and a diastolic value 8 mmHg lower than values obtained by an indirect method.

BP waveforms in common with all waveforms encountered in biology are basically *compound sine waves*, i.e. they can be resolved (by Fourier analysis) into a series of *simple sine waves* of differing frequencies. Thus the arterial pressure waveform is an amalgam of sine waves of frequency range 0–40 Hz. The sensing apparatus itself may have a *natural frequency*, if this occurs within the range 0–40 Hz then *resonance and distortion* may result. Resonance can be avoided by designing a system whose natural frequency is 10× the frequency range being measured. Conversely, damping of the wave form may occur, if there are air bubbles in the liquid column in the connecting tubing, or if the tubing is kinked. To minimise waveform distortion, all connecting tubes should be of low compliance and large diameter, and should be primed with a fluid of low density.

Measurement of cardiac filling pressures

In relation to stroke volume (SV) and thus CO, there are three basic determinants namely, preload, contractility and afterload. The most important of these three factors is preload, as it is this factor that will determine the end-diastolic volume, degree of cardiac muscle fibre stretching and, in turn strength of subsequent contraction, according to Frank–Starling's law (Chapter 15).

Preload can be assessed as a *filling pressure* or as a *filling volume* (see later). Preload as a filling pressure can be measured as CVP for the right ventricle (RV), and if necessary pulmonary capillary wedge pressure (PCWP) for the left ventricle (LV).

In normal cardiac function, it is assumed that filling pressures to the left and right heart are essentially equal, therefore it is only

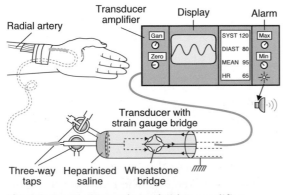

Fig. 9.3 Pressure transducer, bridge amplifier, display and alarm.

necessary to measure CVP. However, there are three circumstances in which this assumption does not hold:

■ significant left-ventricular failure,

■ significant pulmonary hypertension,

■ significant mitral valve disease.

Since it is the LV that determines systemic perfusion, and since in these circumstances filling pressure to the right heart (the CVP) is not a valid approximation, then filling pressure to the left heart must be assessed directly through measurement of the PCWP.

Central venous pressure

In most patients without intrinsic heart disease, measurement of CVP gives a good indication of total intravascular volume. CVP is usually taken in cmH_2O or mmHg.

CVP refers to the pressure of venous blood within the thoracic cavity. It corresponds to the filling pressure of the RV and the tip of the catheter is best placed in the superior vena cava (SVC). This catheter is filled with saline forming a continuous fluid 'bridge' with the measuring device. The insertion of the catheter into the SVC is a skilled manoeuvre and carries considerable risk to the patient (Chapter 8). There are several approaches.

Via the median cubital vein in the elbow

This is the route that should be used by inexperienced clinicians, as it is associated with least morbidity. A suitable X-ray opaque 60-cm catheter is selected and advanced through a previously inserted i.v. cannula under sterile conditions. Advancing the catheter may be difficult due to obstruction in the vein, particularly at the shoulder region. It may be necessary to abduct the arm at 90° while the cannula is advanced into the central vein. In some cases, it may be impossible to reach the central vein by this route. Correct positioning of the catheter is determined clinically by estimating the length inserted and observing a swing in the pressure in phase with the breathing movements. The only reliable method of confirming the correct placement using this approach is with a CXR.

Via the internal jugular vein or subclavian vein

For more details see Chapter 8.

Obtaining the CVP reading

Once catheter tip placement has been confirmed, a saline manometer or a pressure transducer is connected to it. This is arranged as in Fig. 9.4. Zero should be taken as the level of the manubrio-sternal joint with the patient lying horizontally, a spirit level often being used for accurate alignment. There should be a respiratory fluctuation of pressure, confirming that the catheter is in free communication with the SVC. Failure to observe the respiratory fluctuation means that the reading tip is not in free communication with the intrathoracic cavity and the reading will be inaccurate. The patency of the catheter should be maintained with a continuous flow of fluid between readings.

The manubrio-sternal joint is often used as a surface marker for the level of the right atrium (RA) because it is the simplest anatomical reference site. In the supine position, it is above the atrial level by between 5 and 10 cm, and thus values obtained may be negative in the normal patient. The CVP gives important information about the patient's blood volume, particularly with regard to fluid therapy. Fluid depletion may not be reflected as hypotension if the patient is awake, anxious and tachycardic.

Pulmonary capillary wedge pressure

In patients with poor left-ventricular function the close correlation between CVP and left-atrial pressure is lost, i.e. raising the CVP by giving fluids does not produce a satisfactory increase in CO. Left-atrial pressure should be measured but there are no simple techniques for percutaneous insertion of a catheter into the left atrium (LA). Instead, PCWP can be measured by means of a pulmonary artery catheter made to 'wedge' in a fine branch of the artery.

A special 'flow-directed' or 'floating' catheter was developed by Swan and Ganz in the 1960s which is provided with a balloon at

123

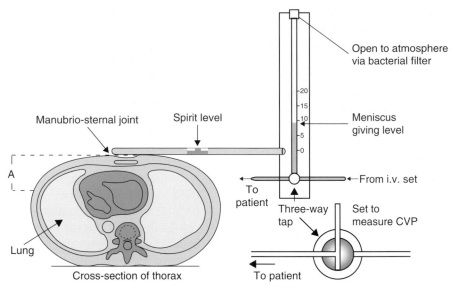

Fig. 9.4 Arrangement of CVP-measuring system. As shown, CVP zero is conventionally taken from the manubrio-sternal joint, whereas the actual level is lower. This difference, which is shown as (a) on the diagram, is about 5–10 cm of water. Thus, in some normal subjects, CVP may have a negative value (*see text*). The insert shows the position of the three-way tap while the CVP is being measured.

its tip; the balloon is inflated with air when the catheter tip is near the RA and this 'floats' the catheter into the RV and then into the pulmonary artery; here the catheter tip can be wedged into one of the small branches of the artery. Once the catheter is wedged, it no longer measures the pressure in the pulmonary artery, but it measures the backpressure from the left atrium via the pulmonary capillaries. This indirect measurement of left-ventricular filling pressure is used to assess left-ventricular function. Most flow-directed catheters have three lumens and are equipped with a temperature sensor at the tip for thermodilution CO estimation. Some catheters are also provided with a thin optic fibre, which allows continuous recording of mixed venous blood Hb oxygen saturation (Fig 9.5(a)).

Measurement of cardiac filling volumes

As previously stated, preload can be expressed in terms of filling 'pressure' or filling 'volume'. The recently developed pulse contour cardiac output (PiCCO) machine measures filling volumes as an index of preload.

Basically, the PiCCO machine performs two measurements. Firstly, cardiac output/blood flow by the conventional thermodilution method (see below). Secondly, 'transit time', the time taken for the injected bolus of cold saline to transit between its injection point in a central vein to its detection point at the tip of the detector located in the descending aorta.

Since flow rate multiplied by time equates to volume, by multiplying the measured CO (flow) by the measured transit time (across the thoracic compartment) the machine derives 'intrathoracic blood volume' (ITBV). This volume is taken as an index of the volume status of the patient. The theoretical advantage of measuring volume rather than pressure as an index of preload is that measured volume in contrast to measured pressure is unaffected by transmitted changes in intrathoracic pressure. (IT BVI is the ITBV index i.e. ITBV ÷ body surface area in m^2)

Invasive measurement of cardiac output

In 1870, Fick described a method of estimating CO derived from arterio-venous oxygen concentration difference and oxygen consumption. This test was difficult to perform in a clinical setting, and so an 'indicator dilution' technique was developed.

Today the standard method for measuring CO is by the thermodilution technique. The principle of operation is based on injecting a small volume fluid (at a different temperature from the flow to be measured) into the flowing stream within a closed pipe and recording the temperature trace distally to the point of injection with a rapidly responding thermistor.

There is an inverse relationship between the flow within the closed pipe and the area under the curve (AUC) of temperature deviation, i.e. the *higher* the flow the *smaller* the AUC. This is expressed mathematically in the Stuart–Hamilton equation:

$$CO = \frac{(t_b - t_i) \times V_i \times K}{\Delta t_b \times dt}$$

where

t_b, the baseline blood temperature,
t_i, the temperature of injectate,
V_i, the volume of injectate,
$\Delta t_b \times dt$, the AUC thermodilution,
K = a constant.

In the real situation, the pipe is the pulmonary artery, the flowing fluid is venous blood and the injectate is cold saline. In practice, the thermodilution technique requires the insertion of a flow directed catheter (see earlier) into the pulmonary artery, provided with a proximal port and a temperature sensor (usually a small thermistor) located at the tip (Fig. 9.5).

Assumptions and errors in thermodilution technique

- Low volume of injectate *overestimates* CO.

- High temperature of injectate *overestimates* CO.

- Intra-cardiac shunts, e.g. atrio-septal defect will cause erroneous values for CO.

- As much as 10% variation in measured value for CO occurs depending on what point in the respiratory cycle injection occurs.

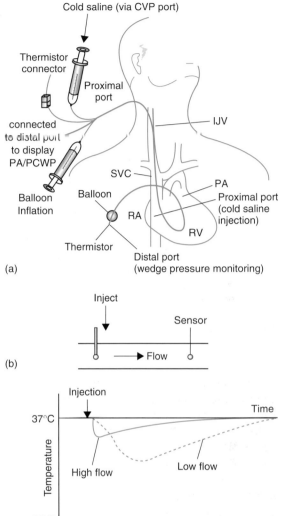

Fig. 9.5 (a) Diagram of the flow-directed, triple-lumen catheter inserted into a branch of the pulmonary artery via the right IJV, SVC, RA, RV and pulmonary artery; (b) shows the principal of the thermodilution method to measure CO applied to a simple, straight pipe with flowing water; (c) shows two curves of temperature changes, at high and low flow, as measured at the tip of the flow-directed catheter. The practical instrument is provided with a small computer that calculates the AUC and displays a value of CO.

Historically dye dilution was the original method of measuring CO. Here a bolus of dye of known volume and concentration was injected on the venous side of the circulation and its concentration/time curve

9

was obtained in a similar manner to the thermodilution technique. The area under the dye concentration/time curve was then used to compute the CO. The basic problem with the dye-based technique were the errors in measurement arising from 're-circulation' of the dye bolus.

The 'dye-dilution' technique has recently been revisited in the form of the LiDCO machine. Here a bolus of isotonic lithium chloride is injected via either a central or peripheral vein, and a concentration/time curve is obtained generated by an ion-sensitive electrode attached to an existing radial arterial line. The basic attraction of this system lies in the fact that it does not require positioning of a CVC.

Continuous cardiac output monitoring
Both PiCCO and LiDCO machines provide the facility of continuous (beat-to-beat) monitoring of CO. This is achieved through 'pulse contour analysis', which involves correlating the arterial pressure waveform obtained from a transducer located in a peripheral artery (usually femoral with PiCCO and radial with LiDCO), with measured CO.

A single 'calibration' of an arterial pressure pulse is carried out either using thermodilution as in the PiCCO system, or dye dilution as in the LiDCO system. Subsequent beat-to-beat measurements of CO are then derived from the pressure pulse waveform measured at the peripheral artery. The basic concern with these methods involving calibration and derivation is the possibility of the derived values 'drifting' from the underlying calibration value. Experience suggests that these machines should be recalibrated 4–6 hourly.

Non-invasive measurement of cardiac output

Deltex CardioQ®
Non-invasive measurements of cardiac output can be obtained utilising the principle of the Doppler effect. Velocity of blood flowing in the descending aorta is obtained by measuring the Doppler shift in

frequency of sound waves bounced off moving RBCs.

The probe tip is positioned in the oesophagus at a depth of about 35–40 cm corresponding to the anatomical level T5/T6. The sound wave frequency employed is set at 4 mHz. CO is calculated from the AUC velocity/time curve and a factor of 30% is added for ascending aortic blood flow. 'Peak velocity' is taken to be an indication of *contractility*, and the 'corrected flow time' to be an indication of *preload*.

The basic advantage of this system is that it is non-invasive (although there is still the risk of oesophageal trauma). The disadvantages include difficulty in positioning the probe tip, and shifting of the probe tip over time leading to a sub-optimal trace.

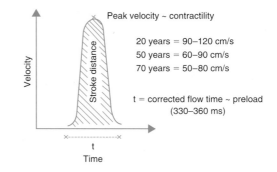

NICO®, non-invasive cardiac output
The NICO obtains non-invasive cardiac output using the Fick principle (see above). Although this is normally calculated using oxygen, carbon dioxide can also be used, as here.

The overall formula is that CO is equal to CO_2 production divided by the difference between mixed venous and arterial CO_2 content.

Thus:

$$CO = VCO_2/(CvCO_2 - CaCO_2)$$

For a non-invasive method, the need to measure $CvCO_2$ is eliminated and this can be done by utilising the differential Fick equation. Thus, there needs to be two measurements taken with different $CaCO_2$ levels in the blood. We get this difference by adding dead space, thereby reducing CO_2 elimination and increasing $CaCO_2$ (and its surrogate, $EtCO_2$).

The increase in dead space is applied for a short enough time for there to be only a negligible change in mixed venous CO_2 or $CvCO_2$.

The machine thus needs to do two things:

1. Accurately integrate CO_2 with gas flow. This seems quite easy to do on the face of it. The machine has to be presented with the right flow and concentration at the same time. Thus we get a CO_2 volume waveform and the area represents the volume of CO_2 passing through the airway.

2. A method of automatically introducing dead space. This is done by introduction of a valve switched loop of added dead space.

The NICO works on a 3-min cycle. A baseline for 60 s, rebreathing 35 s to avoid changes in $MVCO_2$ concentration and stabilisation for 85 s to allow return to normal.

NICO is actually measuring pulmonary blood flow so NICO has to calculate the shunt to get a true reading of Q. There is a need to enter FiO_2 from another instrument and saturation from the integrated SpO_2 monitor. From these values estimation is made of shunt using Nunn theoretical shunt curves. Many human clinical trials have showed good correlation with traditional methods of measuring CO using NICO, an aortic flow probe and thermodilution. NICO will not work, if the $EtCO_2$ is above 10 kPa, following $NaHCO_3$ administration, other non-steady-state conditions and failure of $EtCO_2$ to plateau.

Assessment of cardiac function

CO alone is not a particularly useful measure of cardiac work, as it does not take into account heart rate (HR). Thus a CO of 5 l/min with an HR of 60 bpm is good, a CO of 5 l/min with a HR of 160 bpm is very poor.

A more useful method of assessment is the left-ventricular stroke work index (LVSWI). Now,

work done (see above) = force $\times$ distance
$\qquad$ = pressure $\times$ volume

Thus,

$$LVSWI = (MAP–PCWP) \times (CI/HR) \times 0.136$$
$$\text{(pressure)} \quad \times \text{(volume)}$$
$$= \sim20–50 \, g/m^2$$

(NB: CI = cardiac index = CO/Body surface area in m^2)

Decision-making in cardiac assessment

Observed reduction in CO could be for one of three reasons, reduced preload or contractility, or increase in afterload, the appropriate management of a low output state is to correct whichever of the three factors is deficient. Errors in diagnosis could potentially be catastrophic, e.g. treating a low CO state arising from reduced contractility (ventricular failure) as a preload deficit.

A useful aid to objective diagnosis and treatment is the 'Balooki Box', which basically plots ventricular work against ventricular filling pressure (Fig. 9.6).

Box A: Low LVSWI and low PCWP – require a cautious fluid challenge to raise preload. Try 200 ml bolus of colloid and look for a progressive increase in CO as you move up the Frank–Starling curve. Towards the plateau region of the curve the increase in CO per unit fluid challenge will decrease, until a sudden rise in PCWP indicates that the optimum filling point is passed. Any further fluid administration beyond this point constitutes fluid overload.

Box B: High PCWP but low LVSWI – probably the most difficult type of case to treat. The aim here is to increase contractility and simultaneously reducing afterload. This

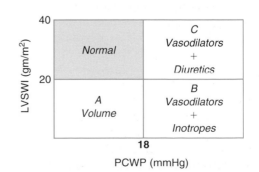

Fig. 9.6 Balooki box.

9

could be achieved with an inodilator such as dobutamine.

Box C: Normal LSWI but high PCWP – suggesting fluid overload, the appropriate treatment would be a diuretic with/or without a venodilator such as GTN to increase capacitance.

The monitoring of metabolic-function–oxygen balance, carbon dioxide elimination and body temperature

Central to the concept of managed pre-optimisation is the maintenance of oxygen balance – oxygen supply equals (or is greater than) oxygen demand, and the avoidance of oxygen stress. The technique of oximetry allows us to measure the oxygen content of blood in real time. Sampling readings from the arterial and venous sides of the circulation allows us to measure arterio-venous difference in oxygen content, and thus in turn oxygen consumption.

Oximetry

Basically an oximeter measures the relative concentrations of oxy-Hb and Hb in circulating blood (Fig. 9.7). From the percentage oxygen saturation derived from these readings, the oxygen content of the blood can be calculated.

The principle of operation of the oximeter is based on spectrophotometry, which involves shining radiation through a sample and measuring how much is absorbed. In the oximeter, light of various wavelengths is transmitted through the blood and a photocell detects the absorbances so that oxygen saturation can be calculated. The absorbencies of three particular wavelengths are of interest, the latter two being used in the oximeter pulse:

- wavelength 805 nm (infrared) – absorbed equally by oxy-Hb and Hb (*isobestic point*);

- wavelength 660 nm (red) – absorption by Hb > absorption by oxy-Hb;

- wavelength 940 nm (infrared) – absorption by oxy-Hb > absorption by Hb.

From the latter two values the concentration of oxy-Hb and thus the oxygen saturation can be calculated. Fibre-optic light guides incorporated into percutaneous vascular catheters positioned either in the arterial or

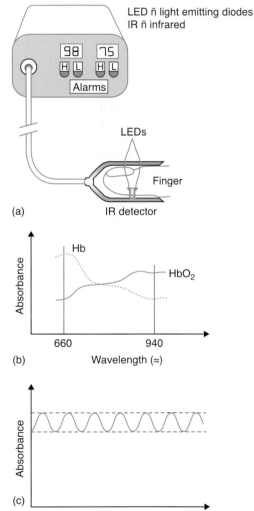

Fig. 9.7 Principle of operation of a pulse oximeter: (a) shows the finger probe with two LEDs and one single IR detector. The diodes emit light at 860 and 940 nM wavelengths where oxy-Hb (HbO$_2$) and reduced Hb (HHb) display different absorbances (b). The diagram in (c) shows how the non-pulsatile portion of the IR absorbance is separated from the pulsatile portion containing oxygen saturation information about the arterial blood only (see text).

venous blood flow allow these devices to monitor oxygen saturations in circulating blood in real time. Each gram of Hb will carry 1.34 ml of oxygen when fully saturated at atmospheric pressure. Thus, oxygen content of blood depends on Hb concentration, and Hb saturation (Chapter 16).

Capnography

This is the measurement of carbon dioxide in the airway. The instrument most widely used is the infrared (IR) absorption capnograph. These are devices with a fast response time (±0.1 s), and are, therefore, able to follow variations with the respiratory cycle. A conventional off-line capnograph, as used in the operating theatre, is shown in Fig. 9.8.

The development of in-line devices with the sampling chamber positioned in the main gas flow to and from the patient has removed the need for long sampling tubes with their potential for occlusion.

The gas flow passes through a sampling chamber, which is crossed by an IR beam. An IR detector, placed on the opposite side of the chamber measures absorption at wavelengths known to be absorbed by carbon dioxide – around 4.2 μm (far IR), and thus derives the concentration of carbon dioxide in the expired gases in real time.

These devices are also used in the postoperative recovery ward in patients whose extubation after operation has been delayed pending assessment of ventilatory function on full anaesthetic reversal, and who are thus breathing spontaneously through an ondotracheal tube. The percentage concentration derived from absorption is converted to a partial pressure in kPa. Thus, a measured concentration of 6% would be displayed as a partial pressure of 6.0 kPa there being 100 kPa in one atmosphere.

End-tidal carbon dioxide concentration, which equates with alveolar carbon dioxide concentration is a good indicator of ventilatory function. Persistent carbon dioxide retention of >8 kPa with corresponding respiratory acidosis would be taken as an indication to re-institute mechanical ventilation (Chapter 17).

Measurement of body temperature

Temperature can be sensed either using a device placed directly in contact with the

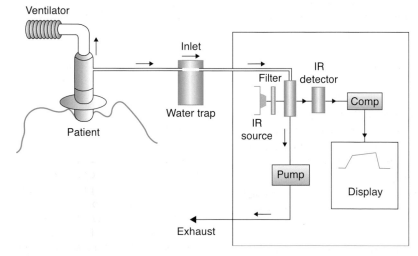

Fig. 9.8 Principle of operation of the capnograph. A sample of gas from the airway is drawn through a water trap and a special minute chamber with quartz walls by a suction pump. An IR light beam is directed through the chamber and detected by a sensor. The output of the sensor depends on the amount of carbon dioxide in the chamber and the signal is processed by an integral computer (comp) before displaying on a screen.

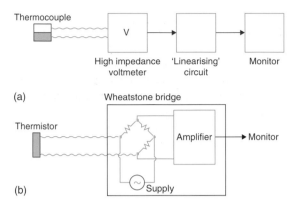

(a)

(b)

Fig. 9.9 Diagram that illustrates the difference in the principles of operation of a thermocouple (a) and the thermistor (b). The latter requires an energising supply and a Wheatstone bridge to operate. Therefore, thermocouple and thermistor probes are not interchangeable.

subject being measured or using a remote device which senses radiation emitted by the subject. Several physical principles are used for the measurement of temperature (Fig. 9.9).

Expansion
It can be either expansion of a fluid or a metal.

Liquid expansion within a sealed tube
This was the first method employed and remains the most commonly used in medical applications. The most commonly used liquid is mercury because of its useful range between freezing and boiling points (−40 – 375°C). The clinical mercury thermometer normally has a range from 34°C to 42°C and an accuracy of about 0.2°C; its response time is of the order of 1.5 min and it is designed to 'hold' the highest reading by means of a constriction at the bulb–capillary junction. The main disadvantages of the clinical thermometer are fragility and slowness of response.

Metal expansion
The usual arrangement is based on a bimetallic strip. The two strips of metal with different temperature expansion coefficients are bonded together in the form of a coil

having one end firmly fixed such that changes in temperature cause the device to coil or uncoil in proportion to the temperature change. The free end of the coil is attached to a dial from which, after calibration, the temperature reading can be taken.

Electrical
Electrical devices are based on wire resistors, on semi-conductors (thermistors) or on the Seebeck effect (thermocouple).

Wire resistors
It was Humphrey Davy who in 1821 reported that the electrical resistance of metal wires varies with temperature and it is still the most stable and accurate thermometer available for reference purposes. The resistance increases linearly with temperature. Wire resistor thermometers are relatively bulky devices with slow response times and have little application in clinical medicine.

Semiconductors
These are usually composed of metal oxides (thermistors). Thermistors have a negative temperature coefficient, i.e. the resistance falls as the temperature increases. The relationship between temperature and resistance is not linear, but dedicated electrical circuits are available which give a linear output over the biological range of temperatures. Thermistors can be made very small and are, therefore, able to respond quickly to temperature changes, and are thus ideal for thermodilution catheters.

Thermocouple
The principle of operation of the thermocouple is based on the voltage generated at a junction between two different metals, which is temperature dependent, the Seebeck effect. As the temperature increase so the voltage increases, and in turn current increases, these changes in current do not occur in a linear fashion, but linearising circuits are available. Thermocouples can be made very small, have a fast response time, and are very cheap and robust.

Liquid crystals

Cholesteric liquid crystals indicate temperature by changing colour in a reversible way. The resolution can be as good as 0.1°C and the crystals may display a range of colours for different temperatures. Several commercial devices are available for clinical use, mostly to indicate skin temperature

Radiation

The temperature of a body can be estimated from the type and intensity of the radiation it emits. This approach is used in clinical thermography, to produce maps of the surface of the body which indicate relatively 'hot' and 'cold' areas which may have clinical significance (e.g. vascular changes or the presence of a tumour).

Table of normal values

CO	Direct	4.0–6.0 l/min
CI	Direct	2.5–4.2 l/min/m^2
CVP (RV preload)	Direct	5.0–10.0 cmH$_2$O
PCWP (LV preload)	Direct	5.0–12.0 mmHg
ITBVI (PiCCO preload)	Calculated	850–1000 ml/m^2
Corrected flow time (Doppler preload)	Direct	350–450 ms
LVSWI	Calculated	40–60 g/m^2
RVSWI	Calculated	5–10 g/m^2
RV pressures	Direct	25/5 mmHg
PA pressures	Direct	25/10 mmHg
SVR	Calculated	700–1600 dyn/s/cm^2
SVRI	Calculated	1700–2400 dyn/s/cm
PVR	Calculated	20–130 dyn/s/cm^2
PVRI	Calculated	150–260 dyn/s/cm

KEY: ABBREVIATIONS ARE EXPLAINED IN TEXT
    RVSWI = Right ventricular stroke work index
    PVR(I) = pulmonary vascular resistance (index)
In all cases I is index and is calculated by dividing the value obtained by body surface area in m^2. See text.

10

Acute pain relief and local anaesthetic techniques

10

Aims

The aims of this chapter are to

- discuss the mechanisms of pain transmission and interpretation in clinical situations;

- discuss the use of the three main classes of 'analgesics', non-steroidal anti-inflammatory drugs (NSAIDs), opioids and local anaesthetics (LAs) and adjuvant drugs in perioperative pain control;

- present the view that perioperative pain management is a multidisciplinary subject;

- discuss the way that regional techniques may be used to provide additional pain relief in selected cases.

Objectives

After reading this chapter, you should be able to

- understand the mechanisms of pain to develop a rational approach to the perioperative pain patient;

- rationally use the available analgesics and adjuvant drugs and LA techniques to optimise pain management in the perioperative period;

- know when to refer the patient to a specialised pain team, if basic pain medication is inadequate.

Introduction

Pain has been officially described as 'an unpleasant sensory and *emotional* experience associated with actual or potential tissue damage, or described in terms of such damage'. It is important to distinguish then between *pain perception threshold*, which is relatively constant (approximately 44–45°C applied to the skin is recognised after a short period of application as painful by most subjects) and the *pain tolerance threshold*,

which is the maximum amount of pain that the subject is prepared to tolerate and is very variable. It is the latter that is most important in the patient's perception and attitude to pain, and thus whether he or she will seek treatment.

Pain pathways

The experience of pain requires four distinct stages: *transduction* (via nociceptors), *transmission* (via sensory nerves and ascending nociceptive tracts), *modulation* (via local spinal pathways and descending inhibition, which reduce pain and peripheral and central sensitisation, which make it worse) and *perception* (including the higher centres, memory of previous events and the motor and neural response to pain such as tachycardia and the stress response).

Transduction

The sensation of pain is transduced by nociceptors, which are receptors on free nerve terminals of sensory nerves at the body surface. They may respond to thermal, mechanical or chemical stimuli. Any stimulus, provided it is strong enough, may produce the sensation of pain, including traumatic and surgically induced injury, excessive heat or chemical injury. Following the 'acute pain' of the skin incision (fast pain), inflammation occurs in the injured tissue, a process which is induced by substance P (SP) and autacoids (e.g. histamine, bradykinin and 5-hydroxytryptamine) release from damaged cells. The nociceptive nerve endings continue to be stimulated by these autacoids (slow pain) a process which is sensitised by prostaglandins. NSAIDs work by inhibition of prostaglandin production.

Transmission

Impulses from the nociceptors travel in two distinct fibres in sensory nerves to the dorsal horn of the spinal cord. The acute, sharp pain is transmitted in the small, myelinated A-δ (fast pain) fibres, while the prolonged pain due to inflammation and tissue damage is transmitted by unmyelinated C-fibres (slow pain). A-δ fibres exist on the surface of the body (including mouth and anus) while C-fibres can originate from all parts of the body outside the central nervous system (CNS) itself. The latter also transmit visceral pain sensation (e.g. from nociceptors in the mesentery and heart) in fibres that run with other C-fibres of post-ganglionic sympathetic nerves.

The biological value of the localised 'fast pain' is to induce a localised reflex resulting in flexion withdrawal of the affected part away from the injury-causing stimulus, thus limiting tissue damage. Anaesthetists spend most of their time ablating this response to surgery with general anaesthetics and neuromuscular blockers or regional blockade with LAs! C-fibre pain is not well localised and is often 'referred' to somatic afferents on the body surface (see later). Being associated with pain and swelling, immobility is induced which forces rest and promotes healing of the affected part.

In the spinal cord A-δ- and C-fibres synapse in dorsal horn laminae such as lamina II, the substantia gelatinosa (SG), decussate and then pass up the contra lateral spinothalamic tract (STT) and spinohypothalamic tract (SHT) to the thalamus. The synaptic transmitter involved in many C-fibres (not A-δ) is SP whose release can be pre-synaptically inhibited by enkephalins and opioids (see later). Thus, opioids have relatively little effect on A-δ- pain (except in overdose where central effects predominate) but act very specifically to ease the pain associated with C-fibre activity.

Modulation

Opioids interact with the two important pain-modulating pathways present in the CNS:

- *A centrally activated, descending pathway*, the descending anti-nociceptive tract (DANT) originates in the periventricular grey (PVG) and periaqueductal grey (PAG) areas of the hypothalamus and midbrain and terminates in laminae I, II (SG) and V where pre-synaptic inhibition of SP production is mediated by the release of enkephalin, an endogenous opioid peptide. Opioid receptors are concentrated in the PVG, PAG

and the spinal laminae. Electrical stimulation or opioids applied in the location of the PAG results in increased activity in the DANT and prolonged analgesia in rats and humans. This central pain inhibitory pathway also mediates the effect that changes in mentation, mood, anxiety state and so on can have on the perception of pain. The presence of naturally occurring morphine-like neurotransmitters (enkephalins, endorphins and dynorphins) and receptors in the CNS underlines the central actions of opioid analgesics.

- *A spinal mechanism* whereby opioids, especially when applied directly to the spinal laminae by intrathecal or epidural injection, result in inhibition of SP release directly.

In addition, mechanoreceptor input from large A-β-fibres can also inhibit pain transmission and thus provide an explanation for analgesia induced by 'rubbing' the affected part and for techniques such as transcutaneous electrical nerve stimulation (TENS). The latter involves placing pads over the nerve distribution of the pain and applying a small electric current through the pads. This sets up electrical activity in the large fibres that cause inhibition of pain transmission through the posterior horn. Subsidiary spinal inhibitory pathways also involve catecholamines and this may explain the augmentation of analgesia achieved by concomitant use of the tricyclic antidepressants in both acute and chronic pain.

The 'gate theory' of pain by Melzack and Wall ties all these facts together by proposing that pain transmission through the spinal laminae is not an 'all or none' phenomenon but can be modulated centrally and locally. Both A-δ- and C-fibre pathways can be blocked by LAs (see later).

The means by which peripheral and central sensitisation is produced by tissue injury is discussed later.

Perception

This occurs in the thalamus and sensory cortex. The STT segregate into two pathways as they approach the thalamus. The medial STT

10

projects to the medial thalamus and reticular formation and is concerned with the autonomic and emotional response to pain. The axons of the lateral STT arise from cells in laminae I to V that have small receptive fields. Having synapsed in the lateral thalamus they project to the sensory cortex in a highly organised manner that corresponds to distinct topographical parts of the body. This allows sensory discrimination and localisation of pain, especially from A-δ-fibres. The SHT is a newly discovered pain pathway that travels to the region of the hypothalamus associated with autonomic function such as stress, arousal and neuro-endocrine release, as well as the reflex response to painful stimuli.

Pathophysiology of acute clinical (surgical) pain

The main distinction between acute clinical pain and experimental pain is that the former leads to

- *tissue damage* leading to inflammatory changes (sensitising soup),
- *nerve damage* leading to neuropathic pain.

This can leads to peripheral *and* central sensitisation of pain.

Mechanisms of peripheral and central sensitisation

Sensitisation is a decreased threshold and a heightened response to a stimulus and leads to the injured area being spontaneously painful (as after a surgical procedure) as well as *more sensitive* to painful and ordinarily non-painful stimuli.

- *Peripheral* sensitisation is caused by a nociceptor 'sensitising soup' of inflammatory mediators released by tissue damage as part of the inflammatory process. This is exacerbated by other mediators such as nerve growth factor (NGF) and neuropeptides as well as increased sympathetic nervous activity in the affected area.

- *Central* sensitisation results from an increased excitability of neurones in the spinal cord due to formation of abnormal connections between A-β- and A-δ- and C-fibres due to neuro-anatomical re-organisation following nerve injury. This leads to an increased duration and area of response to both painful and non-painful stimuli. 'Wind-up' is a phenomenon occurring in the situation where repetitive stimuli from normal or hyperalgesic cutaneous areas give rise to pain. Both these phenomena are associated with n-methyl-d-aspartate (NMDA) receptor activation.

Clinical implications of peripheral and central sensitisation

The result is as follows:

- *Spontaneous pain:* this is the most obvious outcome of tissue damage and is exacerbated by movement and coughing and is responsive to opioids, NSAIDs and LA block.

- *Primary hyperalgesia:* a hyper-responsiveness to noxious stimuli in the injured area.

- *Secondary hyperalgesia:* a spread of hyper-responsiveness to surrounding non-injured tissue.

- *Allodynia:* a reduction in the intensity of stimuli necessary to induce pain so that stimuli not normally producing pain (e.g. touch or pressure) now do so.

Prolonged neuropathic pain unresponsive to opioids

Although neuropathic pain is often associated with pain occurring weeks or even months after surgery (e.g. post-thoracotomy pain due to intercostal nerve damage and neuroma formation) it may occur within hours or days and is particularly difficult to treat. Antidepressants, LAs and NSAIDs may be more effective than opioids.

Pre-emptive analgesia

There is some evidence in animals that the central and peripheral effects of tissue damage and nerve injury that lead to prolonged peripheral and central sensitisation following tissue damage may be modified by drugs such as opioids, NSAIDs and LAs provided they are given prior to the injury. Unfortunately, there is as yet very little firm evidence of a definite beneficial effect in humans.

Opioid receptors

Types

Opioid analgesic receptor subtypes are conventionally divided into mu (μ), delta (δ) and kappa (κ) and these are activated by an endogenous group of peptides that were discovered in the 1970s: the *endogenous* opioids are so named as their action is mimicked by *exogenous* opioids such as morphine. Endogenous ligands for μ-, δ- and κ-receptors are β-endorphin, enkephalins and dynorphin, respectively, although they do not show 100% specificity. Morphine is an agonist at all three receptors and the exogenous antagonist is naloxone (see later). Although some experimental evidence suggested that the receptors may be subdivided, this has not been fully substantiated. It is, therefore, proposed that opioid receptors should be re-classified as OP1 (δ), OP2 (κ) and OP3 (μ).

Mechanisms

These are G-inhibitory protein coupled and activation by opioids results in increased K^+ conductance (hyperpolarised), inactivation of calcium channels (N-type) and inhibition of adenyl cyclase (Chapter 3). This reduces neurotransmission by pre-synaptic inhibition of transmitter (e.g. substance P) release and thus reduces pain.

Analgesics

These are substances that raise the pain threshold but, unlike LAs, they do not specifically block sensory nerves. Analgesics may be divided into four main groups, the NSAIDs or simple analgesics, the opioid agonists and high-efficacy partial agonists, the opioid

agonist–antagonists and miscellaneous drugs whose site of action is unclear.

It should be remembered that these drugs, as a rule, do not attempt to cure the condition causing the pain, but are purely symptomatic, e.g. following surgery, where natural healing processes eventually remove the cause of pain. Other drugs may produce analgesia by actually removing the pain causing condition, e.g. steroids in rheumatoid arthritis, nitrates in angina, carbamazepine in trigeminal neuralgia, amitryptylline and gabapentin in post-herpetic neuralgia and ergot in migraine. In addition, general anaesthetics like nitrous oxide can achieve analgesia *without* loss of consciousness.

Non-steroidal anti-inflammatory drugs

These include aspirin, paracetamol (although not a peripherally acting anti-inflammatory drug), and the newer drugs, such as diclofenac, ketorolac and celecoxib. Their analgesic action is complimentary to opioids, being particularly effective in pain produced from bony injury, inflammation or movement, an area where opioids are relatively ineffective. However, unlike the opioids, C-fibre pain arising from hollow viscera is usually *not* relieved. Given the fact that perioperative pain is often a combination of these two broad categories it is not surprising that NSAIDs are now combined with opioids (and LAs) in perioperative pain management for selected patients.

Mechanism of action

Tissue injury results in activation of lipo-oxygenase and breakdown of cell wall phospholipid to arachidonic acid. Release of autacoids such as histamine and bradykinin initiate inflammation and stimulate receptors (such as bradykinin receptors) on nociceptive nerve endings causing pain, a process which is sensitised by prostaglandins (see earlier). NSAIDs limit the conversion of arachidonic acid to the unstable cyclic-endoperoxide PGG2, which is an intermediate in prostaglandin production, by inhibition of the enzyme cyclo-oxygenase (COX). Thus, inhibition of prostaglandin production by

10

137

NSAIDs results in their analgesic action. The reaction with COX is dependent on the NSAID involved, aspirin having a particularly profound effect as it irreversibly acetylates the enzyme. Other drugs, such as diclofenac, act as competitive blockers. Formation of NGF as a result of tissue injury also causes sensitisation of nociceptors that can be inhibited by NGF inhibitors. A promising area of research!

Side-effects and contraindications of NSAIDs

These side-effects do not apply to paracetamol.

- *Bleeding tendency:* platelets have a high concentration of COX, necessary for the generation of the potent aggregating and constricting agent, thromboxane. Once released from the bone marrow they are non-nucleated and unable to regenerate new enzyme, so aspirin (but not other NSAIDs), even in the small doses used in myocardial infarction prophylaxis, inhibits the enzyme for the life of the platelet (7–11 days). As this can result in a pronounced bleeding tendency following major surgery, aspirin should be stopped for about 10 days prior to major surgery to allow for the production of adequate numbers of unaffected platelets. Where the risk of stopping outweighs the risk of bleeding, e.g. prior to carotid endarterectomy (CEA), then it may be continued right up until the time of surgery. A mild increase in bleeding time has been noted with diclofenac and ketorolac when used intra-operatively but an overt bleeding tendency is unusual.

- *Gastric and intestinal ulceration and bleeding:* inhibition of the cytoprotective gastric prostaglandins, prostacyclin PGI_2 and PGE_2 result in decreased gastric secretion of protective, acid-inhibiting mucous and this renders the stomach more susceptible to injury. This can lead to ulceration, occult blood loss and anaemia. Although this is more of a problem in chronic usage, they are generally contraindicated in patients with known gastric or duodenal ulcers. In selected patients with ulcers, these drugs may be combined with a PGE_2 analogue,

misoprostol, which markedly reduces the incidence of ulcer formation and allows continuation of NSAID use in those patients in whom it is essential (e.g. severe rheumatoid arthritis).

- *Renal impairment and failure:* vasodilator prostaglandins are responsible for optimising the amount and distribution of renal blood flow in hypovolaemia, chronic renal and heart failure and ascites by opposing the effects of vasoconstrictors such as angiotensin and noradrenaline. Inhibition by NSAIDs can result in a severe decrease in renal function and may even precipitate renal failure. NSAIDs should be avoided in these patients and in those in whom major bleeding cannot always be avoided, e.g. major aortic surgery. Ability to excrete a water and sodium load may also be affected resulting in a decreased urine output in the perioperative period.

- *'Allergic' reactions:* ranging from rhinorrhea to full-blown asthma or anaphylaxis occur in a small percentage of patients. Although bronchospasm may be due to an imbalance in production of dilator versus constrictor prostaglandins, the actual mechanism is unknown. Affected individuals may react to any NSAID. Up to 25% of atopic or asthmatic individuals are susceptible, so these drugs should probably be avoided in this group of patients unless they have known uncomplicated exposure to the drug being used.

Use and doses used in perioperative pain

Apart from the contraindications above, NSAIDs can be employed throughout the perioperative period alongside opioids and LAs. They are particularly useful as adjuncts in day surgery where long-acting opioids should be avoided. In the immediate postoperative period, gastric emptying is delayed so either a large loading dose is given pre- or intra-operatively to cover this period (e.g. diclofenac 100 mg by suppository in the adult (12.5–25 mg in the child, an unlicensed use) or parenterally, e.g. 1 mg/kg diclofenac i.v. diluted in 100 ml of normal saline or

0.15 mg/kg ketorolac i.m.). Subsequently, the oral preparation can be given, e.g. (in the 60 kg adult) 50 mg diclofenac b.d. or ketorolac 30 mg q.d.s. The rectal route is useful throughout the perioperative period.

In less severe pain, paracetamol is the drug of choice, as it does not have the side-effects of other drugs in this group, e.g. gastric irritation and bleeding or platelet dysfunction. It is given in a dose of two tablets (1 g) 6 hourly. In children, it may be given as an elixir of 120 mg in 5 ml in a dose of 15 mg/kg b.d.

Recent evidence supports the proposition that there are two distinct types of COX, types 1 and 2 (COX 1 and COX 2). COX 1 is the constitutive enzyme that is normally present in tissues and results in the formation of prostaglandins that are protective (as seen above). COX 2 is the inducible form that is produced following injury and is responsible for the formation of abnormal amounts of prostaglandins that sensitise nociceptors. Specific COX 2 inhibitors have been developed which it was hoped would relieve pain without the side-effects of COX 1 inhibition as described above. The evidence available so far suggests that substantially improved safety is possible with these drugs. However, they are much more expensive than the non-selective NSAIDs such as ibuprofen. It should also be remembered that since these selective COX 2 inhibitors drugs lack anti-platelet activity they do not provide protection against ischaemic cardiovascular events. Recently, parenteral COX 2 inhibitor NSAIDs have become available and may be useful for patients in whom conventional non-selective NSAIDs are definitely contraindicated, e.g. following transurethral resection of prostate. NB: COX 2 is normally present in the kidney and thus these drugs should still be used cautiously in patients with renal impairment.

Opioid agonists and high-efficacy partial agonists

History of the use of opium
The use of opium dates from time immemorial and is well described in ancient civilisations.

The first reference to its use was found on a Sumerian tablet (4000 BC). In Egypt, the juice of *Papaver somniferum* (the white poppy) was recognised as an efficacious analgesic and indeed poppy fields existed around Thebes (from which the name thebaine is derived). In Ancient Greece, it is interesting to note that Morpheus was Ovid's God of Dreams and is where the name morphine is derived. The juice of the white poppy was called 'Opion'. The first written reference to opium was by Theophrastus in the 3rd century BC. In Ancient Rome, the specific use of opium as a pain killer and sedative was known and described by Galen and Dioscorides. Much of this knowledge was lost during the dark ages and opium was re-popularised in Europe by Paracelsus (1493–51). Thomas Sydenham introduced 'laudanum' or 'tincture of opium' in the 17th century. He wrote that 'Among the remedies which it has pleased Almighty God to give to man to relieve his sufferings, none is so universal and efficacious as opium'. Its widespread use in the American Civil War led to a major spread of addiction. The development of the syringe by Pravaz in 1853 and the hollow needle by Wood in 1855 allowed it to be employed parenterally. The increased efficacy of giving these compounds in this way (bypassing the problems with absorption, decreased gut motility, high first-pass metabolism and nausea and vomiting) lead to an increased incidence of side-effects.

The alkaloid content of opium
Naturally occurring opium consists of the following:

Morphine	9–17%
Noscapine (narcotine)	2–9%
Codeine	0.3–4%
Thebaine	0.1–0.8%
Papaverine	0.5–1%

Note: Papaveretum is standardised to contain 50% morphine with no noscapine (genotoxic) with 15.6 mg/ml.

Only morphine and codeine should, strictly speaking, be referred to as opiates (naturally occurring in opium). Other analgesics in the same class such as diamorphine and pethidine should be referred to as opioids. Although morphine can be synthesised it is still obtained from opium commercially.

Present-day opioids
These include morphine, buprenorphine (high-efficacy partial agonist), diamorphine, pethidine, papaveretum and the intra-operative analgesics fentanyl, alfentanil and remifentanil.

Actions
They work both spinally and in areas of the brain stem rich in naturally occurring opioid peptides (see above). Beneficial actions, apart from analgesia, include euphoria and anxiolysis.

Problems with conventional opioids
They have many side-effects that limit their effectiveness for the treatment of severe pain, e.g.

■ *Respiratory depression* that is usually dose related and means that the drug cannot be prescribed regularly except in a high-dependency area or ICU. In addition, although respiratory depression is usually maximal within 10–15 min of administration of an opioid by the i.v. route, it may take up to 24 h when the same drug (e.g. morphine) is given spinally. This is less of a problem with buprenorphine.

■ *Short duration of action*, which means that these drugs are relatively ineffective when given by intermittent i.m. injection (methadone and buprenorphine are exceptions).

■ *Nausea and vomiting*, especially in the ambulant patient limits their use for day surgery.

■ *Tolerance and addiction* potential leading to proscribed use.

■ *Sphincter of Oddi spasm*, especially with morphine and its congeners makes them unsuitable for alleviating the pain of biliary colic (not so with pethidine and buprenorphine).

■ *Constipation and adynamic ileus* is a serious problem in the chronic pain patient and the ICU patient on i.v. opioids for sedation (except buprenorphine).

■ *Side-effects* not directly associated with opioid activity such as histamine release (morphine and pethidine) and chest wall stiffness (e.g. fentanyl).

All these result in limitations being imposed on the amount of analgesics that patients are prescribed and actually receive. This is justifiable when related to their tendency to cause respiratory depression but not as regards their addictive potential in acute usage. However, the latter does impose logistic restrictions on drug administration (*vide infra*). In particular, the great variability in pain perceived and effectiveness of opioids between patients requires that they are conventionally prescribed 'on demand' (see later). Patients have to be told that they must ask for the drug when they are in pain. Most other drugs are prescribed regularly.

Nausea and vomiting are very common side-effects, which means that they are usually prescribed with anti-emetics. There is little evidence to suggest that one opioid is superior to another in this respect.

Administration of opioids for postoperative pain
There is evidence that prescribing habits result in patients receiving less analgesia than they need. But, patients are usually uncomplaining, so just because they do not make a fuss does not mean that they are not in pain! Various methods of drug delivery are available in the postoperative period. It is important to note that opioids are mainly effective against steady, dull pain and are less consistently effective against the pain on movement and coughing.

Nurse administered

P.r.n. (pro re nata) prescription of an i.m. opioid
This may seem simple to the prescriber but in practice it may be fraught with difficulties.

Unfortunately, to give a controlled drug on a general ward may take up to 30 min involving:

- complicated protocols and extra staff due to controlled drug regulations;

- the use of syringes and needles (adding to expense, time and patient discomfort);

- if the drug is short acting (e.g. 2 h for pethidine), then up to 25% of the nurses time may be engaged in administering postoperative pain relieving drugs;

- the onset time of an i.m. drug (30–60 min) may be too slow to catch up with the rapidly declining analgesia of a short-acting intra-operative opioid (*vide infra*).

The result is that the patient ends up in pain! In addition, doctors often underprescribe analgesics and nurses reduce these doses still further.

Pharmacokinetic and pharmacodynamic principles dictate that it is impossible to expect 3–4 hourly p.r.n. i.m. regimes of parenteral opioids (except buprenorphine and methadone) to produce consistently good postoperative analgesia. A better solution is to use either a long-acting (due to pharmacodynamics) analgesic such as buprenorphine which consistently gives equivalent (or better) analgesia to controlled drugs with less administrative effort, or to titrate i.v. a long-acting (due to pharmacokinetics) analgesic such as methadone.

Although oral absorption of opioids on demand is feasible following surgery, delay in gastric emptying and ileus may result in loss of effectiveness initially, followed by overdosage when motility returns. The s.l. administration of buprenorphine avoids these difficulties but is unlikely on its own to compensate for the rapid decline in analgesia in the immediate perioperative period when fentanyl has been used as the primary intra-operative analgesic. Thus, slow absorption from the s.l. route may fail to produce adequate analgesia *unless* it has been preceded by a loading dose of a long-acting opioid.

Regular pre-emptive opioids

Excellent analgesia is obtainable by *regular* (pre-emptive) use of opioids in the postoperative period. This has included a variety of techniques and agents, such as by i.m. injection, s.l. or by nurse controlled i.v. infusion. The results are good, with both s.l. buprenorphine and i.m. morphine proving equally satisfactory to patient-controlled analgesic (PCA, see next section). However, these techniques, particularly i.v. infusion, have the inherent danger of respiratory depression and *must only be carried out in a high-dependency environment* with nurse/patient ratios much higher than is to be found on a normal ward.

Patient-controlled analgesia

This was first introduced in 1970 into obstetric practice where the patient simply controlled the administration of i.v. pethidine by operation of a spring loaded clamp on an infusion set! In a way, it mimics the use of the patient-controlled analgesia (PCA) 50:50 nitrous oxide/oxygen gas mixture (Entonox®, see later). The rationale of PCA is that an improvement in analgesic efficacy is obtained by allowing the patient (rather than the nurse) to manage analgesic requirements. Although the availability of custom made apparatus with in-built safety features have increased the popularity and applicability of the technique, the cost of the apparatus remains high. The normal route of administration is i.v., but the i.m., s.c. and epidural routes are also used. The patient must be given clear instructions on how to use the apparatus for maximal benefit. To avoid inadvertent toxicity, the following parameters must be correctly pre-set by the operator:

- *Dose and concentration* of opioid used is set-up in the machine, this allows calculation and storage of doses administered to the patient. A common regime is 100 mg diamorphine in 50 ml 0.9% saline, or 2 mg/ml.

- *Demand dose* administered (e.g. 1 ml (2 mg) for diamorphine).

10

141

■ *Lockout interval* is the interval from an administered dose until the next dose is given by the machine, despite patient requests (e.g. 8 min for diamorphine). This prevents repeated doses at short intervals and thus limits toxicity but also the amount of drug the patient can receive.

■ *Maximum hourly or 4 hourly dose* (e.g. 5 mg/h for diamorphine) and, less commonly.

■ *Background infusion* of opioid, if required. This may be fixed or interactively adjusted according to the frequency of patient demands.

Much effort has been expended on coming up with suitable doses of analgesics and the time intervals of administration. For maximum efficacy a loading dose of the appropriate analgesic must be administered before allowing the machine to take over as these regimes only cater for maintenance requirements. Once the apparatus is satisfactorily set-up, the great advantage claimed for PCA over techniques of postoperative analgesia, such as opioids by infusion, regular administration and by spinal techniques, is absence of need to monitor the patient in a high-dependency environment, always providing that a background infusion is *not* used. Administering the PCA opioid s.c. rather than i.v. increases safety and acceptability without apparent reduction in efficacy.

Although the technique has proved acceptable, poor results for PCA can occur and may be explained by

■ failure to adequately explain the apparatus to the patient;

■ failure to give a loading dose (Chapter 3). It should be remembered that the PCA regime above is a maintenance regime and relies on a titrated, loading dose being administered prior to the PCA being started;

■ the patient chooses to have pain rather than suffer the adverse effects of opioids, e.g. nausea and excessive sedation;

■ excessive pain following a period of sleep during which there has been no administration of analgesic, during the 'catching up' period, the patient will be in pain.

The latter problem is partially addressed by utilising apparatus that has the ability to provide a background infusion of opioid, but this is not entirely effective and leads to increased opioid consumption and need for high-dependency care.

PCA techniques have only recently come into widespread use for two reasons:

■ the expense and complexity of the original apparatus.

■ the introduction, at about the same time, of spinal opioid techniques which were 'automatically' assumed to be more efficacious. This view has been questioned.

It is only in the late eighties that direct comparison was made between PCA and epidural opioids, the former being found to be slightly less efficacious but equally, if not more, acceptable to the patient (see later). Is PCA the ideal way to administer opioids for postoperative pain relief? The very narrow dividing line between serious respiratory depression, good analgesia and no pain relief at all, suggests that it might be. However, it must be said that some studies have shown the much simpler regime of regular sublingual buprenorphine or i.m. morphine give equivalent analgesia to i.v. PCA.

Spinal opioids

The discovery of endogenous opioid receptors and ligands in the brain and spinal cord (see above) led to the feasibility of their use spinally. Intrathecally applied narcotics produced a long lasting elevation in the nociceptive threshold in animals. Use of this technique in man followed in 1979. At the outset, it is most important to establish the rationale for the spinal administration of opioids. There must be firm evidence that this route is preferable, in terms of analgesic effectiveness, without an increase in side-effects such as respiratory depression, when compared with simpler and less invasive routes of administration. If questioned, patients may not wish to accept increased risks for the possible benefit of improved analgesia. It should also be remembered that *none of the opioids are specifically licensed for use by the epidural or intrathecal route.*

Crucial to the subsequent popularity of spinal opioids was the observation that the effects were seemingly limited to pain perception, so-called *selective spinal analgesia*, with little effect on motor, sensory (e.g. touch *and* pin prick) and autonomic function as occur with LA. Adverse effects of spinal and parenteral opioids are similar and hopes that respiratory depression and nausea and vomiting would be lessened have not been fulfilled. This is due to the fact that, by the epidural route, systemic uptake of both morphine and particularly the more lipophilic agents such as fentanyl, is as great as if given i.m. or i.v., so blood levels are similar. In fact, depending on the opioid used, side-effects may be more severe, especially when using morphine intrathecally. In addition, pruritus and urinary retention are more common.

Intrathecal opioids

Although large individual series of intrathecal opioids have been reported, there has been little work comparing their use with more conventional techniques in randomised, double-blind, prospective studies. Diamorphine and low-dose intrathecal morphine (0.1–0.3 mg) are effective and may be less prone to respiratory depression than larger-dose techniques. This route is much less popular than the epidural route.

Epidural opioids

Morphine has a slow onset and a long duration of action. The contribution from systemic uptake is modest. *Diamorphine* is more lipophilic than morphine with a faster onset of action and a large (early) contribution from systemic uptake. Duration of action is less than with morphine although its conversion to morphine makes it longer than would be expected from the physical properties. *Fentanyl* has a very rapid onset of

action, mainly due to systemic absorption. Recent evidence suggests that it is as effective by the i.v. route so the use of the epidural route has been questioned.

Monitoring

Whenever spinal administration of opioids is used, the patient is at increased risk from opioid-induced respiratory depression, thus diligent monitoring must be employed, e.g.:

- *Frequent measurement of BP, pulse rate, respiration and pulse oximetry (SpO$_2$)*: Clear instructions must be available indicating who to call if defined limits are exceeded (e.g. systolic BP <80, respiratory frequency <8 breaths/min, SpO$_2 <90\%$).

- *What to do in an emergency:* For example, use of naloxone and oxygen if respiratory embarrassment occurs; use of fluids, ephedrine and tipping the bed head-down if hypotension occurs.

- *Whom to call if there is inadequate pain control:* It is most important that the nurses have a straightforward and reliable line of communication, particularly to the anaesthetic resident on duty. Bleep numbers (and alternates) should be left with the ward staff. Many patients endure hours of needless suffering due to inadequate communication between nurses and medical staff. This is particularly important as, for safety reasons, no alternative i.m. opioid regime is usually prescribed.

Close monitoring of these patients is essential and is often carried out in an HDU or ICU, although some units have dispensed with this requirement. This is best achieved by production of a special chart with all the details alluded to above, thus facilitating patient management and acceptance of the technique if it is used on general wards. Nurses and resident surgical staff must be fully aware of possible complications and be able to initiate treatment if they should occur.

Conclusion

The effectiveness of opioids on their own by the epidural route (versus parenteral) has

10

10

increasingly been questioned. They are now administered more frequently by infusion in *combination* with LAs with which the effects appear synergistic. A suitable regime is to mix 5 or 10 mg of diamorphine with 50 ml of 0.25% bupivacaine in a 50-ml syringe driver. A rate of 1–6 ml/h is usually sufficient (following a loading dose to obtain satisfactory analgesia).

Other uses of opioids

As they are addictive (less so for buprenorphine), their use is restricted to severe pain, such as with myocardial infarction, renal colic and cancer. Their euphoric side-effects make them useful premedicants, and, together with the tendency to depress respiration, have led to their use in ICU for sedating patients undergoing mechanical ventilation (Chapter 12).

Opioid agonist–antagonists

Actions

The side-effects of conventional opioid agonists led to the development of a new class of compound, the antagonist analgesics. They were so called because they originated from the morphine antagonist nalorphine, which was only later discovered to have analgesic properties of its own. Due to its unfortunate propensity to cause dysphoria it was not clinically useful as an analgesic, but it did not seem to produce as serious respiratory depression or addiction as the conventional opioids such as morphine. It led to the development of more clinically useful compounds such as pentazocine and nalbuphine.

Their ability to antagonise opioid agonists, and yet have analgesic properties of their own led to the original proposition, initially on clinical grounds, of the three different types of opioid receptors described above. Conventional opioids are agonists and produce analgesia at the μ or mu (named after morphine) receptor at which pentazocine and nalbuphine are antagonists. The latter are thought to produce analgesia at the κ or kappa (keto-cyclazocine) receptor and

dysphoria at the σ or sigma (named after the Smith Kline and French drug, normetazocine) receptor. This would explain why nalorphine is unable to antagonise the respiratory depression of pentazocine, but naloxone (a pure μ- and κ-antagonist) is. Side-effects include dysphoria, nausea and vomiting (pentazocine more than nalbuphine) and respiratory depression. They are not as efficacious as the opioid agonists.

Uses

These are similar to the opioid agonists. However, pentazocine is not recommended for myocardial infarction, as it tends to increase right heart work. The alternating use of the opioid agonists and the agonist–antagonists is not advised. Nalbuphine is not a CD and is classified as a prescription-only medicine (POM).

Miscellaneous drugs

Nefopam and meptazinol are unique strong analgesics whose site of action is less clear than with other opioids, but there appears to be a reduced tendency to produce respiratory depression. Other side-effects are unpredictable. Ketamine is a powerful analgesic in sub-anaesthetic doses of 20–40 mg; it causes sympathetic stimulation and marked hallucinations (probably via the receptor) which can be attenuated with diazepam. Inhalation of a 50:50 mixture of nitrous oxide and oxygen (Entonox) is a very useful analgesic which is given `on demand' by the patient placing the mask on the face and actuating a demand valve by taking a breath in. If the patient becomes drowsy, the mask falls away and gas delivery stops. It is particularly useful for use in ambulances and for the intermittent pains of labour but can still be utilised postoperatively for manoeuvres associated with acute pain such as physiotherapy and dressing change.

Tramadol is a recently available opioid in the UK with a potency and efficacy very similar to pethidine. However, it has a lessened tendency to cause respiratory depression, it is much less addictive (it is not a controlled drug and is available as a POM) and is available orally. Its main effects are as a μ-agonist but it also has spinal effect on 5HT receptors. The significance of the latter is not entirely clear. As a POM it is obviously easier to prescribe for day surgery patients than pethidine or morphine although like other opioids, nausea and vomiting may be troublesome.

Miscellaneous techniques

TENS, hypnosis and acupuncture have been used with success in some patients but have never been widely employed for acute pain relief.

Use of opioid antagonists

Severe respiratory depression is an ever-present problem when opioids are used for postoperative pain relief. In most cases this can be avoided by careful patient assessment prior to administration of opioid by whatever route. A respiratory rate below 6–8 in the adult or 10–15 in the child necessitates withholding further drug until the rate increases. Supportive measures such as additional oxygen, together with assessment of BP, pulse and oxygen saturation are all that are usually necessary. If the respiratory rate falls to below 6, the specific antagonist naloxone should be administered in a dose of 2–6 μg/kg i.v. bolus. The effects are immediate but short lived so the dose may need to be repeated. A dose-related reversal of analgesia occurs so the smallest effective dose should always be administered. Non-specific respiratory stimulants such as doxapram (1–2 mg/kg i.v. bolus) cause arousal and improve ventilation without reversing analgesia.

Strategies for effective postoperative analgesia

Introduction

Many recent reports have emphasised the inadequacies of postoperative analgesic regimes. Up to 70% of patients complain of moderate to severe pain in the postoperative period following major surgery. What has gone wrong?

Problems

The reasons for inadequate pain relief are multifactorial and include the following.

Patient expectations

These are often conflicting as to the amount of pain that they should expect to have in the postoperative period. This ranges from the patient who expects to be totally pain free to the patient who expects to have moderate to severe pain and is thus 'prepared to put up with it'. They may not be informed that postoperative analgesics are often only given 'on demand'. Patients also vary in the analgesic response to a given level of opioid in the plasma, some studies showing a 10-fold variation in drug level to produce the desired analgesic effect.

Nurse expectations

These are also conflicting as to the amount of pain a patient should be expected to suffer. Some feel that any pain is bad while others are more cautious and try to help the patient cope with the 'inevitable' pain of the postoperative period.

Operating surgeons

They often do not concern themselves enough with the issue.

Anaesthetists

They are often only concerned with a smooth intra-operative course and a rapid awakening of the patient so that he or she can be expeditiously returned to the ward. This often involves the use of ultra-short-acting potent opioids, ideal for obtaining smooth operative conditions, but *guaranteeing* that the patient will be in severe pain very early on in the postoperative period. Add this to the problem of limited efficacy of i.m. opioid administration 'as required' on the ward and one has the perfect scenario for inadequate postoperative pain control!

Resident surgical staff

They do not fully understand the pharmacology of opioids, expect them to be a panacea, and generally just 'leave it all up to the nurse'!

10

Although this represents the 'worst possible' case, it is not unusual to find these attitudes engrained in clinical practice. Putting matters right does not require vast expenditure on time and equipment. Acute pain teams, use of epidural catheters and administering opioids and LA or expensive PCA computers, although effective, do not address the problems of the majority of patients. They have tended to divert our attention away from a more rational approach that must include *all* patients.

Finding a solution

This approach includes the following and emphasises that close co-operation must be maintained between all the parties involved.

Patients

They must be educated to appreciate the effects of the operation in producing pain (especially on movement and coughing) and the effect this will have on their mobility and recovery. The types of pain relief available and how it can be obtained must be explained (usually by the anaesthetist in the preoperative visit) and a strategy outlined.

Nurses

They must be aware of the methods chosen and must be fully supported by the medical staff, particularly, if methods such as epidural infusions of opioids are to be used.

Operating surgeons

They can contribute by utilising nerve blocks and LA infiltration that may significantly reduce the requirement for opioid analgesics in the postoperative period.

Anaesthetists

They should employ techniques that allow a smooth transition from good operative to good postoperative analgesia. This can involve *either* careful titration of longer-acting opioids so that there is not a sudden offset of analgesia just as the patient is leaving the operating room *or* insertion of epidural catheters that can be used in the postoperative period.

Resident surgical staff

They must form the link between all these parties and should be fully informed of the techniques used and the problems that may be encountered. Familiarisation with some of the pharmacology of analgesics explained in this chapter would be a good start!

Recording postoperative pain

It is perhaps surprising that so little attention is given to recording postoperative pain. While BP and pulse rate are meticulously charted, the patient is writhing in agony without a quantitative record being made! A pain chart also indicates to the resident staff when a regime is ineffective and the possibility of involving the acute pain team in problem cases at the earliest possible time.

Pain assessment methods

Visual linear analogue scale

This is a 10 cm horizontal line drawn on a piece of paper with one end indicating 'no pain' and the other 'the worst possible pain that the patient could imagine'. From this scale, a score of 0 indicates 'no pain' and 10 'worst possible pain'. This is presented to the patient who is asked to make a mark on the line corresponding to the pain being experienced. Although the line has no gradations, a rough score can be obtained from the patient's mark by use of a ruler with 1 cm. gradations. A score of 2–3 is acceptable while a score of 7–8 is obviously not.

Nominal five-point scale

On a nominal five-point scale, 0 = no pain, 1 = slight pain, 2 = moderate pain, 3 = severe pain and 4 = very severe pain. A score of 0 or 1 is ideal whereas 3, 4 or 5 are not. In practice, the commonest score is 2!

Analgesic effectiveness

The effectiveness of the prescribed analgesic should also be recorded on a nominal scale as: no relief = 0, slight relief = 1, moderate relief = 2, good relief = 3 and complete relief = 4. This allows the doctors and nurses to assess the effect of the prescribed analgesic and will indicate whether a change in dose, dosage interval or type of analgesic is required.

Postoperative pain record

The above should be amalgamated into a single record that can be reviewed alongside the BP, pulse and temperature chart at frequent intervals so that action can be taken if pain control is inadequate.

Analgesic techniques for a few common procedures

The following is a simple guide to achieving good postoperative analgesia. It is assumed that the patient is a 60 kg fit adult and that there are no contraindications to the drugs suggested.

Major abdominal surgery

An NSAID, e.g. diclofenac 100 mg p.r. or 100 mg p.o. is given with the premedication or 75 mg administered i.v. during the procedure. The anaesthetic technique will often include a short-acting analgesic such as fentanyl or remifentanil. To compensate for rapidly declining analgesia at the end of the procedure (especially with the latter), a long-acting i.v. opioid such as morphine (10–20 mg), diamorphine (5–10 mg) or buprenorphine (0.3–0.6 mg) is given. This may be combined with LA infiltration of the wound with up to 40 ml of 0.25% bupivacaine at the end of the procedure prior to skin closure. The anaesthetist ensures that sufficient analgesia is present at the end of the procedure and, on awakening, the patient is comfortable and able to take deep breaths to command. This often involves further small increments of the opioid, e.g. morphine 2.5 mg, diamorphine 2 mg or buprenorphine 0.15 mg in theatre or the recovery room. This regime is followed by p.r.n. morphine 10–15 mg i.m., diamorphine 5 mg or buprenorphine 0.3–0.6 mg i.m. (or s.l.) 4 hourly. The dose of diclofenac is repeated

the following day. This regime provides good to excellent analgesia in the majority of patients.

Alternatively, a PCA regime (see above) or an epidural infusion of opioids and LA can be considered for more difficult patients.

Inguinal herniorrhaphy and varicose veins

Analgesia is achieved by NSAIDs, such as diclofenac 100 mg by mouth or suppository (p.r.) 1 h preoperatively or 75 mg i.v. intra-operatively, together with LA infiltration and block with bupivacaine by the surgeon at the operative site. Short-acting opioids can be given intra-operatively but long-acting opioids have little place in postoperative analgesia, the majority of patients being day cases. If necessary, a small dose of opioid (e.g. 50–75 mg i.m. pethidine with an anti-emetic, or PCA fentanyl) may be given in the early postoperative period. Diclofenac 50 mg p.o. b.d. is continued from the following day for 3 more days.

Cystoscopy, dilation and curettage

Analgesia is achieved by perioperative use of NSAIDs. A short-acting opioid is used for the operative procedure but plays no part in the provision of postoperative pain control.

Local anaesthetics and techniques in regional anaesthesia

Local anaesthetic drugs

Of all anaesthetic agents, LAs are perhaps those most widely used by non-anaesthetists. Serious and fatal complications associated with their use have escalated in recent years.

Lidocaine

Pharmacological properties

Lidocaine is the most frequently used drug in this group. It works by blocking the inward Na^+ current necessary for propagation of nerve impulses along sensory, motor and

10

147

10

autonomic nerves (see Chapter 3). It may be used as an LA or as an anti-dysrhythmic agent.

1. As an LA, lidocaine may be used as a 4% cream, or fluid for topical application, as a 2% solution for nerve blocks, 1.5% solution for epidurals, 0.5–1% solution for local infiltration of tissues and as a 0.5% solution for i.v. regional anaesthesia (Bier's block). With the exception of the i.v., epidural and topical application, it is usually given mixed with adrenaline in the strength of 1:200 000 or 5 μg in 1 ml. Adrenaline significantly reduces the absorption of lidocaine from tissues, therefore delaying uptake and prolonging its local effect.

   As an infiltration LA, the total amount administered over 1 h must not exceed a maximum of 200 mg when given as a plain solution in the fit average 70 kg adult (i.e. about 3 mg/kg). With adrenaline, the maximum dose of lidocaine can be doubled to 400 mg (6 mg/kg). Proportionately smaller maximum doses apply to smaller BW, and great caution should be exercised with its use in the elderly and the very ill.

   Duration of action depends on the type of block and on the total amount given. It averages approximately 1 h for plain lidocaine and 2–3 h if used with adrenaline.

2. As an anti-dysrhythmic agent, lidocaine is given i.v. as a 1–2% solution. It is indicated in the treatment of ventricular dysrhythmias. Initially, 1.5 mg/kg can be given as a bolus injection, followed by half this amount 10 min later if necessary (see Chapter 3). If effective, a continuous i.v. infusion (0.8%, 4 g in 500 ml) may be set up at a starting rate of 30 μg/kg/min (2 mg/min in a 70-kg patient). A maximum rate of 50 μg/kg/min should not be exceeded because of the likelihood of inducing cardiac and neurological toxicity.

Pharmacokinetics
The distribution and elimination of lidocaine is probably one of the best studied. The half-life of the redistribution phase is approximately 10 min, but the half-life of the slower elimination phase is nearly 2 h (see Chapter 3).

Side-effects
The main side-effects of lidocaine are due to an exaggeration of its therapeutic effects upon excitable tissues, namely depression of the CNS and of the conductive tissue of the heart, as outlined above. Depression of the CNS may be preceded by excitation.

The first sign of overdose in the awake patient is usually the sensation of tingling in the tongue and lips. Shortly afterwards the patient looks pale, and feels anxious and nauseated. Unconsciousness may soon follow, or may be preceded by an epileptiform convulsion. At this point the full skills of a trained anaesthetist are required. The patient may have a very low BP and respiratory depression; full resuscitation measures are needed.

Bupivacaine (marcaine)
Bupivacaine is second to lidocaine in frequency of use. It is about four times more potent and four times more toxic than lidocaine. The duration of action is much longer, and for this reason it is often preferred; in nerve blocks its effects normally lasts 4–6 h. It is not associated with tachyphylaxis, unlike lidocaine. However, it has a greater potential to cause cardiac toxicity with a propensity, unlike lidocaine, to cause sudden cardiac arrest. This has led to great circumspection in its use and dosage. Although it is no longer used for *intravenous regional anaesthesia* (IVRA), it still retains its popularity. Newer similar drugs such as the L isomer of bupivacaine (levobupivacaine) and ropivacaine are probably less toxic than bupivacaine.

Bupivacaine is used for epidural analgesia in obstetrics for two additional reasons: first, it crosses the placental barrier at a much slower rate, reaching the foetus in lesser amounts; and secondly, it causes a smaller degree of motor paralysis than lidocaine or any other LA agent for the same amount of sensory blockade. This is an important advantage in analgesia for vaginal delivery.

It is used as 0.25%, 0.5% or 0.75% plain solutions. In labour, the 0.25% solution or an intermediate 0.375% are used initially. The side-effects of bupivacaine are similar to those of lidocaine; the occurrence of convulsions due to overdosage has been claimed to be more frequent.

Prilocaine (citanest)

Prilocaine is only slightly less potent than lidocaine, but much less toxic (higher therapeutic index as an LA). It has a duration of action in between lidocaine and bupivacaine. In high doses (more than 600 mg) it may cause methaemoglobinaemia. Due to its low toxicity, prilocaine is recommended for i.v. regional anaesthesia in the strength of 0.5%; volumes up to 40 ml can be safely used in the average fit adult. It is also of value as a surface anaesthetic, in 2% solution, for fibre-optic bronchoscopy in the awake patient.

Other local anaesthetic agents

The following are also used for special purposes:

- *Cocaine* in topical anaesthesia of the nasal mucosa and conjuctiva; it has a marked vasoconstrictor effect.

- *Amethocaine*, mostly used as a topical analgesic in the UK and as a spinal analgesic in the US.

- *EMLA cream*®, which is a eutectic mixture of lidocaine 2.5% and prilocaine 2.5% (Chapter 3). This combination 'melts' above 16°C. The droplet concentration in the emulsion is high enough (greater than 80%) to enable surface analgesia of the skin to be obtained provided that the cream is applied beneath an occlusive dressing for a period of about 1–5 h. It is ideal for removing the pain of venepuncture (especially in children) and prior to small skin graft sites.

Note: The concentration of LAs is usually given as '% weight to volume (w/v) solution'. To avoid toxicity it is necessary to limit the dose of these agents on a mg/kg basis. 1% (1 in 100) solution means that there is 1 g of the substance in 100 ml or 10 mg/ml. Thus, 10 ml of 1% lidocaine = 100 mg. A concentration of

solution less than 1% is often expressed as, e.g. 1 in 1000, 1 in 10 000 and so on. 1 in 1000 is 1 g in 1000 ml or 1 mg/ml, 1 in 10,000 is 1 g in 10,000 ml or 1 mg in 10 ml. Thus, if the toxic dose of bupivacaine is 1.5 mg/kg, then a 70-kg patient can have a maximum of 100 mg. This would allow 40 ml of 0.25% (2.5 mg/ml) or 20 ml of 0.5% (5 mg/ml) bupivacaine.

Regional blocks should be carried out with resuscitation equipment and expertise immediately available. A few of the relatively safe and easy blocks, which have a high rate of success are described. i.v. regional anaesthesia is discussed with emphasis on avoiding its complications.

In addition, the technique of epidural and spinal anaesthesia (which should only be performed by the specialist) are outlined, as they are often the method of choice for some types of surgery.

Intercostal nerve blocks

Indications

Few therapeutic measures receive as much patient gratitude as intercostal nerve blocks following rib fractures. It is also useful following insertion of a chest drain.

Preparation

Intercostal nerve blocks can be done with the patient sitting or lying on the side. Bupivacaine (or the newer variants, see above) is the LA of choice because of its prolonged action. A 20 ml syringe is filled with anaesthetic and a 21G (green) or 23G (blue) needle attached. A sterile technique is used.

Technique

Intercostal nerves are best blocked at the angle of the rib as this ensures that the lateral cutaneous branch is included. The rib is palpated 7–9 cm from the midline with the second and third fingers of the left hand. The needle is inserted in a cephalad direction (as shown in Fig. 10.1), until it hits the rib. This gives an unmistakable inelastic feeling like

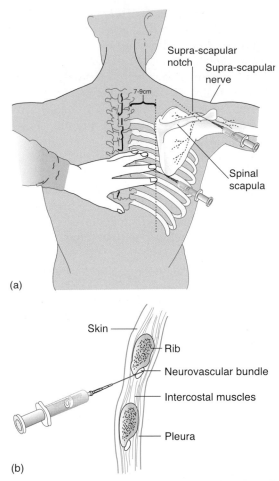

(a)

Supra-scapular notch
Supra-scapular nerve
7-9cm
Spinal scapula

Skin
Rib
Neurovascular bundle
Intercostal muscles
Pleura

(b)

Fig. 10.1 (a) Shows supra-scapular nerve block and insertion point for intercostal nerve block (b) shows intercostal nerve block in detail.

hitting hard wood. The needle is withdrawn a few mm and advanced in a more caudal direction until it meets the rib again and this procedure repeated until no bone is felt. The needle is then advanced a further few mm until a sudden 'give' or 'pop' is felt as the needle enters the sheath of the neurovascular bundle running along the lower edge of the rib. Following aspiration to ensure that the needle is not in a blood vessel, 3–4 ml of LA are injected. There should be little resistance as the LA is going into the loose tissue surrounding the neurovascular bundle (Fig. 10.1). The needle should not be advanced any further as there is a risk of entering the pleural cavity and causing a pneumothorax.

The block is then repeated at other intercostal spaces as necessary. Systemic absorption of anaesthetic is very rapid after intercostal block, so great care must be taken not to exceed the maximum dose of 20 ml of 0.5% bupivacaine (100 mg in the 70-kg patient). Pain relief usually lasts up to 12 h when the block may be repeated.

Complications
These include:

- accidental intravascular injection of LA and subsequent cardiac and neurological toxicity;

- excessive absorption of LA from perivascular tissues (intercostal nerve blocks produce the highest systemic concentration of LA per amount injected of any regional block);

- pneumothorax due to accidental pleural puncture.

Supra-scapular nerve block
This block is very simple and safe to perform and provides rewarding relief of shoulder pain (e.g. after trauma or after manipulation or reduction of dislocated shoulder under general anaesthesia).

It is best done with the patient sitting; the spine of the scapula is palpated and its mid-point marked on the skin with a pen. A long (6 cm or more) 21G or 23G needle is inserted through the skin one finger width above the pen mark, pointing slightly medially and downwards, until the bone of the supraspinatus fossa is met. This should be very close to the supra-scapular notch where the supra-scapular nerve passes (see Fig. 10.1a). Paraesthesia, experienced as pain at the tip of the shoulder, may sometimes be elicited. At this point 5–10 ml of 0.5% bupivacaine is injected, after pulling on the plunger of the syringe to ensure that the tip does not lie in a blood vessel. Analgesia of the shoulder should last for up to 10–12 h.

Ring block of the finger or toe
Fingers and toes are supplied by two dorsal and two palmar (or plantar) nerves. These can

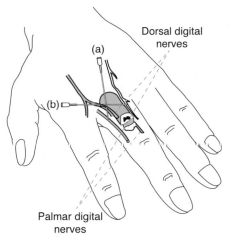

Fig. 10.2 Palmar and dorsal digital nerve anatomy and injection sites for performing a digital ring block.

be blocked effectively for minor surgical procedures. A fine 25G (orange) needle should be used; after preparation of the skin the needle is inserted dorsally at one side of the base of the finger (or toe) and advanced close to the surface of the bone until its tip lies close to the palmar (or plantar) surface. Then, while slowly withdrawing the needle, inject 2–3 ml 2% plain lidocaine.

Before the needle is totally withdrawn, it should be deflected and advanced to the other side and a further 0.5–1 ml injected under the skin at the point where the needle is to be reinserted to block the digital nerves on the other side of the finger. Fig 10.2 sketches this procedure.

The injection of anaesthetic must be done slowly because the distension of the tissue in this region is very painful.

Note: Adrenaline or other vasoconstrictors must *not* be used in this block as they can cause digital ischaemia and even gangrene of the extremity.

Intravenous regional anaesthesia of the arm (Bier's block)

Introduction
This is a unique regional technique as it relies on the nerves being blocked by diffusion of LA from the venous system. Exactly how this occurs is not known but it is presumed that the LA gains access via the venous drainage of the nerve roots by back diffusion. The technique involves total isolation and drainage of the venous network in the arm via use of an Esmarch bandage and tourniquet. The former empties the veins while the latter prevents further influx of blood. The veins are then filled with LA and within minutes the arm below the tourniquet is analgesic and relaxed. It is suitable for most superficial surgery of the arm and for bony manipulations, e.g. following a Colles fracture of the wrist.

Technique
It cannot be emphasised enough that this block must *not*, under any circumstances, be undertaken without having full resuscitation facilities and expertise at hand. It should be noted that, if the dose of LA injected i.v. for the procedure should gain rapid access into the systemic circulation, it will produce toxic side-effects ranging from convulsions to a state of general anaesthesia with respiratory and cardiovascular depression (see above).

The patient should lie supine and comfortably, with the affected arm supported by an arm board. A suitable tourniquet (type used for orthopaedic surgery of the arm, or a specially devised double cuff tourniquet) is put round the affected arm over cotton wool padding, and carefully secured to prevent accidental deflation or detachment.

A 20–22G cannula is then inserted into a vein of the dorsum of the hand (if this location interferes with surgery or is inconvenient, it may be inserted into any other superficial vein of the arm as distally as possible), and the arm raised vertically for 3 min to reduce the volume of blood contained within the venous compartment. Another cannula is inserted into the other arm so that an open vein is available during the procedure for the injection of adjuvant drugs such as opioids and benzodiazepines as well as drugs for the treatment of toxicity (see later). A special tourniquet with pressure gauge and pump attached is wrapped around the upper

10

arm over a generous layer of cotton wool padding. Most tourniquets include an automatic inflation device but some still employ a bicycle pump to inflate the cuff.

If the lesion to be treated surgically is not painful, a flat rubber bandage is tightly applied round the whole limb, starting distally, draining the blood away into the general circulation. If the bandage cannot be applied, a pneumatic device may be applied or the brachial artery may be compressed with the fingers (without obstructing venous return) for 30 s while keeping the arm upright. The tourniquet is then inflated rapidly to a pressure about 50 mmHg above the patients systolic BP and maintained throughout the procedure. The pressure in the tourniquet must be carefully observed throughout the whole procedure and not allowed to fall.

With the tourniquet inflated, 40 ml of 0.5% lidocaine or prilocaine (up to 3 mg/kg) is then injected very slowly through the cannula with the arm horizontal, watching for signs of venous distension (Fig. 10.3). If veins appear distended, the rate of injection must be reduced or stopped, because pressures may be generated within the venous system sufficient to cause leakage of anaesthetic into the general circulation.

The patient soon feels paraesthesiae and within 5–10 min a complete sensory and motor block should ensue, lasting for as long as the tourniquet is applied (up to 1 h). If a double-cuffed tourniquet is used, the proximal cuff is first inflated. When analgesia of the arm is established, the distal cuff (lying on anaesthetised skin) is inflated to the same pressure and the proximal one deflated. This usually relieves the discomfort associated with the pressure of the cuff.

The tourniquet must not be let down for at least 15 min after the injection of the LA. This time interval ensures that enough anaesthetic has diffused out of the vascular compartment, such that the amount entering the circulation as a 'bolus' is not sufficient to cause toxic effects.

Advantages
■ The only expertise required is ability to cannulate the vein and a rigorous technique.

■ Extremely high (>95%) success rate, higher than any other block.

Disadvantages
■ Not suitable for deep operations as analgesia is not sufficiently intense.

■ Tips of fingers are often missed and an additional ring block may then be necessary (*vide infra*).

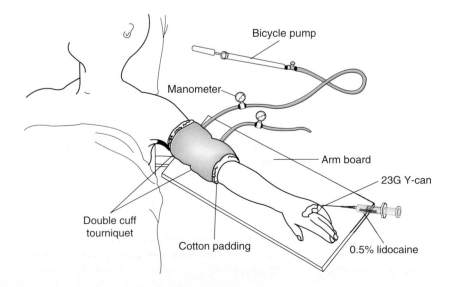

Fig. 10.3 Intravenous regional analgesia (Bier's block).

- The tourniquet may become extremely uncomfortable and thus limit the duration of surgery (using a second tourniquet together with the judicious use of adjuvant drugs may overcome this problem).

- Surgical time is limited to about 1 h due to the tourniquet that *must not be released* during the procedure.

- Postoperative analgesia is extremely short lived.

Complications

Should the tourniquet be accidentally deflated less than 15 min after injection of lidocaine the patient must be closely monitored for side-effects; paraesthesiae of the tongue and lips is usually the first symptom of systemic overdose.

Should an epileptiform fit occur, 10 mg of diazepam should be injected i.v. through the cannula in the opposite hand, and 100% oxygen given through a face mask until the convulsion is over. The dose of diazepam may be repeated twice if necessary, but it must be remembered that it will potentiate the respiratory depression caused by lidocaine. An i.v. infusion should be set up in the 'free' arm.

The first toxic symptom may be loss of consciousness. If respiratory depression occurs (also following a convulsion) manual ventilation with 100% oxygen must be started immediately and monitoring of pulse, BP and ECG instituted. The P–Q interval of the ECG is likely to be prolonged, the HR slow, and the BP low. If systolic pressure is below 60 mmHg, 3–5 mg boluses of ephedrine may be given i.v. (up to 30 mg total). If the BP is unrecordable (no pulses felt in the carotids) external cardiac massage must be started (Chapter 15).

Epidural and subarachnoid anaesthesia

Introduction

Epidurals may be performed at any level of the cervical, thoracic, lumbar or sacral spine. Lumbar epidurals at L2–3 or L3–4 level are the commonest, followed by the sacral (or caudal) approach. Lumbar epidural or subarachnoid blocks are suitable for most surgery of the lower abdomen and lower limbs.

Both are effective, firstly upon the sympathetic and then upon the sensory and motor fibres. This is more marked with subrachnoid block (differential block) as it works directly on the nerve sheaf in the CSF. Epidurals work principally on the nerve roots as they traverse the epidural space and the para-vertebral foramina, only subsequently penetrating the dura. This indirect action, combined with the large volume of distribution of the epidural space, means that much higher doses of LA are required as compared with the subarachnoid route (five times the amount). Sympathetic blockade always causes vasodilation in the lower half of the body and a variable fall in BP.

The discovery of opioid receptors in the spinal cord has led to the use of opioids either separately or in combination with LAs, both intra-operatively or for postoperative analgesia. This is discussed in more detail in the section above on postoperative pain.

Advantages and disadvantages

The following advantages are claimed for epidural and subarachnoid anaesthesia with LA and/or opioids:

- *reduced stress of surgery* due to sensory and autonomic blockade (Chapter 13);

- *decreased effect on respiratory function* and intereference with ventilation both during surgery and in the postoperative period (Chapter 17);

- *reduced incidence of postoperative* DVT in major orthopaedic surgery (Chapter 7);

- *relief of postoperative and labour pains* by use of continuous infusion techniques (see above);

- *increased cardiovascular stability* in patients with IHD and good left-ventricular function (Chapter 15).

10

There are also disadvantages and these include:

- *technical difficulties and time* taken to complete the block and get it working (up to 1 h in some cases).

- *sympathetic block* with LAs may produce catastrophic falls in BP, especially if the patient is hypovolaemic.

Contraindications

- *Patient refusal*, despite adequate assurance and explanation. However, the patient must be informed of the risk of haematoma and paralysis when consenting to the procedure, even though it is a very rare (but devastating) complication.

- *Abnormal anatomy or infection* at the site of the proposed block.

- *Coagulopathy*, this also includes the relative contraindications of DVT prophylaxis with mini-dose heparin.

Complications

- *Epidural haematoma or abscess* rarely occurs post epidural block but may have disastrous consequences, such as paraplegia.

- *Inadvertent dural tap*.

- *Sympathetic block* leading to hypotension and depressed response to sudden blood loss and hypovolaemia can cause severe hypotension which is difficult to reverse.

Despite some of the advantages alluded to above, there is little evidence, except in orthopaedic surgery, of an overall reduction in morbidity or mortality using epidural/subrachnoid block versus general anaesthesia. In fact, the techniques are often combined.

Epidurals

Firstly, decide that there are no contraindications to the technique and ensure that the patient has given informed consent for the technique (Chapter 5). Set up an i.v. infusion and (subject to acceptable cardiac function) administer 15 ml/kg of Hartmann's solution or colloid. This reduces the incidence of hypotension on production of the sympathetic block.

Technique

The patient is turned onto the left side and the site chosen, usually L2/3 to L3/4. The skin is cleaned with an antiseptic solution and a small skin wheal is made with LA. A 16G or 18G Tuohy needle is inserted through the skin in the mid-line and advanced through the supraspinous ligament and then between the spines of the vertebrae into the interspinous ligament. At this stage, the stylet is removed and it will be noticed that the needle is firmly gripped by the ligaments. If not, the needle is still in subcutaneous fat and should be advanced further. A well-lubricated glass syringe is attached to the hub of the needle and air or normal saline injected. A 'bounce' is detected with air if the needle is in the ligament. If saline is used there will be almost total resistance to injection. The patient is then asked to flex the back by bringing the chin onto the chest and the knees up to the abdomen. This opens up the space between the spines and adjacent lumbar laminae, the position is maintained by an assistant. As the needle is advanced further it penetrates the ligamentum flavum, a firm, rubbery ligament with a characteristic 'solid' feel. Still checking for resistance to injection of air or saline, the needle is further advanced through the ligamentum flavum and thence into the epidural space (Fig. 10.4b). This is not a true 'space' but contains nerve roots, blood vessels and fat. It offers very little resistance to injection of air or saline and thus a 'loss of resistance' is felt as the needle enters this space. The needle is detached and a check made for leakage of fluid (due to inadvertent dural tap). The injected saline can sometimes confuse the operator at this stage but a dural tap is usually quite noticeable.

The anaesthetic solution is slowly injected into the epidural space (Fig. 10.4b). Volumes ranging from 8 ml of 0.5% bupivacaine (for relief of pain in labour or postoperatively) to 30 ml of 0.5% bupivacaine or 1.5% lidocaine (for lower abdominal or hip surgery) may be injected, it will take from 20 min (1.5% lidocaine) to 40 min (0.5% bupivacaine) to fully establish the sensory block, which then lasts up to 90 min with bupivacaine. Occasionally, the block produced is unsatisfactory for surgery because one side or a particular segment remains resistant to the effect of the drug regardless of repeated top-ups or repositioning of the catheter.

Caudals are a form of epidural analgesia, but the epidural space is reached through the sacrococcygeal membrane. The nature, rate and seriousness of complications is the same as in lumbar epidurals. Single-shot caudals with 0.5% bupivacaine are often given for postoperative pain relief after perineal surgery (e.g. circumcision in children).

10

Top-ups

Topping up epidurals through the indwelling catheter carries identical risks to the initial administration. The risk of injecting the wrong drug is always present, and it cannot be emphasised enough that only specially trained personnel, fully aware of (and able to deal with) the possible complications, should perform this technique (e.g. by specially trained midwives in labour wards). The BP must be monitored at 5 min intervals for 20 min after topping-up. A well-drilled routine should be established to deal with complications such as a precipitous fall in BP or total paralysis.

Subarachnoid (intrathecal) analgesia

The patient is similarly positioned (or sitting, see Fig. 10.4a) and the subarachnoid space is reached with a fine needle (22–27G) by advancing a few mm beyond the epidural space and through the dura and arachnoid mater as for a diagnostic lumbar puncture (Fig. 10.4 a and b). The correct position of the tip of the needle is confirmed by obtaining clear CSF dripping off the hub. Only 1.5–3 ml of anaesthetic is injected to produce a block equivalent to that obtained with 20–30 ml in the epidural space, the effect being obtained within 5–10 min.

Subarachnoid analgesia is very reliable in its effects; patchy blocks are very rare, an

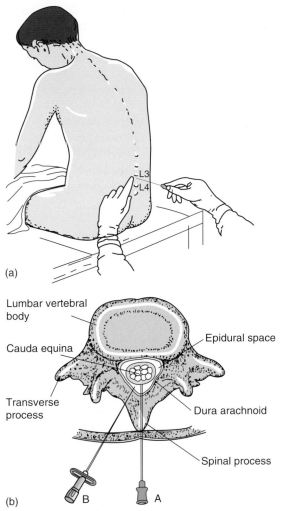

(a)

Lumbar vertebral body

Epidural space

Cauda equina

Transverse process

Dura arachnoid

Spinal process

(b)   B   A

Fig. 10.4 (a) Shows the patient in the sitting position prior to the insertion of the spinal needle. The sitting position is often adopted for a subarachnoid (intrathecal) block; otherwise the patient is placed on the left side. (b) Shows the tip of the intrathecal needle A in the CSF while the tip of the epidural needle B is in the epidural space. B is shown at an angle for clarity but in fact takes the same direction as A.

injected directly through a needle or through a fine plastic catheter. The plastic catheter has the advantage of allowing top-ups if left in situ (usually 2–3 cm inside the epidural space).

Complications

Note that the doses are close to those causing systemic side-effects. Once the anaesthetic is

advantage over epidurals. Although it is traditionally a single-shot procedure, top-ups are possible using a very fine 32G catheter threaded through the spinal needle. A percentage of young patients, varying from 1% to 3%, complain of headaches postoperatively due to leakage of CSF through the hole made by the needle in the dura. The incidence is lowest with very fine 25–27G needles, elderly patients seeming relatively resistant to this complication. The anaesthetic solutions used are normally mixed with 6–9%

glucose to make them hyperbaric (heavier, or more dense than CSF), such that by positioning the patient appropriately a more localised block (e.g. one-sided) may be obtained.

The most commonly used anaesthetic solutions is heavy bupivacaine 0.5% in 8% glucose.

Late complications of epidural and subarachnoid blockage may occur, such as persistent paraesthesia or weakness, often of a patchy nature. Their management is beyond the scope of this book.

11

Surgical infections and their management

Aims

The aims of this chapter are to

- define the terminology associated with infection;

- describe the preoperative, intra-operative and postoperative factors that can lead to infection;

- detail the signs, symptoms and investigation of surgical infection;

- discuss which pathogens are likely to cause infection;

- provide a rationale for antibiotic prescription, whether as prophylaxis or after established infection (either before or after microbiological diagnosis).

Objectives

After reading this chapter, you should be able to

- identify patients at risk of perioperative surgical infection,

- recognise and investigate the presence of infection in patients,

- make an educated guess as to which organisms are causing infection,

- treat the systemic manifestations of infection,

- formulate a rationale for 'blind' antibiotic therapy.

Introduction

Perioperative infection of the surgical patient is common. Lifestyle factors, such as diet and smoking, together with the presenting disease process (e.g. cancer), predispose patients to infection. Endogenous microbial colonisation of tissues can occur as a consequence of the course of a disease (e.g. perforation of an intra-abdominal viscus) or as a result of

operative intervention. Exogenous infection of the patient may occur through non-sterile surgical technique or simply by failure to maintain an acceptable standard of cleanliness on wards or between each patient contact. The *prevention* of infection is of paramount importance and may be achieved by antiseptic/aseptic precautions, together with the judicious use of prophylactic antibiotics. The management of established infection involves general interventional care of the patient combined with antibiotic therapy. Occasionally, a surgical procedure may be required. Communication with, and the involvement of, microbiologists facilitate rational antibiotic therapy. Indiscriminate use of antibiotics can lead to both microbial resistance and superadded infection, resulting in increased mortality rates, particularly amongst immuno-suppressed patients.

Some definitions

There is often confusion amongst medical practitioners over what is meant by the various terms used to describe infection and its systemic effects. Currently, the most commonly accepted definitions are those formulated by the American College of Chest Physicians and the Society of Critical Care Medicine (1992):

- *Infection*. Microbial phenomenon characterised by an inflammatory response to the presence of micro-organisms or the invasion of normally sterile host tissue by those organisms.

- *Bacteraemia*. The presence of viable bacteria in the blood.

- *Systemic inflammatory response syndrome (SIRS)*. The systemic inflammatory response to a variety of severe inflammatory insults. The response is manifested by two or more of the following conditions:

  - temperature outside the range 36–38°C;

  - heart rate (HR) above 90 bpm;

  - respiratory rate more than 20 bpm or $PaCO_2$ lower than 4.3 kPa;

11

- White blood cell (WBC) count outside the range of 4–$12 \times 10^9/l$, or more than 10% immature forms.

- *Sepsis*. The systemic inflammatory response caused by infection, i.e. the presence of the above physiological parameters in response to the presence of an identifiable infective agent.

- *Severe sepsis*. Sepsis associated with organ dysfunction, hypoperfusion or hypotension. Hypoperfusion and perfusion abnormalities may include, but are not limited to, lactic acidosis, oliguria or an acute alteration in mental status. Hypotension describes a systolic BP of less than 90 mmHg or a reduction of more than 40 mmHg from baseline, in the absence of other causes for hypotension.

- *Septic shock*. Sepsis with hypotension, despite adequate fluid resuscitation, along with perfusion abnormalities that may include, but are not limited to, lactic acidosis, oliguria, or an acute alteration in mental status. Patients who are on inotropic or vasopressor agents may not be hypotensive at the time that perfusion abnormalities are measured.

- *Multiple organ dysfunction syndrome (MODS)*. Presence of altered organ function in an acutely ill patient such that homeostasis cannot be maintained without intervention.

Note that the above definitions describe a progression of worsening disease from infection to MODS. Septicaemia, which inaccurately describes a wide range of infection and its pathophysiological consequences, has been abandoned in the terminology of infection (see also Chapter 13).

In addition, several other definitions are used (Table 11.1).

The pathophysiology of infection

Many pathogens normally reside in or on the human body without causing infection. For example, 35% of family members of patients with *Neisseria meningitidis* infection (meningococcal meningitis) have been found to be asymptomatic carriers. It has been estimated that the adult human intestine contains 2 kg of bacteria. In the non-diseased state, a number of specific and non-specific mechanisms contribute to the host's resistance to infection.

Non-specific mechanisms of immunity

There are a number of physical barriers that prevent host inoculation by pathogens. To gain entrance to the body, organisms must physically breach membrane barriers in the host, including the skin, respiratory tract, mucous membranes or urinary tract. In

11

Table 11.1 **Definitions associated with surgical infection**

Carrier	A person who has been colonised, but who does not manifest infection
Pathogen	An agent with the ability to cause infection
Endogenous infection	Infection of the body by natural host flora
Exogenous infection	Infection of the body by organisms not usually cultured from the host
Nosocomial infection	Infection acquired during hospitalisation
Virulence	The potential of a pathogen to cause infection

11

Table 11.2 **Non-specific host defences**

Behavioural factors
Personal hygiene
Nutrition
Personal contact

Skin
Fatty acids
Low pH

Tear production
Tears contain antibacterial lysozyme and IgA

Respiratory tract
Upper
  Coughing and sneezing
Lower
  Mucociliary escalator
  Bactericidal secretions
  Secretory IgA
  Macrophages

GIT
Stomach acidity
Enzyme production
Hepatic macrophages – Kuppfer cells
Secretory IgA

Urinary tract
Urine flow
Urine acidity

Normal surface flora
Competition for nutrients
Produce antimicrobial agents

Table 11.3 **Host response to infection**

Non-specific mechanisms
Physical barrier
Behaviour
Secretions
Natural flora

Specific mechanisms – immunity
Artificial
  Active – vaccination
  Passive – Ig antiserum
Natural
  Active – humoral, cell mediated
  Passive – maternal transfer of antibodies

---

addition, a number of non-specific host defences operate (see Table 11.2).

Specific mechanisms of immunity

Specific mechanisms of immunity are those that have developed either artificially or naturally, through evolution. Artificial immunity may be provided passively or actively. Passive immunity involves injection of immunoglobulin (Ig) or antiserum to provide immediate protection; immunity declines over the subsequent few months. Active immunity (vaccination) employs inactivated or attenuated organisms (or structural elements thereof) to induce the formation of antibody isotypes. A low-intensity, short-duration phase of antibody formation occurs during the month after vaccination. Subsequent exposure to the appropriate pathogen produces a rapid (3–5 days), larger and more sustained response to the infecting organism.

Similarly, natural immunity may be provided actively or passively. Passive natural immunity occurs due to maternal transplacental transfer of antibodies to the foetus and provides a degree of immunity for the newborn until 6 months of age. Active natural immunity involves a complex interaction between humoral (antibodies, complement), cell-mediated (macrophages, T-lymphocytes and B-lymphocytes) and cytokine components.

Infection, therefore, is likely to result when the host responses described in Table 11.3 are bypassed, circumvented or absent, particularly by a more virulent organism.

Direct inoculation of pathogens into the bloodstream avoids non-specific host responses to infection. This may occur when barriers are absent or damaged:

■ de-epithelialisation:

  ● burns,

  ● trauma;

- gross tissue damage:
  - burns,
  - trauma,
  - infection,
  - surgery;
- medical intervention:
  - intubation and ventilation,
  - iatrogenic (intravenous access, inadvertent tissue damage),
- disease process:
  - perforation intra-abdominal viscus,
  - inflammation (pancreatitis, SIRS).

In addition, and less apparently, the structural and functional integrity of intact barrier mechanisms may be indirectly disrupted:

- alterations in natural flora:
  - antibiotic usage,
  - nosocomial colonisation,
  - malnutrition,
  - use of bowel preparations;
- damage to
  - immobility and pressure necrosis of tissues;
- epithelial cells:
  - irradiation,
  - chemotherapeutic cytotoxins,
  - contact hypersensitivity (to dressings, skin preparations);
- tissue ischaemia/anaemia:
  - hypoxia,
  - hypotension,
  - reduction of arterial flow – internal emboli, external inflammation;
  - cross-clamping.

Specific immunity may be compromised in several ways:

- Overwhelming infection after gross inoculation.
- Genotypic factors.
- Immuno-suppression:
  - cancer;
  - malnutrition;
  - drugs (immuno-suppressants, steroids);
  - HIV infection;
  - blood transfusion.

There may exist considerable interindividual variation in response to bacteraemia. A cohort of patients undergoing the same surgery under similar conditions will exhibit a range of responses to surgical infection. Some patients will not develop infection. Others will exhibit mild infective signs but will recover. A minority may develop fulminant infection, leading to multiple organ failure (MOF) and death. Both a reduction in major histocompatibility complex (MHC)-II expression by monocytes (which effect antigen recognition and presentation) and an excess of CD16 expression on neutrophils have been described in non-survivors, implying that death after infection may occur as a result of both an underactive *and* an overactive immune response.

Preoperative considerations

There are a number of preoperative factors that may predispose patients to surgical infection. Their identification and treatment prior to surgery may greatly contribute to a reduction in the rates of infection and perioperative morbidity. Three groups of preoperative factors are recognised – co-existing diseases, surgical diseases and environmental factors.

Co-existing conditions
This group comprises chronic pathologies or behaviour exhibited by the patient prior to surgery.

Cardiovascular disease
Cardiovascular pathology may effect infection, inhibiting the body's response to infection or

11

limiting the ability of the patient to cope with physiological strain placed upon it by sepsis. Atherosclerosis, venous stasis and cardiac failure give rise to tissue ischaemia, which may be compounded by anaemia. Ischaemia may predispose to infection, inhibit humoral and cell-mediated immune responses and delay recovery from infection. Pulmonary oedema attenuates non-specific lung immune responses. Damaged heart valves may become colonised during episodes of bacteraemia, resulting in bacterial endocarditis. During sepsis and MODS, ischaemic heart disease (IHD) limits cardiac output, which worsens tissue ischaemia.

Respiratory disease

Chest infection is common following surgery, with an increased incidence amongst asthmatics and patients with chronic obstructive pulmonary disease (COPD). Patients who have surgery while suffering from an upper respiratory tract infection (or up to 2 weeks after the infection) have both an increased risk of airway complications during anaesthesia (coughing, laryngospasm) and postoperative chest infection; this is particularly true of children. Chest infection results in relative hypoxia, which can worsen wound healing, and may result in wound dehiscence after bouts of coughing.

Smoking

Smokers are at increased risk of perioperative surgical infection. Smoking is an airway irritant. It results in inflammation, disruption of ciliary function and increased production (with decreased clearance) of respiratory secretions. Chronically, alveolar fibrosis and emphysematous damage occur, disrupting immune and respiratory function. Carboxy-Hb has 100 times greater affinity than oxygen for Hb, resulting in reduced oxygen transport by Hb. Ischaemia is worsened by smoke-related increases in blood viscosity (due to hypoxia-induced polycythaemia) and cardiovascular disease (atherosclerosis and coronary ischaemia). Immune function appears to be inhibited by some of the 4000 chemicals that have been identified in cigarette smoke together with lowered Ig levels and decreased leucocyte function.

Preoperative cessation of smoking should be strongly encouraged, preferably for more than 8 weeks before surgery. Carboxy-Hb has a half-life of 4 h; so even 24 h-cessation allows relative normalisation of Hb oxygen carriage.

Obesity

Several definitions of obesity exist, but the most commonly used describes a person as obese if their body mass index (BMI) is more than 30. Approximately, 33% of the population, therefore, are classed as obese; 1% of the population is morbidly obese – they have a BMI of greater than 40 (Chapter 14):

$$BMI = weight\ (kg)/height^2\ (m)$$

The physiological stresses placed on the body by obesity lead to excessive perioperative morbidity and mortality. Perioperative infection is more common for several reasons:

- the obese have increased chest wall weight and a greater volume of intra-abdominal contents. When placed supine, the compliance of their chest wall decreases, causing the functional residual capacity (FRC, the volume of air in the lungs after tidal expiration) to fall below the closing capacity ((CC) i.e. the volume of air in the lungs when small airways begin to close). This leads to small airway closure, atelectasis and ventilation/perfusion mismatch, which is worsened by anaesthesia and neuromuscular blockade. Being unable to cough as effectively as thinner patients, they are, more prone to postoperative chest infections. In addition, the obese are more prone to gastro-oesophageal reflux, which may contribute to pulmonary colonisation by enteric organisms.

- The resultant hypoxaemia, together with the increased oxygen consumption and IHD associated with obesity, leads to relative tissue ischaemia and results in poor wound healing, with dehiscence and infection.

11

- Suture lines are placed under abnormal strain in obese people resulting in wound dehiscence.

- Diabetes and abnormal glucose tolerance are more common in the obese and are worsened by the stress response to surgery, resulting in poor wound healing and urinary tract infection.

- Pressure sores are more common. Hyperglycaemia and hypoxia play a role, but ischaemia due to body size is of primary importance. Consider two people, one with a body mass of 65 kg (patient A) and the other with a body mass of 130 kg (patient B). If they both have a sacral pressure area of approximately 20 cm^2 (0.04 m^2), the pressure exerted over that area is:

  Patient A
  $P = F/A$
  $\quad = (65 \, kg \times 9.81 \, N/kg)/0.04 \, m^2$
  $\quad = 16{,}000 \, N/m^2 \text{ (approximately)}$
  $\quad = 16{,}000 \, Pa = 16 \, kPa$
  $(16 \, kPa/101.3 \, kPa) \times 760 \, mmHg = 120 \, mmHg$

  Patient B
  $P = F/A$
  $\quad = (130 \, kg \times 9.81 \, N/kg)/0.04 \, m^2$
  $\quad = 32{,}000 \, N/m^2 \text{ (approximately)}$
  $\quad = 32{,}000 \, Pa = 32 \, kPa$
  $(32 \, kPa/101.3 \, kPa) \times 760 \, mmHg = 240 \, mmHg$

  therefore, if the systolic BP of both patients is 130 mmHg, blood will flow to the sacral pressure area of patient A (as the BP supplying the area is temporarily higher than the mechanical pressure exerted on the arterioles of the area by body mass) but will not flow to the sacral pressure area of patient B, resulting in tissue ischaemia and breakdown.

- Increased adipose tissue predisposes patients to wound haematomas, which may become infected.

- Deeper skin folds produce warm, humid conditions for bacterial growth and facilitate bacterial entry to the body through friction damaged skin.

Malnutrition

In the Western world, malnutrition is an often under-recognised condition in patients presenting for surgery. The patient may be undernourished (a pure calorie deficiency) or inappropriately nourished (e.g. obtaining virtually all their calories through the intake of alcohol!). Several groups of patients are at greater risk of malnutrition: babies, the elderly, starved patients, alcoholics and patients with malabsorption, intestinal fistulae, chronic sepsis, previous GI surgery, cancer (particularly if undergoing chemotherapy or radiotherapy) or chronic liver disease. Hypercatabolism, associated with the stress response to surgery, further reduces the nutritional reserves of the patient. Malnutrition results in poor wound healing, increased muscle breakdown (predisposing the patient to chest infection) and reduced immune function. Liaison with dieticians is important. Nutritional support in the perioperative period may be provided by supplemental use of nutritional drinks, nasoenteral feeding or parenteral nutrition (see Chapter 18).

The elderly

Old age is not *per se* an independent variable for perioperative infection, but a number of pathophysiological changes occur in the elderly that increase the likelihood of infection:

- reduced chest and lung compliance, raised CC and reduced autonomic responses to hypoventilation predispose to chest infection;

- atherosclerosis and reduced cardiac function lead to tissue ischaemia, with delayed wound healing, which may be worsened by anaemia;

- increased incidence of occult malignancy;

- obesity;

- malnutrition and increased alcoholism;

- reduced mobility;

- reduced communication and reduced compliance with treatment;

- increased periodontal disease;

- thin skin;

- impaired temperature regulation;

- reduced immune function.

Diabetes

In the perioperative period, several factors alter glycaemic control in the diabetic patient, including fasting, anxiety and the stress response to surgery. Diabetics are more prone to infection than non-diabetics because

- cellular immunity is reduced;

- glycosuria and chronic renal failure predispose to urinary tract infection;

- peripheral neuropathy reduces patient awareness of early infection (e.g. loss of pain sensation);

- autonomic neuropathy reduces sensitivity to hypoxia and hypercapnia, resulting in hypoventilation and reduced blood oxygen carriage. Autonomic neuropathy also produces gastric paresis with an increased incidence of aspiration pneumonia.

Perioperative glycaemic control may be improved by the involvement of the diabetic team, and by using 'sliding-scale' short-acting insulin regimes, for both insulin-dependent and non-insulin-dependent diabetics (Chapter 4).

Steroids

Steroids, although invaluable in the treatment of autoimmune disease, organ transplants and inflammatory disorders, have several side-effects that predispose patients to infection:

- altered body habitus and obesity;

- thinning of the skin, increasing the likelihood of it being breached by minor trauma (e.g. removal of adhesive bandages) and delaying wound healing;

- hyperglycaemia;

- reduced immune function;

- reduced fibroblast function, decreased fibrosis and decreased blood vessel proliferation.

Despite these problems, steroid usage should continue throughout the perioperative period. Cessation may have two adverse effects. Firstly, the condition for which the steroids are being given may worsen; this may not be so problematic in the case of, e.g. polymyalgia rheumatica, but can lead to significant morbidity, for instance, if it enables rejection of a transplanted organ. Secondly, chronic steroid administration causes adrenal suppression. Perioperative cessation of steroids could, therefore, render the patient less capable of dealing with the stress of surgery. Indeed, it may be the case that those on exogenous steroids require perioperative supplementation, particularly for more major surgery, because they are unable to produce the endogenous steroid surge required to enable the body to cope with trauma (Chapter 4).

Surgical conditions

Certain surgical pathologies predispose to perioperative surgical infection.

Gastrointestinal disease

The alimentary canal, from mouth to anus, is colonised with bacteria. Excessive translocation of bacteria from the gut lumen into the circulation or to surrounding tissue can occur quickly if the structural and functional integrity of the gut wall is breached, such as may occur with facial trauma, duodenal and diverticular perforation, or mesenteric infarction. Spillage of large bowel contents into the abdominal cavity bypasses the immune capacity of the liver, and bacteria may translocate into the circulation in the subphrenic area and paracolic gutters. Collection of blood, pancreatic secretions and bacteria can result in abscess formation, particularly in the subphrenic region. This may be prevented to a degree by thorough irrigation of the abdominal cavity, prior to closure.

11

Trauma

Soft tissue injury causes haematoma formation, oedema and tissue ischaemia, which provide ideal growth conditions for bacterial growth and replication. Skin damage promotes wound colonisation. Deeper infections may result due to blunt trauma and penetrating injury, particularly if inoculation of debris (such as clothing, bullets, skin) occurs. Severe trauma leads to massive endothelial damage, with the release of vasoactive substances and inflammatory mediators, resulting in MOF; sepsis is often co-existant (either secondary to the trauma itself or due to enteric bacterial translocation) and mortality is high.

Burns

Burns cause thermal damage to tissue, which has two effects. Firstly, the burnt tissue becomes ischaemic, due to blood vessel damage and oedema. A serosanguinous exudate is produced by skin that is partially burnt which acts as a growth medium for bacteria. Secondly, in a similar fashion to severe trauma, the massive endothelial damage associated with burns effects an inflammatory cascade that results in MOF. Large burns cause extreme hypercatabolism so malnutrition quickly ensues, as does hyperglycaemia, which both favour infection.

Environmental factors

Semmelweiss described asepsis in 1851. Lister described antisepsis in 1867. Both recognised that disease could be transmitted from one person to another; even if the carrier themselves did not show signs or symptoms of disease. Scrupulous hygiene on wards and amongst staff was the main method of infection control until the introduction of antibacterial agents (notably penicillin in the early 1940s). Subsequent reliance on antibiotics to treat infection has produced a degree of indifference to maintaining standards of hygiene in hospitals. The recent evolution of multiple drug-resistant bacteria, however, has reiterated the importance of antiseptic precautions.

The hospital environment

By the nature of their activity, hospitals are prone to the transmission of infection amongst patients. Intrapatient and interpatient infection may occur through patient/patient, patient/relation and patient/staff contacts, as well as through ventilation systems, washing and sanitary facilities. It is, therefore, prudent to minimise patient contact with the hospital environment: investigations and preoperative assessment may be carried out on an outpatient basis and the time between admission and surgery should be minimised. Patient transfer around the hospital and between hospitals should be avoided. The importance of handwashing (and the use of alcohol and glycerine skin lotion) by relatives and staff between patient contacts cannot be underestimated and is to be strongly encouraged. Appropriate protective clothing may be required to nurse some patients. Special areas or wards should be reserved for patients with established infection or particularly virulent forms of infection. Similarly, those patients at particular risk of infection (those with HIV or haematological malignancy) should be isolated onto special wards. An infection control team should be employed to co-ordinate the hospital's infection policy.

The surgical list

Introduction

The order of the surgical list may need to be altered to account for operations or patients with a high risk of infection. Surgical procedures may be stratified into four classes, according to their potential for causing both infection and contamination of the surgical environment (see Table 11.4).

The theatre environment

Theatre design and the conduct of surgery and staff have been designed to minimise the

Table 11.4 **Classes of surgical procedure (GU = genitourinary)**

Parameter	Class of surgical procedure			
	Class I	Class II	Class III	Class IV
GI, GU, tracheobronchial system integrity	Intact	Transection with minor spillage	Transection with major spillage Incision through infected tissue	Dead tissue, direct infection, pus
Sterile technique	Continuous	Minor lapses	Interrupted	Contamination despite sterile technique
Antibiotic prophylaxis	Not required	Single dose	Broad spectrum	Broad spectrum
Wound infection rate	1.5%	<8%	12% 15–25% without antibiotics	>25%
Surgical wound produced	Non-traumatic Uninfected	Mildly contaminated	Grossly contaminated	Contaminated with pus, faeces or extraneous material
Examples	Endocrine Orthopaedics Skin	Elective GI Dental Gynaecological	GI perforation Open fracture reduction	Abscesses Faecal peritonitis Trauma >4 h

likelihood of perioperative infection. These include the following.

List order
This is common sense and means putting a grossly infected patient on the end of the list rather than the beginning!

Area designation
The theatre environment becomes progressively more sterile from the 'front door' to the operating table. The patient initially passes from the ward to theatre reception, beyond which relatives should not be allowed to pass. From reception, or a holding area, they pass to the anaesthetic room. Accompanying ward staff should wear shoe coverings and hats during this transfer, and should leave shortly after handing over the patient. All theatre staff should wear surgical scrubs and theatre shoes, have their hair tied back under theatre hats and avoid the wearing of make-up or jewellery. Staff should never leave the theatre environment in surgical gear; if this is unavoidable, they should always change their scrubs before returning to theatre. Non-sterile non-surgical procedures, such as urinary catheterisation, should be carried out in the anaesthetic room, prior to transfer to the operating theatre. Likewise, blankets and extraneous items should be removed before entering the operating theatre.

Operating theatre design
Operating theatres are ventilated with positive pressure, clean and filtered air, that cycles from the patient to the periphery of the theatre. For

most types of surgery, the air is recycled 20 times an hour. This may be increased to 40 times an hour in the case of prosthetic joint surgery, for which specially designed compartmental airflow systems (e.g. Charnley®) may also be used. The design of entrances and exits is such that laminar airflow is correctly maintained, even when doors are opened. Three separate areas of the operating theatre exist: the operating room proper and the instrument preparation room, both of which are maintained highly sterile, and the scrub area. The operating theatre floor should be cleaned with antiseptic solution between each case, and the whole theatre is more thoroughly decontaminated and sterilised after each surgical list. Ideally, after 'dirty' cases a period of 30 min should elapse before commencing the next case, to allow sufficient time for airborne pathogens to be filtered. Separate areas external to the operating theatre are maintained for the disposal of waste, the storage of equipment and the cleaning of equipment.

Scrubbing

Correct scrubbing technique is essential to maintain a sterile field around the patient. The process should be taught and retaught to surgeons by theatre sisters. The surgeon should wear clean theatre dress, a theatre cap and a surgical mask. A gown pack is opened and surgical gloves placed, opened, next to it. Before the first patient of the list, a 5-min handwash should be performed, using Betadine® or chlorhexidine. Nails should be scrubbed. The hands are dried, and the gown is put on followed by the gloves. A second person ties the surgeon into the gown. Between subsequent cases a 2-min handwash is sufficient, providing the surgeon has not left the theatre environment in the interim, and has not just operated on a dirty case. Regloving is required:

- if the gloves are punctured,
- if a non-sterile area/person is touched,
- during long procedures or
- during dirty procedures.

The patient

Ideally, the patient should be encouraged to shower before surgery. Shaving of the incision site may be required, but should be performed carefully to avoid microabrasions, which encourage infection. Once on the operating table (correctly positioned and prepared by the anaesthetist), the patient's skin should be cleaned with antiseptic solution. Betadine or chlorhexidine are commonly used. Betadine should be applied for at least 3 min prior to incision; it has the advantage over chlorhexidine of clearly demarcating the area cleaned, but excites a higher incidence of allergic reactions. Cleaning should advance from the proposed site of incision outwards. Drapes are applied to leave the incision site exposed, but to cover every other part of the patient, which might come into contact with sterile personnel or equipment. Transparent, adhesive drapes are increasingly used to further limit patient skin exposure.

Adequate care should be taken during the procedure to maintain tissue perfusion and oxygenation. This is mainly the concern of the anaesthetist, who should endeavour to keep the patient normovolaemic, normotensive and normothermic, as well as protecting pressure points and reducing patient stressors (e.g. awareness and pain).

Surgical technique

The practice of surgery has become considerably more refined with the passage of time – speed is no longer the only requirement of a good surgeon. Attention to intra-operative surgical technique can significantly hinder the development of perioperative infection. The following factors should be considered:

- *Attire, scrub technique, patient preparation.*

- *Choice of technique:* For instance, minimally invasive surgery reduces both tissue contamination by skin flora and the degree of tissue trauma. The infection of prosthetic material can be particularly disastrous; therefore, avoidance of

11

prosthetics by the use of autologous tissue may be beneficial.

- *Surgery of infected material:* Adequate debridement of dead and infected tissue is required, together with irrigation (hence the surgical maxim 'the solution to pollution is dilution'). Delayed primary closure or healing by secondary intention may be indicated. More esoteric treatments may be employed, including suction packing, hyperbaric oxygen therapy and the application of maggots.

- *Haemostasis, closure and wound dressing:* Haematomas provide an excellent growth medium for bacteria, so attention should be given to attaining haemostasis at surgery, particularly in patients with coagulopathy, cancer and chronic infection. Expansion of a haematoma may further compromise tissue blood supply. Drains may be used to prevent haematoma formation or the accumulation of infected/infectable fluids, but should be removed shortly after drainage of fluid ceases. Closure of the wound should aim to reconstitute normal anatomy, so as to prevent the formation of tissue dead spaces, in which seromata and bacterial multiplication might occur. Sutures should be applied in such a way as not to compromise the blood supply of the wound (thus avoiding wound breakdown). A range of suture material is available (e.g. natural and synthetic sutures, staples, self-adhesive sutures and tissue glue) and the choice should be made according to the clinical indication. Sutures are removed, if necessary, once the skin has united. Dressings should be clean and applied without compromising blood supply. Postoperatively, dressings should be subject to regular inspection and replacement.

Diagnosis of infection

A number of clinical, haematological and microbiological variables may be assessed in order to both diagnose and monitor the course of an infection.

Wound inspection

Infected wounds may be red, swollen, tender and hot (rubor, tumour, dolor and calor) due to the localised release of endogenous chemicals that cause vasodilation, increased membrane permeability and pain fibre sensitisation. The wound may extrude pus (which is predominantly composed of white cells), and may be malodorous. In addition, there may be a degree of dehiscence or tissue breakdown around drain sites. The efficacy of treatment may be observed by daily inspection of the wound.

Temperature

The wound itself may be hot. The patient may have a raised core temperature (above 37.5°C), due to the systemic release of pyrogens, such as interleukin-6 (IL-6), and the patient may be diaphoretic (sweaty) in an attempt to reduce their body temperature. Hyperpyrexia may lead to rigors, confusion, lethargy and tachycardia. Note that hyperpyrexia may occur in the perioperative phase *without* the presence of infection (e.g. stress response, post-blood transfusion, drug reactions and malignancy), or due to an infection not associated with the wound (e.g. urinary tract infection, chest infection and venous line-related sepsis. Swinging pyrexias are associated with abscess formation, low-grade pyrexia with wound infection (particularly if they occur around 5–6 days after surgery).

White cell count

The white cell count (WCC) is most commonly raised in the presence of infection (i.e. greater than 11×10^9 white cells/l), with a marked predominance of neutrophils on the differential count. However, note that the WCC *may* be either low or normal, particularly in immuno-suppressed patients, leukaemic patients or occasionally when Gram-negative organisms infect the patient.

Other biochemical markers

C-reactive protein (CRP, an acute phase protein) levels, erythrocyte sedimentation rate (ESR) and plasma viscosity may all be increased

11

in the presence of infection. They are reasonably sensitive markers for infection but are very non-specific; and their use, therefore, is limited to monitoring the progress of treatment. CRP levels are mildly raised after surgery, decreasing to normal after 48 h. The ESR and plasma viscosity may be normal after surgery depending on the degree of haemodilution.

Radiology

Radiological tests may be used as an adjunct to thorough clinical examination and appropriate simple investigations. X-rays may be used according to the findings of the clinical examination (e.g. CXR if a chest infection is suspected). Ultrasound scans may be used to detect collections of pus, though abdominal ultrasound is often technically difficult and may prove inconclusive in the presence of excess bowel gas or fat. Computerised tomography (CT) is an alternative to ultrasound scanning, but subjects the patient to a high degree of radiation exposure. A white cell scan uses radiolabelled white cells (indium 111-labelled leucocytes) to identify the site of infections that are difficult to diagnose clinically (e.g. osteomyelitis and vascular graft infection), although there is a real (but small) risk of HIV transmission with this technique.

Microbiology

Microbiological analysis of tissue specimens does not so much confirm the presence of infection as discover what the infecting organism is. Ideally, a specimen of pus or infected tissue should be sent – this may involve needle aspiration or operative retrieval of the specimen. Other samples to consider sending include blood, sputum, urine, faeces and drain contents. Samples should be sent before the commencement of antibiotic therapy. If the patient is already taking antibiotics, the type, dose and length of treatment should be written on the request form. Samples should be collected in a sterile manner to avoid false positive results due to cross-contamination. Blood should be sent for microbiology, culture and sensitivities, if the patient is systemically unwell. Blood should be taken in the normal sterile manner; an alcoholic swab should be used to clean the top of the culture bottles, the aerobic bottle being filled first, to avoid the inadvertent introduction of air into the anaerobic bottle. The results of a Gram stain are available within a few hours. Culture and sensitivity results take 24–72 h. Immunological methods (for viruses) and more elaborate culture methods (e.g. for fungi and tuberculosis) may take longer.

Species of *Spirochaetes*, *Mycoplasma*, *Legionella*, *Rickettsia*, *Coxiella*, *Chlamydia* are termed 'atypical' because they cannot be classified as either bacilli or cocci. They are Gram-negative organisms. Bacteria may be further sub-classified according to oxygen tolerance, i.e. aerobes, facultative anaerobes or strict anaerobes.

Gram staining imparts information concerning the cell wall of a bacterium. Gram-positive bacteria have a peptidoglycan cell wall that envelops the outer wall of the cell membrane. Gram-negative bacteria also possess a peptidoglycan cell wall (though it is thinner), but this is enveloped by an additional outer membrane with surface polysaccharide. This difference suggests that antibiotics that exert their effects on peptidoglycan cell walls, such as penicillins, will be less effective against Gram-negative organisms, in which the cell wall matrix has reduced exposure to antibiotic. Figure 11.1 gives an idea of the efficacy of various antibiotics.

Treatment

General principles

In general, the treatment of perioperative infection involves both the avoidance of cross-infection with other patients and the tailored treatment of the specific infection affecting the patient. Cross-infection may be avoided by barrier nursing, handwashing and use of alcohol and glycerine handrubs between patient contacts, the use of sterile instruments and isolation methods.

11

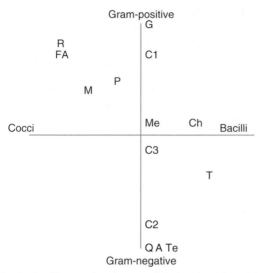

Fig. 11.1 Efficacy of various antibiotics. (R: rifampicin; FA: fucidic acid; G: glycopeptides; C1: 1st-; C2: 2nd-; C3: 3rd-generation cephalosporins; P: penicillins; M: macrolides; Me: meropenem; Ch: chloramphenicol; T: trimethoprim; Q: quinolones; Te: tetracyclines; A: aminoglycosides.) For example, rifampicin (R) is more active against Gram-positive cocci, whereas aminoglycosides (A) are most effective against Gram-negative organisms, cocci and bacilli.

Specific patient treatment involves careful clinical assessment, appropriate investigations, wound care, general treatment (e.g. fluid management, analgesia, physiotherapy, pressure area care), antibiotic treatment and reassessment.

Wound care
Ideally the wound should be kept scrupulously clean. Foreign debris (e.g. drains) should be kept to a minimum, and removed as soon as viable. The wound should be inspected daily and redressed in a sterile manner with an appropriate dressing:

- *light exudates* – non-adherent gauze (e.g. Vaseline® dressing);
- *heavy exudates* – hydrocolloid dressing;
- *mild slough* – hydrogel dressing;
- *heavy slough* – enzymatic desloughing dressing;
- *chronic slough* – vacuum sponge drain, larval therapy.

The wound should be protected until healing is advanced, and the patient should be educated to avoid touching or picking at the wound. Topical antimicrobial agents or antiseptic washes may be employed.

Antibiotics
Without doubt, the discovery and use of antibiotics has saved many lives that would have otherwise been lost due to perioperative surgical infection. However, it is important to reiterate that they should only be used as an adjunct to general hygiene and antisepsis, due to the potential for development of bacterial resistance. There are a seemingly endless number of antibiotics from which to choose. Initially, it is often confusing to know which to use, as they vary in efficacy against different bacteria, in pharmaceutical preparation and in side-effect profiles. The ideal antibiotic would be cheap, easy to produce, stable in a low-volume solution, available and effective in oral, i.v. and topical preparations, be bactericidal against Gram-positive and -negative rods and bacilli, spirochaetes and anaerobes, have a wide therapeutic range with minimal side-effects, be non-allergenic and resilient to the development of bacterial resistance.

In order to understand which antibiotics are appropriate treatment for which bacteria, it is helpful to classify bacterial species into one of four groups, depending on their morphology (bacilli or cocci) and acceptance of Gram stain (Gram positive or Gram negative, Table 11.5).

Atypical bacteria (*Mycoplasma*, *Legionella*, *Rickettsia*, *Coxiella*, *Chlamydia*) are best treated with tetracyclines, spirochaetes with penicillin. Anaerobic bacteria are killed by metronidazole.

Antibiotic prophylaxis
Prophylactic antibiotics reduce the rate of postoperative infection after procedures that produce bacteraemia or wound contamination, and in susceptible patients (e.g. those with valvular heart disease, the immuno-compromised, and patients receiving prosthetic implants). Prophylaxis alone does not prevent infection, but forms part of the

11

Table 11.5 Classification of bacteria by Gram stain and morphology

Cocci	Bacilli
Gram positive	
Staphylococci	Bacillus
Streptococci	Clostridia
	Corynebacteria
	Listeria
	Mycobacterium
Gram negative	
Neisseria	Pseudomonas
	Enterobacteria
	Escherischia
	Yersinia
	Salmonella
	Shigella
	Klebsiella
	Proteus
	Parvobacteria
	Vibrio
	Haemophilus
	Bordatella
	Brucella
	Serratia
	Campylobacter
	Bacteroides

general anti-infection measures taken in the perioperative period.

A number of broad-spectrum antibiotics are used, their choice being dependent on the type of surgery, the likeliest source of bacterial contamination, patient factors (e.g. allergy) and local or regional antibiotic policy. Prophylactic antibiotics are usually administered as a single dose prior to the operation, the aim being to have a high circulating concentration of antibiotic at the site of skin incision (they should, therefore, be administered at least 5 min prior to application of a tourniquet). Prophylaxis may be carried on into the immediate postoperative phase (up to 24 h) after which continued administration is classed as therapeutic. Commonly used prophylactic regimes are shown in Table 11.6.

Specific antibiotic therapy

There is inevitably a delay between taking a microbiology sample and obtaining a culture and sensitivity result. Therefore, the initial treatment of perioperative infections necessitates an empirical, 'best-guess' approach to antibiotic treatment.

This is based on

- clinical assessment of the most likely infecting organism (according to the type of surgery and the site of infection);

- the severity of the infection;

- Gram-stain results;

- local antibiotic policies;

- patient factors (allergy, renal impairment, recent antibiotic administration).

Common empirical regimens include:

- minor surface infections:

  - narrow spectrum: flucloxacillin (if *S. aureus*) suspected,
  - broad spectrum: cefuroxime;

- chest infection:
  - penicillins;

- after GI surgery:

  - cefuroxime + metronidazole ± gentamicin ± antifungal;

- after urological surgery:

  - co-amoxiclav, gentamicin;

- severe sepsis:

  - vancomycin + gentamicin + metronidazole;

- methicillin (i.e. penicillin)-resistant *S. aureus* (MRSA):

  - vancomycin;

- vancomycin-resistant enterococcus (VRE):

  - consult microbiologist;

- *Pseudomonas suspected:*

  - ciprofloxacin.

11

171

Table 11.6 **Commonly used prophylactic antibiotics**

Type of surgery	Likely infecting organism	Prophylactic antibiotic
Cardiac Vascular Prosthesis placement Neurosurgery Thoracic Orthopaedic	*S. aureus* coagulase negative staphylococci	Cefuroxime 750 mg i.v. or Vancomycin 15 mg/kg i.v. (if cephalosporin sensitive)
Gastro-intestinal	G− bacilli, *S. aureus,* *S. faecalis* anaerobes,	Cefuroxime 750 mg i.v. + Metronidazole 500 mg i.v. ± Gentamicin 5 mg/kg i.v. (3 mg/kg in renal disease)
Obstetric/gynaecological	G− bacilli, *S. aureus,* group B streptococci, anaerobes	
Head and neck (including dental)	*S. aureus* streptococci, anaerobes	
Urological	G− bacilli, *S. faecalis*	Gentamicin 120 mg i.v. Amoxycillin/clavulanic acid 1.2 g i.v.

Subsequently, therapy should be guided by the appropriate antibiotic sensitivities obtained after microbiological culture. The main types of antibiotics currently used are listed in Table 11.7.

Antibiotic resistance

Bacteria may be naturally resistant to antibiotics, or may acquire immunity by a number of mechanisms. What is clear, however, is that antibiotic resistance is increasing: species that were formerly sensitive to certain antibiotics have mutated into resistant forms. Examples include MRSA and VRE. The development of antibacterial resistance is primarily due to the indiscriminate use of current antibiotics, such that inadequate doses of broad-spectrum antibiotics are being administered for an inadequate time period.

Natural bacterial resistance may occur due to

- natural impermeability to antibiotic molecules,

- lack of target-binding sites,

- lack of target metabolic pathway,

- the production of antibiotic-destroying enzymes (e.g. β-lactamases).

Combinations of β-lactam antibiotics with β-lactamase-inhibiting drugs (e.g. amoxicillin + clavulanic acid − co-amoxiclav) may be effective against β-lactamase-producing bacteria.

Acquired resistance may result from

- alteration in cell wall/membrane permeability;

- alteration in target-binding site (e.g. penicillin-resistant *S. pneumoniae*);

- alteration in metabolic pathway (e.g. trimethoprim resistance);

Table 11.7 **The main groups of antibiotics**

Antibiotic	Site of action	Effective against	Side-effects
β-lactams (penicillins, cephalosporins)	Bacterial cell wall	Broad spectrum or narrow spectrum	Hypersensitivity Nausea, vomiting, diarrhoea (NVD)
Antimetabolites (sulphonamides, trimethoprim)	Bacterial tetrahydrofolate production (→purine synthesis)	Urinary infections	Blood dyscrasias Rashes
Glycopeptides (vancomycin, teicoplanin)	Bacterial cell wall	Severe G+ infections	Blood dyscrasias Renal impairment
Quinolones (e.g. ciprofloxacin)	Bacterial DNA gyrase	G− infections *Pseudomonas*	NVD Cytochrome P450 inhibition
Rifampicin	Bacterial DNA-dependent RNA polymerase	G+ cocci *Mycobacteria*	Liver enzyme induction Deranged liver function tests (LFTs) Orange urine
Protein synthesis inhibitors Macrolides (erythromycin) Chloramphenicol	Bacterial 50S ribosomal subunit	G+ cocci Bacilli	NVD Cholestatic jaundice Blood dyscrasias Grey baby syndrome
Tetracyclines	Bacterial 30S ribosomal subunit	G− bacteria (especially, gynae flora)	Adsorbs onto growing bones and teeth
Aminoglycosides (gentamicin)	Bacterial 30S ribosomal subunit	G-organisms	Ototoxicity Nephrotoxicity
Metronidazole	Forms high-energy bactericidal free radicals due to low redox potential	Anaerobes	NVD Antabuse effect Taste Neuropathy
Azole antifungals (e.g. fluconazole)	Fungal membrane	Yeasts *Candida*	Mild liver enzyme induction
Polyene antifungals (e.g. amphotericin B)	Membrane sterols (bacteria and humans)	Many fungal species	Deranged K^+, Mg^{++} and LFTs Nephrotoxicity Anaemia NVD

11

11

- gene activation to produce antibiotic-destroying enzymes (e.g. aminoglycoside resistance);
- New gene acquisition to produce antibiotic-destroying enzymes.

HIV infection

The HIV is a retrovirus that infects CD4 (helper) lymphocytes (amongst others), with the result that cell-mediated immunity to infection is compromised. Up to 30,000 people are infected with HIV in the UK, a third of whom remain undiagnosed; 1.3% of the hospital patient population is infected with HIV. People with HIV infection are surviving longer due to earlier diagnosis and effective antiretroviral therapy. However, antiretroviral therapy, usually taken as a combination (triple therapy) of two nucleoside analogues and a protease inhibitor (e.g. zidovudine – AZT), can have marked side-effects including pancreatic, hepatic and renal dysfunction, peripheral neuropathy, bone marrow suppression and gastrointestinal (GI) disturbances, all of which may debilitate the patient prior to operation.

The normal CD4 count is 0.6–1.5 $\times$ 10^9 cells/l, but falls progressively after infection.

Symptomatic disease typically occurs below 0.2 $\times$ 10^9 cells/l, and is associated with susceptibility to opportunistic and postoperative infections (the latter occurring in up to 60% of cases) (Table 11.8). Opportunistic infections may include bacteria, viruses (especially herpes simplex (HSV) and varicella zoster (VZV) viruses, and cytomegalovirus (CMV)), fungi and protozoa, and there is a greater risk of these being multidrug-resistant. Immuno-suppression may be further worsened by major surgery, anaesthesia, malnutrition, malignancy, concurrent organ failure and drug abuse.

HIV infected patients may present for any type of surgery. In the absence of any ethical or practical screening programme, all hospital patients undergoing surgery are effectively treated as if they might be infected, i.e. universal precautions are employed for every patient. These precautions include:

- avoidance of contact between the patients' body fluids and health care workers' skin or mucous membranes (gowns, gloves, masks/goggles, avoidance of hollow needles and aerosolisation of fluids);

Table 11.8 **Potential postoperative infections in HIV-infected patients**

Site of sepsis	Causative organisms
Superficial wounds/venous access	*S. aureus, S. epidermidis,* Coliforms, *Bacteroides* spp., *Psuedomonas aeruginosa,* HSV, VZV
Deep wounds/prostheses	*S. aureus, S. epidermidis,* Coliforms, *Bacteroides* spp.
Respiratory tract	*S. aureus, Pneumocystis carinii, Mycobacterium tuberculosis, S. pneumoniae, Legionella pneumophilia,* fungi
GI tract	Coliforms, *Bacteroides* spp., *Pseudomonas aeruginosa, Candida albicans, Cryptosporidium parvum, Clostridium difficile*
Urinary tract	Coliforms, Enterococci
CNS	CMV, HSV, *Toxoplasma gondii, Cryptococcus neoformans*
Septicaemia	All of the above organisms, if immuno-suppression is severe

- use of electrocautery, blunt dissection and stapling guns, instead of scalpels and sutures;
- use of intermediate receptacles for the handling of sharps;
- guidelines for splash or direct inoculation injuries.

All doctors are obliged to avoid infecting themselves *and others*. Surgeons and anaesthetists should seek advice perioperatively from HIV specialists and microbiologists. In addition, doctors should adopt practices which reduce exposure of the patient to opportunistic infections. Measures include the use of skin preparation and scrupulous aseptic technique, microbiological screens prior to surgery, prophylactic antibiosis and early treatment of suspected infection

11

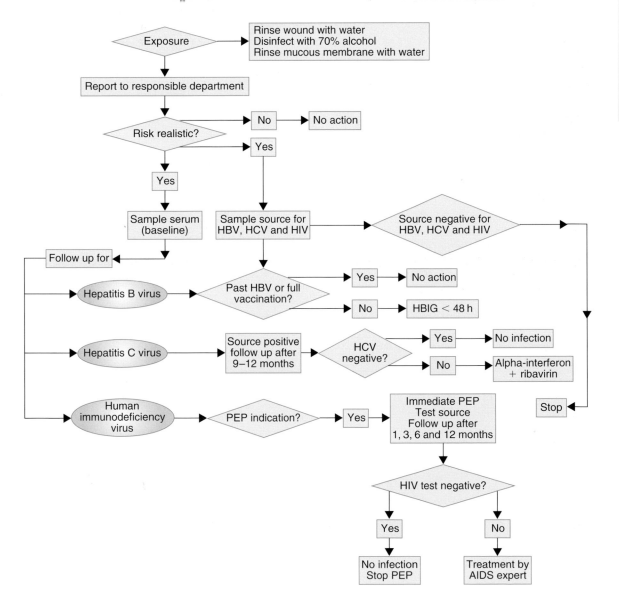

Fig. 11.2 The course of action to be taken by a health care worker after suspected inoculation from an HIV-, hepatitis B- or C-infected patient (HBIG, hepatitis B immune globulin; PEP, post-exposure prophylaxis). (Source for copyright, World Organisation of Gastroenterology, website http://www.omge.org/guides/guideline2.htm#action)

and appropriate perioperative isolation procedures including barrier nursing. Surgery may be deferred until the patient overcomes a concomitant infection, or until the CD4 count has recovered to an appropriate level (e.g. above 0.5 × 109 CD4 cells/ for contaminated surgery).

Postoperative pulmonary infections may be reduced by the appropriate use of regional anaesthesia, together with chest physiotherapy and early mobilisation.

The risk of transmission of HIV from a patient to a health care worker is reported as 1/450,000 to 1/1.3 billion. The risk of transmission of HIV from an infected surgeon to a patient is 1/130,000. Approximately 6/100 operations are associated with percutaneous injury to the surgeon. The seroconversion rate after percutaneous exposure is 0.3%. The flow chart (Fig. 11.2) details the course of action to be taken by a health care worker after suspected inoculation from an HIV-infected patient.

12

The role of ICU/HDU in the management of high-risk surgical patients

Aims

■ To define the basic concepts of critical care both ICU and HDU.

■ To explore the limitations of critical care.

■ To establish the proper roles of critical care, both pro- and re-active in the management of high-risk surgical patients.

Objectives

■ To promote the proper use of what is essentially a resource that is both scarce and costly.

■ To avoid inappropriate admission to critical care areas.

12

Introduction

The practice of intensive care medicine in general, and the management of the high-risk surgical in particular occur in an ever-changing environment, with shifting hues of a political, scientific, moral and social nature. The consideration of the potential place of critical care in the planned or unplanned care of the high-risk surgical patient invokes many factors beyond the simple technical feasibility of the surgery and the immediate postoperative management. The purpose of this chapter is to briefly outline these wider issues and establish their role in informing sound clinical judgement.

Definition of intensive care

In May 2000, the Department of Health published a document entitled '*Comprehensive Critical Care*'. The core of this document was a definition of the various levels of health care provided to patients in hospitals across the UK:

■ Level 0: normal ward care.

■ Level 1: acute (e.g. surgical) ward care.

■ Level 2: *high-dependency care* – involves detailed observation and support of *one* failing organ system, including *basic* respiratory support.

■ Level 3: *intensive care* – involves *advanced* respiratory support or basic respiratory support in combination with support to *two or more* failing organ systems.

This specification was also supported by a recommendation that all hospitals providing elective surgery should be able to provide Level 2 care, and the facilities for safe transport to Level 3 care either within the same institution or to an adjacent hospital. Typically, within any institution in the UK, between 1% and 2% of all hospital beds should be supported as critical care beds. This is a much lower percentage than in other countries. In the USA, up to 10% of beds may be designated as critical care beds.

The cost of intensive care

Intensive care is both a highly costly, and limited clinical resource. In an average North American Hospital, between 20% and 30% of the entire acute hospital budget may be allocated to intensive care services alone. In the UK, this figure is, typically, only between 1% and 2% of the acute hospital budget; however, at the time of writing this still works out to a running cost of about £1200 per bed, per day.

Measuring clinical performance in intensive care

The fact that intensive care is so severely demanding of resources, many audit tools have been developed to measure both efficacy and efficiency of delivered care.

Physiological scoring systems are used to determine clinical *efficacy*. Probably, the most commonly used physiological scoring system is the acute physiology and chronic health scoring system (APACHE 2), first devised by Knauss and published in 1985. The basic premise of this system is that severity of illness is defined by degree of physiological disturbance. Scores are assigned to 12 physiological variables reflecting the degree of departure from the normal value for each of the variables. Scores are also assigned for pre-existing medical conditions, and for age. Day 1 APACHE scores are used to define the presenting severity of illness together with a predicted mortality. APACHE scores on subsequent days are used to assess the patient's response or otherwise to treatment. In audit terms, the patient episode is *stratified* according to the severity of presenting illness, and the standard mortality ratio (for that stratum) calculated:

$$\text{standard mortality ratio} = \frac{\text{observed mortality rate}}{\text{predicted mortality rate}}$$

Intervention scores are used to determine clinical *efficiency.* These scoring systems are based on the hypothesis that the intensity of intervention defines the severity of illness by proxy. A common example of such a scoring system is the therapeutic intervention scoring system (TISS). This system was first devised by Cullen and published in 1974. Basically, a score of 1–4 is assigned to each of 70 medical and nursing procedures on a daily basis.

As with many aspects of medical science, clinical applications can be used for purposes beyond which they were originally intended. There is a great drive today in political and managerial circles to assess 'quality' of care delivered, and clinical scoring systems are increasingly being utilised as indices of quality. However, these systems have significant limitations when applied within the context of critical care:

- Problems with data quality.
- Lead-time bias.
- The significance of age.
- Limitation of outcome assessment.

Problems with data quality

The quality of the database is only as good as the human agent that collects it. Errors occur through recording errors, omissions and errors of interpretation.

Lead-time bias

This term originates from the science of systems management, and refers to the fact that in a system built of multiple components, the function of one component can affect the function of another. Thus in intensive care, does the quality of patient care on the ward, prior to admission, impact on subsequent outcome in intensive care, independently of the quality of intensive care treatment? Or again, are the APACHE scores captured before or after initial resuscitation? If it is captured after resuscitation, then the score may not accurately reflect the severity of illness. This is a particular problem if resuscitation has been attempted on the ward prior to admission.

The significance of age

As discussed below, age may be regarded as a physiological variable that impacts *directly* on outcome. However, age is also an *ethical* and *social* variable that can impact *indirectly* on patient outcome through its subjective influence on the responsible clinician.

Limitation of outcome assessment

This factor, above all others, points to the severe limitation of clinical scoring systems. These scoring systems record only a simple binary outcome, either 'death' or 'survival'. This then begs the questions:

- Is survival always a positive outcome or is death always a negative outcome?

- How about the *quality* of survival or how about the *quality* of dying?

Thus, although at first glance, clinical scoring systems provide a completely objective solution to assessing the quality of delivered care, there are, in point of fact, elements of subjectivity in both their derivation and interpretation. Perhaps, 'quality' like beauty yet remains ultimately in the eye of the beholder.

Clinical outcomes in intensive care

In 50 years of the practice in intensive care medicine, overall mortality has remained fairly

12

constant at between 20% and 30%. Further, more recent studies have suggested that up to 50% of admissions to intensive care are inappropriate. Significant resources are expended on patients who, by reason of severity of illness, cannot possibly benefit from intensive care, and who are destined to die. In point of fact, it may cost twice as much to die on intensive care as it does to survive. Studies also indicate that up to 60% of intensive care admissions are effectively preventable. Given the significant resource implications of intensive care, these figures highlight important problems of both a financial and ethical nature. The observation that intensive care outcomes have not significantly improved in 50 years of practice may at least partly be explained by the following factors:

- Cost constraints on clinical practice.

- Advancing surgical techniques.

- An ageing population.

- Genetic factors.

- Lack of an evidence base.

Cost constraints in clinical practice

There is a constant imbalance between demand and supply for intensive care beds within the UK through lack of appropriate funding. In a recent review, this factor was identified as the primary reason that the UK has one of the most severely ill intensive care populations. Typically, patient admission to intensive care is delayed until it becomes an absolute necessity. The inevitable consequence of this approach is that by the time the patient reaches intensive care, their disease process has progressed to such a stage that the chances of preventing or reversing multiorgan dysfunction have become remote. The reviewer rightly observed that this re-enforces cost-ineffective practice, by concentrating scarce resources on patients who may no longer be able to benefit, and whose death is then deferred at great emotional and financial cost.

Advancing surgical techniques

The technical possibilities of surgical technique are constantly expanding; supported in turn by ever-more sophisticated methods of anaesthetic monitoring and support. The risk/benefit equation seems to be shifting inexorably towards increasing surgical intervention, not simply for 'curative' procedures, but for the burgeoning 'palliative' or 'bridging' or 'salvage' procedure! There seems to be an increased willingness to intervene despite the almost certain knowledge that the patient will not survive. The gentle remonstrance that 'more may in fact be less' has little credence in the literal 'cut and thrust' of modern interventional surgery and anaesthesia.

An ageing population

Here, we venture onto almost forbidden territory. Yet, many years ago population biologists predicted a 'rectangularisation' of the survival curve (survival versus age). Basically, an ever-increasing proportion of the population would live to old age in a relatively fit state, their final demise occurring late in life would be a sudden, rapidly evolving, and consistent decline, as underlying physiological reserves were finally expended.

This view is in accord with basic principles of pathophysiology. Cell biologists suggest that all cells (and by turn, tissues and organs) have an in-built limitation to their working life. Hayflick's principle states that virtually all mammalian cells undergo a fixed number of divisions (~50) after which they are programmed to self-terminate, query through apoptosis. This principle makes sound teleological sense, since each time a cell divides inevitably minor errors occur in transcription (transmission) of genetic information to the 'daughter' cells. Single errors are probably of little import, but errors accumulating through many generations could potentially become highly significant, affecting the cell's ability to function normally. Conceivably, 'immortal' cell lines that divide an unlimited number of times progressively mutate through many generations to become unrecognisable.

12

The practical import of this is that all tissues and organs have an in-built functional time limit, and that physiological reserve necessarily declines with age. Given the increasing age of the population overall, and the rectangularisation of the survival curve, more and more therapeutic interventions will be applied in aged patients whose organ reserves are limited and often exceeded. Thus, it will become increasingly difficult, as we push back the limits of age as constraint to intervention, to make those interventions without triggering major upsets in the patient's physiology, leading in turn to varying degrees of organ dysfunction and even MOF.

The service implications of these simple biological facts are profound, and one fears not being currently addressed. Doctors will have to confront the basic physiological truth that in an ever-increasing proportion of the population (the aged), they will be deprived of the luxury of being able to make specific acute interventions in an entirely and controlled manner without having to carry the physiological consequences of their action. Simply stated, they must have the ability (and be willing) to manage all the consequences of their actions, i.e. to learn to look after *whole* patients again!

This, of course, flies in the teeth of received wisdom about medical and nurse training. We live in an age of the 'specialist' doctor and the 'specialist' nurse. Doubtless, these individuals are supremely skilled in their chosen field of interest, and able to focus in on the diagnosis and treatment of a specific problem very efficiently. However, in the real (and often unforgiving) world of aged whole-patient physiology, these individuals may be able to initiate, albeit unwittingly, a chain of physiological events by their specific intervention, but are unable to recognise, far less treat the consequences of that action.

To any conscientious medical practitioner working at ward level, the most obvious change occasioned by the highly 'specialised' and 'time-constrained' systems of training that now prevail, is the gradual disappearance of the acute general surgeon or the acute general physician. With their demise has gone the clinical experience necessary to properly co-ordinate, prioritise, and yes in some cases even limit, the care of sick patients at ward level.

Genetic factors

As discussed in Chapter 13, the role of genetic predisposition in the initiation and propagation of the acute phase response (APR) is being increasingly understood. The moral and ethical issues relating to this relatively recent insight have yet to be fully explored in depth. After nearly 50 years of wrestling with the APR and consequent MOF, it is humbling to reflect that to a significant degree, the ultimate outcome of the critically ill patient (death or survival) occurs *despite*, rather than *because* of, medical intervention, and goes someway to explaining the persistent mortality rate.

Lack of evidence-based practice

Paradoxically, for a speciality that relies so very heavily on scientific theory and technology, very little, if any, of the 'day-to-day' practice of the average ICU is rooted in an evidence base. The reason for this is really very simple, the single intervention/single outcome case-controlled study model widely deployed in most other areas of medicine is simply not applicable in the intensive care setting.

Firstly, the fact that each patient in unstable MOF presents an almost unique constellation of physiological variables, precludes any real form of case control. Secondly, the patient in MOF presents a positive melee of pathophysiological checks and balances, some ordered and some disordered, tracking the outcome of any single intervention in this complex and highly regulated system is well nigh impossible. There remains, therefore, no 'standard' practice in intensive care medicine from which to even begin to benchmark.

12

Key points in clinical practice

- Critical care beds are a limited commodity, costly in both money and human resource.

■ Patients should only be admitted to a critical care bed with some reasonable expectation of a *functional* recovery.

■ Critical care areas are not the appropriate setting to deliver *palliative* care or to simply defer death.

■ The fact that a surgical procedure is technically possible is not a sufficient justification for its application.

■ The risk/benefit analysis of a given intervention should extend beyond the first postoperative day to embrace *all potential outcomes*, and to pro-actively address the problem of the appropriateness or otherwise of treatment *escalation,* if it becomes necessary to the further maintenance of life.

■ To date, one of the few areas in which intensive care knowledge and technology have had a clear benefit on outcome is in the management of 'high-risk surgical patients'. In this group, relatively simple interventions, such as the maximising of oxygen delivery, have consistently reduced mortality and improved survival. The fact that similar interventions applied later in the course of established sepsis multiorgan dysfunction appear to confer no benefit, strengthens the argument for a pro-active approach to intensive care.

12

13

Sepsis, trauma and the acute phase response

Aims

The aims of this chapter are to

- understand the concepts of adaptive reduction,
- understand the basics of the acute phase response (APR),
- understand the role of oxidant stress and the function of anti-oxidants,
- understand the potential role for genetics and cell kinetics in the APR,
- understand the potential role of 'immunonutrition'.

Objectives

The objectives of this chapter are to

- provide a conceptual framework as the basis of understanding the APR,
- provide a rational basis on which to plan management of patients manifesting APR.

13

Understanding the basics of the acute phase response

The function of the APR is best understood when viewed in the context of its teleology.

Teleology is defined as the explanation of phenomena by the purpose they serve, rather than by postulating causes.

So what is the purpose of the APR?

All vital processes, locomotion, mechanical work, mentation, digestion, immune surveillance, require the consumption of free energy. That free energy is derived from the oxidation of various metabolic substrates namely, fats, carbohydrates and protein. In health a precise balance (homeostasis) is maintained between demand and supply of free energy through careful regulation of substrate intake, storage, mobilisation and oxidation.

The constraining circumstances of acute prostrating illness or polytrauma markedly disturb the balance between energy demand and supply. On the one hand, substrate intake from the environment is severely curtailed. On the other hand energy requirements are increased (basal metabolic rate + 30%) jointly by the demands of an activated immune system directed towards containment and elimination of microbial invasion, and by the demands for repair or replacement of damaged tissue.

The APR functions to restore the balance between energy demand and supply within the context of severe acute illness, through the process of *adaptive reduction* (see below).

In simple terms, the APR, once initiated, is a balance between a *pro-inflammatory* cascade of cellular and humeral elements, and an *anti-inflammatory* cascade. Survival is ultimately dependent on achieving a balance between the two. Excessive *pro-inflammatory* activity gives rise to the systemic inflammatory response syndrome (SIRS). Excessive *anti-inflammatory* activity gives rise to the compensatory anti-inflammatory response syndrome (CARS). Both conditions represent the extreme ends of the same spectrum of disordered physiology, and are associated with significant morbidity and mortality. The ability, or otherwise, to achieve a balance consistent with survival is probably an issue of genetic determination.

It may seem strange when faced with a patient in fulminant septic shock that the body can manifest such potential for seeming self-destruction. However, when viewed from the evolutionary context, i.e. considering the species as a whole rather than an individual, it is an entirely appropriate response. Given a species exposed to an infective agent, the APR acts to ensure that:

- those individuals destined to survive, survive better;
- those individuals destined to die, die quicker.

Thus, conserving to the species as a whole nutritional resource to those best able to usefully survive, within the constraint of prostrating infective disease.

The concept of adaptive reduction

Implicit in the concept of adaptive reduction is a re-ordering of the physiological melee around a new homoeostatic set point.

Two decades of applying various 'goal-directed therapies' and targeted pharmacology to the patient *in extremis* have yielded no significant success. In study after study, the common observation is that although clinical end points were achieved in treatment groups, and normal physiological values (commonly directed at oxygen balance) were restored, the ultimate outcome (mortality) remained unchanged between treatment and control groups.

Such accumulated evidence raises the question – are values considered 'normal' in health, appropriate in the established APR?

We now recognise that in all probability the physiology of states of extreme illness is very different from that of health. In the APR, the body's physiology moves to a new homoeostatic position, with a different profile of 'normal' parameters.

Again evolutionary biology may help to clarify the point. In the natural environment, an individual prostrated by extreme illness is not in a position to feed or even to process complex nutritional substrate, all the available free energy being directed to tissue repair and the mounting of an immune response.

In a state of prostration the body must defer to mobilising stored metabolic substrates, lipids in adipose tissue, proteins and carbohydrates in functional tissue. The process of mobilisation itself must incur the minimum of energy expenditure. Simple pre-processed substrates are the preferred fuel.

Clinical observation identifies the following four primary metabolic characteristics of the APR:

- a net negative nitrogen balance (nitrogen flux);

- loss of lean body mass despite presentation with appropriate calories either via the enteral or parenteral route;

- a marked resistance to insulin;

- in the conscious patient the paradoxical development (intriguingly) of anorexia.

Can we tie these simple clinical observations into some coherent explanation?

We are already familiar with the concept of shock in cardiovascular physiology, and the compensatory reflexes aimed at maintaining oxygen delivery to 'vital' tissues such as brain and myocardium, at the expense of 'non-vital' tissues such as kidneys and gut.

Oxygen of course is just one half of the basic oxidation reaction that underpins the mobilisation of free energy from any metabolic substrate. For the 'vital' tissues to survive requires that oxidisable substrate – the other half of the oxidation reaction – is also conserved and delivered to them in a similar preferential fashion.

There is mounting evidence that in states of extreme illness, just as oxygen is conserved to 'vital' tissues, so too are corresponding amounts of simple oxidisable substrate (primarily glucose).

Prostration itself is an integral part of the APR, the resultant reduction in mechanical work goes someway to redressing the balance between energy demand and supply. However, more significantly, the onset of insulin resistance effectively isolates the skeletal muscle mass from access to the circulating pool of plasma glucose, the muscle must then fall back on its own stores of energy for maintenance. The main source of energy substrate in muscle is protein, which, unlike fat substrates in adipose tissue, is 'stored' as functional tissue. Thus, mobilisation of energy rich substrate in muscle is necessarily at the expense of functional muscle mass. This accounts for the observed nitrogen flux, and reduction in lean body mass.

In these circumstances, tissue glutamine not plasma glucose becomes the primary metabolic substrate for muscle. Glutamine, which constitutes two-thirds of the free amino pool in skeletal muscle, is pivotal to

13

many vital functions at cellular level. From glutamine can be synthesised:

- the metabolic substrate glycogen;
- the ubiquitous anti-oxidant glutathione;
- the NO donor arginine (via citrulline), important in the modulation of vascular competence.

Glutamine in health is regarded as a *non-essential amino acid*, in that daily requirements for glutamine are well within the body's capacity for synthesis. However, in the APR where massively increased demand for glutamine (particularly, in skeletal muscle) outstrips the capacity to re-supply via synthesis, it thus becomes a *conditionally essential amino acid.* There is accumulating evidence that glutamine supplementation in the diet of severely ill patients, sufficient to restore normal plasma levels, reduces loss of lean body mass and improves outcome.

Further evidence for substrate 'conservation' comes from the proposed role of lactate in the APR. Established teaching on the metabolism of glucose divides it into *aerobic* and *anaerobic* metabolism.

In essence, the process of aerobic metabolism, located in the mitochondria involves the full oxidation of glucose (via pyruvate) to carbon dioxide and water with the generation of 38 molecules of ATP per glucose molecule oxidised.

The process of anaerobic metabolism in contrast, located in the cell cytoplasm (hexose monophosphate shunt (HMS)), involves the partial oxidation of glucose to lactate with production of only two molecules of ATP per glucose molecule utilised.

As the terminology indicates, classical physiology suggests that whether the available glucose is fully oxidised via the *aerobic* route, or only partially oxidised via the *anaerobic* route, is in fact determined by the ambient availability of oxygen. Anaerobic glycolysis and consequent lactic acidosis is then a direct result of tissue hypoxia or ischaemia.

Classical physiology further states that given aerobic metabolism yields 38 molecules of ATP per molecule of glucose, compared to a yield of only two molecules of ATP per molecule of glucose metabolised anaerobically, then aerobic metabolism is thus deemed *more efficient* than anaerobic metabolism.

However, for many years two types of lactic acidosis have been recognised clinically. Type 'A' lactic acidosis occurs in the presence of recognisable tissue hypoxia. Type 'B' lactic acidosis, on the other hand, occurs in the presence of normal ambient oxygen levels.

More recent work suggests that in point of fact it is *not* ambient oxygen tension that determines the route of glucose oxidation, *but* ambient circulating levels of catecholamine. The switch to lactate-based metabolism being associated with significantly elevated levels of circulating catecholamine.

What possible survival advantage could be conferred by utilising the apparently inefficient HMS as the preferred route of glucose metabolism in the APR?

A single molecule of glucose can only pass once through the aerobic pathway, since on being fully oxidised its constituent carbon atoms are effectively volatilised in the form of carbon dioxide and subsequently lost to the environment via ventilation. In contrast, a molecule of glucose having passed through the HMS is converted to a molecule of lactate. That molecule of lactate can then be returned to the liver and reconverted to glucose through gluconeogensis.

Thus, a molecule of glucose being fully oxidised in the aerobic pathway produces 38 molecules of ATP in a single pass, before being effectively irreversibly destroyed. But a molecule of glucose passing through the HMS, although only generating two molecules of ATP per pass, can be recycled via the liver and back through the shunt in an infinite number of passes, generating two molecules of ATP at each pass, dependent only on a functional liver.

Thus, the survival advantage of switching from aerobic to anaerobic glucose oxidation is that, despite the reduction in energy efficiency, carbon chains are conserved to the individual, and not lost to the

13

environment – carbon conservation. Lactate in this context acting as a 'redox shuttle' between metabolising tissues on the one hand, and the liver on the other.

There remains to consider the interesting observation that acute phase reaction is often accompanied by *anorexia* in the conscious patient. The immediate result of anorexia is the reduction of substrate intake from the environment. This raises the question why in times of significant increase in metabolic demand is there survival advantage in limiting substrate intake?

Ingestion of substrate from the environment in itself increases BMR and thus energy demands. There is an obligatory energy expenditure that occurs during substrate assimilation into the body, this energy expenditure is referred to as the *specific dynamic action* (SDA). Thus, for every 100 kcal of protein assimilated, 30 kcal of that energy is actually expended on the process of assimilation. The equivalent values for fat and carbohydrate are 4 kcal/100 kcal and 6 kcal/100 kcal, respectively.

In extremis there is a demand for maximum substrate availability at minimum metabolic cost, in the short term this demand is best met by mobilising the existing pool of glycogen, fats and amino acids stored in body tissues, rather than engaging in the costly process of assimilating environmental substrate.

Micronutrient deficits in acute illness may also contribute to the problems of environmental substrate assimilation. The body cannot utilise fat, carbohydrate and protein fully when vitamin deficiencies limit metabolic processing. The result is that intermediate products of metabolism accumulate in the circulation, and are probably directly responsible for stimulating the sensation of anorexia.

It is now recognised that it is not necessarily the absolute amount of a given macronutrient presented to the body in 24 h that is important, *but the rate at which it is administered.* In a similar way to drug handling, the body's ability to metabolise a given macronutrient (particularly lipid calories) becomes severely diminished in acute illness. In pharmacokinetic terms it marks the transition from '*first-order/non-saturable*' kinetics to '*zero-order/saturable*' kinetics (Chapter 3).

Thus, the onset of anorexia during the acute prostrating illness is probably an adaptive response directed to preventing overloading of the body's capacity to assimilate environmental substrate, through a negative feedback loop. Our ability to administer substrate (enterally or parenterally) to patients in such circumstances, effectively overriding this feedback loop, raises the potential for harm. Evidence suggests that the dangers of overfeeding patients in such circumstances are probably as great if not greater than the dangers of underfeeding, see Chapter 14.

The acute phase response

As discussed above the APR basically serves three functions:

- the containment and elimination of microbial invasion,

- the repair and replacement of damaged tissue,

- the diversion of free energy to effect these functions.

Essentially, the APR is made up of two elements:

- an *inflammatory response*, innate and non-specific mediated via humoral factors (cytokines), neutrophils, granulocytes and monocytes;

- an *immune response*, adaptive and specific mediated by 'T'- and 'B'-lymphocytes.

Two distinct phases can be distinguished in the APR:

- an *early phase*, which the inflammatory element predominates, thus termed *pro-inflammatory/immuno-suppressive*;

- a *late phase*, in which the immune element predominates, thus termed *anti-inflammatory/immunoproliferative*.

13

187

The early innate inflammatory response

The primary mediators of the inflammatory response are the cytokines produced from monocytes activated by damaged tissue, or structural fragments of micro-organisms. The cytokines function to recruit granulocytes to the area of damage or invasion firstly via chemotaxis and secondly via interaction with local vascular endothelium. Cytokines stimulate vascular endothelium to express adhesion receptors ensnaring granulocytes from the circulation and facilitating their passage across vessel walls and subsequent migration on to the site of inflammatory activity (margination).

Of the 20 known pro-inflammatory cytokines, only three produce specific *metabolic* effects:

- interleukin 1 (IL-1),
- interleukin 6 (IL-6),
- tumour necrosis factor (TNF) α.

The other 17 pro-inflammatory cytokines produce immuno-modulatory effect only.

There are three key factors that modulate the intensity of the early inflammatory response:

- oxidant/anti-oxidant balance,
- genetic factors,
- cell kinetics.

Oxidant/anti-oxidant balance

Free radical oxidants are the final effectors of the inflammatory cascade, killing cells by disruption of the lipid component of their outer membranes. Indiscriminate damage of invading cells and host tissue cells leads to further stimulation of cytokine production and the creation of a positive feed back loop.

However, a negative feedback loop also operates to moderate the intensity of oxidant action, through the simultaneous up regulation of the synthesis of the anti-oxidant glutathione. Production of glutathione requires the presence of certain dietary cofactors – micronutrients.

Reserves of anti-oxidant are depleted if micronutrients are not present. The following conditions are associated with reduction in micronutrient reserves:

- surgical stress,
- ARDS,
- inflammatory bowel disease,
- cirrhosis,
- type-2 diabetes,
- HIV infection,
- age.

Genetics and the inflammatory response

Between individuals there is an observed tendency to possess a constant ability to produce cytokines at high, medium or low levels, it would thus seem the individuals are 'hard wired' for cytokine production. The production of the pro-inflammatory cytokine TNFα is a case in point.

TNFα production is located on the short arm of chromosome 6, the locus has two regions designated TNFα and TNFβ, the α region specifies the molecule, and the β region controls the amount of production. Each region has two alleles:

TNFα region = alleles TNF1 and TNF2

TNFβ region = alleles TNFβ1 and TNFβ2

The presence of TNFβ1 is associated with low levels of TNFα production. Conversely, the presence of TNFβ2 is associated with high levels of TNFα production. Thus, the homozygous condition TNFβ2/TNFβ2 is associated with the worst outcomes in sepsis.

The presence of the TNFβ2 allele is associated with

- increased mortality in sepsis.

The presence of the TNF2 allele is associated with

- increased mortality in severe meningitis,
- rapid progression in HIV infection,
- increased morbidity in chronic hepatitis C,

- increased susceptibility to lepromatous leprosy,

- increased incidence of cardiac and renal transplant rejection.

Sexual dimorphism: Gender is now recognised to be a significant factor in outcome of the APR. In laboratory tests, female rats were more tolerant than male rats of lethal levels of circulatory stress, with a reduced propensity to develop acute lung injury. This survival advantage is lost following ovariectomy, but restored again with subsequent treatment with oestradiol. Oestrogen is known to enhance 'T'-cell function, conversely androgens are known to depress 'T'-cell function.

Observational work in human populations suggests that pre-menopausal women are more tolerant of sepsis than men of compatible age, but this survival advantage disappears after the menopause. Increased levels of oestrogen are known to depress production of the pro-inflammatory cytokines IL6 and TNFα. Further, immune cells are known to display receptors for sex hormones and prolactin. Prolactin reverses the 'T'-cell depression observed in overwhelming sepsis.

Cell kinetics and the acute phase response
In simple terms granulocytes, having fulfilled their function at the site of inflammation, need to be removed before the damage they cause becomes irreversible. Several lines of experimental evidence have emerged that support the hypothesis that, by contrast with necrosis, *apoptosis* (programmed cell death) provides the granulocyte clearing mechanism that functions to limit tissue injury.

Apoptosis occurs in response to pre-determined internal or external signals at cellular level. The important functional difference between apoptosis and necrosis is that the resultant cell detritus does not itself provide a focus to further amplify the inflammatory response.

Hypoxic conditions, when occurring in damaged tissue, tend to inhibit apoptosis, however, nitric oxide (NO) and high levels of TNFα tend to promote apoptosis. This may go some way to explain the beneficial effects of nitric oxide in inflammation.

The late adaptive immune response
At about 4–5 days the production and activity of pro-inflammatory cytokines wanes through a combination of inhibition by the anti-inflammatory cytokine IL-10, and the rising levels of the anti-oxidant glutathione, respectively. This is also a time of significant clonal proliferation of various 'T'- and 'B'-lymphocytes as an adaptive response. This massive proliferation of cells involves consumption of high levels of nutritional substrate, most notably glucose and glutamine.

Do analgesics and catecholamines administered to the unstable patient modify the acute phase response?
There is the intriguing possibility that drugs administered to the patient as part of a general supportive strategy have the potential to indirectly modify the APR.

Consider inotropes and vasoconstrictors administered to support BP in the patient in shock or cardiac failure. There is evidence that, for instance, β2 agonists have an anti-inflammatory effect and promote apoptosis. Dopamine agonists may potentially have an anti-inflammatory effect through the production of prolactin. In contrast, α1-agonists are known to up-regulate the production of pro-inflammatory cytokines.

Of particular interest is the apparent close relationship between the immune system and the nervous system reflected in the well-established links between opioid neuropeptides on the one hand, and the cytokine cascade on the other:

- Chronic opioid administration is known to have an immuno-suppressive effect in laboratory mice through depression of lymphocyte proliferation and γ-interferon production, an effect reversed by naloxone.

- Endorphins inhibit the production of the pro-inflammatory cytokine IL-6.

13

- Opioid μ-receptors modulate TNFα production in macrophages.

- Enkephalins released by pain fibres at the site of tissue injury cause instantaneous local up-regulation of cytokine production. Providing an immediate 'stop gap' response until the immune system can be fully activated.

Conversely,

- opioid μ-, δ-, and κ-receptor transcription in glial cells appears to be cytokine modulated;

- genes coding for endorphins are present in the genome of 'T'-lymphocytes, activated 'T'-cells migrating to the site of inflammation, release endorphins – a natural example of targeted analgesia.

Thus, there is very intimate relationship between the neural and immune systems, typified by the anatomical proximity of the two basic components of the CNS – neurones and glial cells. Glial cells are basically immunocytes that have taken up permanent residence in the CNS. The neuropeptides that support communication between these two cell populations are phylogenetically very ancient. There is a clear sequencing homology between both invertebrates and vertebrates divergent by several million years of evolution.

This has led Sebriakoff to postulate that cognitive neurological function has in fact evolved from the immune system. The early mechanisms of recognition and processing inherent in the immune system evolved through pain perception and associated avoidance strategies, to sentient processing of environmental information.

It may be that the opioids that we administer to patients to control the pain of tissue injury, are in point of fact a form of cytokine refined by millions of years of evolution!

The concept of immunonutrition
The forgoing discussion serves to illustrate that the clinical onset of the APR marks a profound change in underlying physiology and metabolism. Changes in metabolism in turn, lead to changes in substrate requirements. The concept of the 'Nutriceutical' aims to address the specific substrate requirements necessary to support an active immune response, by supplementing the 'conditionally essential' elements of a normal diet. Examples of these added elements include the following:

- *Glutamine:* an amino acid that provides the main metabolic substrate for activated immune cells, and is also thought to improve gut barrier function.

- *Arginine:* an amino acid necessary for the synthesis of NO donors, and thus in turn linked to vascular competence.

- *Sulphur-containing amino acids:* necessary for the synthesis of the anti-oxidant glutathione.

- *N3 polyunsaturated fatty acids:* promote the synthesis of anti-inflammatory cytokines and enhance lymphocyte function.

- *Nucleotides:* improve 'T'-cell function.

Trials of enteral and parenteral feed preparations containing theses added elements have yet to demonstrate significant benefit in outcome.

Key points in clinical practice

- The APR may constitute an evolutionary adaptive response to debilitating illness.

- As such it may be defined by a new set of 'normal' values that differ from the normal values pertaining to health.

- This may go some way to explain the failure of 'goal-directed therapies' when applied to patients in the established APR.

- The APR is in essence a complex cascade of cheques and balances, tampering with single (proximal) elements of this cascade, e.g. targeting TNF, may simply upset the balance and worsen outcome.

13

- However, studies on activated protein C suggest that therapies targeted at specific physiological endpoints in the (distal) cascade may improve outcome in certain circumstances.

- In extremis, it would appear that the body defers to utilisation of endogenous sources of nutritional substrate in preference to exogenous sources.

- In practical terms, this results in a reduction in the bodies ability to handle administered nutrition, particularly, lipid calories.

- Genetic predisposition plays a pivotal role in the genesis of the APR, and adapt ion to its metabolic consequences.

- For diagrammatic summary of the acute phase response please see below.

Diagrammatic summary of the acute phase response (APR)

The *early* acute phase response

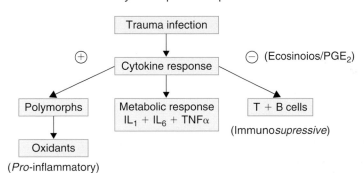

The *late* acute phase response

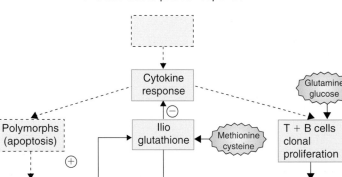

14

Principles of nutrition in perioperative medicine

Aims

This chapter attempts to give a very basic outline of the physiology relevant to nutrition and the practical aspects of clinical nutrition relevant to the practice of perioperative medicine. In particular, it outlines:

- the concepts of free energy, oxidation and combustion;
- the tri-carboxylic acid (TCA) cycle and the hexose monophosphate shunt (HMS);
- the concept of basal metabolic rate (BMR);
- the basic substrates utilised for free energy – fat, carbohydrate and protein;
- the balance between anabolism and catabolism;
- nutritional assessment;
- metabolic assessment – indirect calorimetry;
- the concept of a balanced diet;
- the process of enteral feeding;
- the process of parenteral feeding.

Objectives

After reading this chapter, you should:

- have a basic overview of relevant physiology;
- understand the prevalence of malnutrition in clinical practice;
- be able to make an objective clinical assessment of nutritional status;
- be able to identify nutritionally 'at-risk' patients presenting for surgery;
- appreciate the importance of feeding up patients prior to elective surgery;
- understand the impact of nutritional status on clinical outcome following surgery;
- formulate a basic plan for nutritional intervention in the perioperative period;
- be able to communicate relevant details when referring cases to clinical nutritionists and biochemists.

14

Introduction

The issue of nutrition in perioperative care highlights an emerging problem in the practice of modern hospital medicine in the UK. Much energy is directed at the high profile aspects of surgical intervention, refining surgical techniques in respect to access, extent of resection, and intra-operative imaging. However, the *basic* details of patient management – fluid and nutritional optimisation are often overlooked.

Anyone who doubts this assertion should take careful note of recently published data suggesting that within the NHS, 40% of elective surgical cases are admitted to a surgical ward in a pre-existing clinical state of malnutrition, and further, that 60% of patients leaving an NHS hospital following treatment are discharged in a worse nutritional state than when they were admitted.

As long ago as 1936, Studley observed that in patients presenting with perforated peptic ulcer, those who were clinically underweight (20% or more by predicted values) on admission, had an overall postoperative mortality of 33%, compared to a postoperative mortality of 3% in those whose weight on presentation was within the normal range.

Studies indicate that failure to maintain normal cell turnover, including the delayed healing of surgical wounds can occur when an individual looses as little as 5–10% of body weight (BW). Evaluation of the economic impact suggests that clinical malnutrition increases the cost of a single surgical episode by as much as 50% through increased length of stay and number of infected episodes.

Basic physiology

All vital processes, mechanical work, mentation, digestion, immune surveillance, require the consumption of free energy. Chemical free energy is firstly released from the oxidation of nutritional substrates,

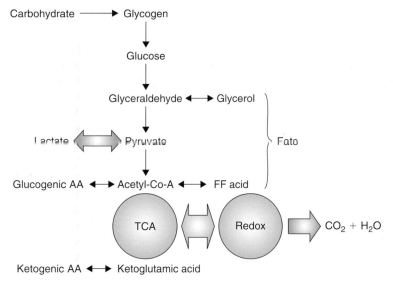

Fig. 14.1 Basic physiology of nutrition.

namely fats, carbohydrates and proteins, and subsequently stored in the form of high-energy phosphate bonds.

Thus, in simple terms, the currency of biological free energy is the phosphate bond. Various nutritional components may be processed either through the HMS which is located in the cell cytoplasm, or the TCA cycle which is located within mitochondria. The central intermediate product of metabolism is pyruvate. Pyruvate is metabolised via the HMS to lactate (partial oxidation) yielding two phosphate bonds per molecule. Pyruvate metabolised via the TCA (full oxidation) yields 38 phosphate bonds per molecule, the end products of full oxidation being carbon dioxide and water. Different nutritional components feed into the system via different intermediate metabolites and are summarised in Fig. 14. 1.

If the total free energy contained in each molecule of glucose was released instantaneously the result would be an explosive reaction – combustion, which would be catastrophic for the cell. Thus, the energy is released in a controlled stepwise fashion through a series of paired reduction/oxidation reactions known as a redox chain (Fig. 14.2).

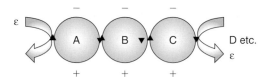

Fig. 14.2 The Redox chain and extraction of free energy.

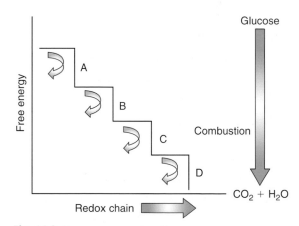

Fig. 14.3 Free energy extraction.

Thus, the free energy of oxidation/combustion is extracted in small manageable amounts (Fig. 14.3):

■ the *oxidation* of 'A' is exothermic;

■ the *reduction* of 'B' is endothermic;

14

- the oxidation of 'A' is more exothermic than the reduction of 'B' is endothermic;

- there is thus a small net release of free energy in this redox pairing;

- this is repeated B/C, C/D, etc.;

- free energy released is stored in phosphate bonds.

Basal metabolic rate

The minimum energy requirement to sustain normal bodily function is known as the BMR. This equates to approximately 2000 kcal/day (30 kcal/kg) in an average man, but can be calculated from the Schofield/Harrison–Benedict equation, which accounts for age, sex, and weight.

Schofield/Harrison–Benedict equation:

15–18 years = 17.6 × weight + 656
13.3 × weight + 690

18–30 years = 5.0 × weight + 690
14.8 × weight + 485

30–60 years = 11.4 × weight + 870
8.1 × weight + 842

60+ years = 11.7 × weight + 585
9.0 × weight + 656

The Schofield/Harrison–Benedict equation calculates BMR, actual calorie requirements in 24 h depend on level of activity thus:

- low physical activity = BMR × 1.4,

- moderate physical activity = BMR × 1.5,

- heavy physical activity = BMR × 1.6.

It seems almost counter-intuitive that the difference in calorific requirement between low and heavy physical activity is only 0.2 BMR. This leads to the question: Where does the calorific requirement for BMR come from? – The main components of calorific demand are as follows:

- mechanical work = 50% BMR,

- membrane transport = 25% BMR,

- cell turnover = 25% BMR.

The significant calorific consumption of membrane pumps, particularly Na^+/K^+-ATPase accounts for the generalised shift of fluid into the intra-cellular compartment with resultant tissue oedema that occurs in critical illness and malnutrition. The relative lack of calories leads to shut down of membrane pumps with consequent influx of sodium and water into cells. Rapid nutritional replenishment is associated with the re-feeding syndrome, which is simply a clinical manifestation of the re-activation of membrane pumps (see later).

Tissue calorie utilisation divides up as follows:

- brain ~ 25% BMR,

- liver ~ 25% BMR,

- muscle ~ 25% BMR,

- other ~ 25% BMR.

In relation to stores of free energy, an average man will carry 2000 kcal of carbohydrate calories and 120,000 kcal of fat calories, given the daily requirement of about 2000 kcal, this constitutes enough stored energy for about 60 days.

As in oxygen delivery, a balance exists between nutritional demand and nutritional supply. Demand results primarily from the requirements of free energy for active function on the one hand, and tissue repair and maintenance on the other. As discussed in the chapter on the APR, an activated immune system imposes a considerable increase in demand for free energy, which if unmet constitutes 'nutritional stress' entirely analogous to the concept of oxygen stress.

The precise balance between storage and utilisation of free energy is controlled by a balance between 'anabolic' and 'catabolic' hormones.

The principle *anabolic* hormones are as follows:

- Insulin:
  - increases glucose phosphorylation and glycogen synthesis;
  - increases esterification of free fatty acids;
  - increases protein synthesis.

- Growth hormone:
  - increases glucose transport into muscle;
  - decreases glycogen synthesis in the liver;
  - increases protein synthesis.

The principle *catabolic* hormones are as follows:

- Glucagon:
  - increases glycogenolysis,
  - increases hepatic uptake of amino acids,
- Cortisol:
  - increases mobilisation of free fatty acids,
  - increases proteolysis,
  - increases gluconeogensis.

Basic principles of perioperative nutrition

Management of perioperative nutrition involves three basic stages, namely:

- determining which patients need nutritional support through *nutritional assessment*,
- selecting the *appropriate level of nutritional support* and appropriate substrate,
- *obtaining access* for the delivery of the substrate.

Nutritional assessment

There are basically two components to nutritional assessment, evaluation of *body composition*, and evaluation of *body function*.

Body composition

There are three basic elements in assessing body composition, collectively referred to as *anthropometric measurements*, namely:

- BW,
- lean body mass,
- fat stores.

BW is properly expressed in relation to body height, the so-called body mass index (BMI):

$$BMI = \frac{weight\ in\ kg}{height\ in\ m^2}$$

Overweight BMI = 25–30; obese BMI = 30–40; severe (morbid) obesity BMI > 40.

Lean body mass is assessed clinically as *mid-arm muscle circumference*; however, this parameter tends to overestimate lean body mass.

Fat stores are assessed clinically as *triceps skin-fold thickness*; however, this parameter tends to underestimate fat stores.

Body function

There are three basic elements in assessing body function namely measurement of

- dynamometric function,
- synthetic function,
- metabolic function.

Dynamometric function is assessed as *grip strength* in the non-dominant hand.

Synthetic function is assessed as a laboratory assay of the levels of various synthesised proteins in the plasma. For example, retinal-binding protein, thyroxine-binding protein and transferrin. The utility of measuring these plasma proteins is that (unlike albumin) they have a short half-life and rapid turnover, thus any sudden cessation in synthesis will manifest rapidly as falling plasma levels.

Metabolic function or calorific requirement can be assessed through the principle of 'indirect calorimetry'.

14

Theory of indirect calorimetry

Indirect calorimetry relies on the fact that all substrates are utilised through the same mechanism, i.e. oxidation. Four basic assumptions underlie its practical application:

- *Assumption 1:* that the amount of energy produced is directly proportional to the volume of oxygen consumed.
- *Assumption 2:* that each substrate has a given calorific yield per litre of oxygen consumed:
  - fat = 4.6 kcal/l oxygen consumed,
  - carbohydrate = 5.0 kcal/l oxygen consumed,
  - protein = 4.3 kcal/l oxygen consumed.

197

■ *Assumption 3:* that each substrate has a characteristic respiratory quotient, i.e. the unit volume of carbon dioxide produced per unit volume of oxygen consumed.

■ *Assumption 4:* that in normal function the calorific contribution of protein substrate is minimal.

Firstly, measure the respiratory quotient for the patient. It will lie somewhere between the extreme values of 0.7 (fat) and 1.0 (carbohydrate) depending on what particular combination of substrates is being metabolised. Secondly, from the nomogram read off the corresponding calorific value for oxygen. Thirdly, measure the oxygen consumption.
Energy requirements (consumption, Kcals/min) can be calculated from the product of

oxygen consumption (l/min) × calorific value
    = Kcals/min

The basic limitation of this technique is the assumption that protein catabolism is not a source for free energy, this assumption may hold true in health, but is not valid in critical illness where protein catabolism correlates with severity of illness (Fig. 14.4).

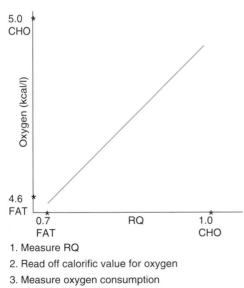

1. Measure RQ
2. Read off calorific value for oxygen
3. Measure oxygen consumption
4. Oxygen consumption × calorific value = energy requirement (see text)

Fig. 14.4 Assessment of energy requirements – theory of indirect calorimetry.

Clinical features of malnutrition

As in all aspects of acute medicine, the monitoring of physiological and biochemical parameters should be used to support, not replace, clinical observation. The clinician managing patients for major surgery should be ever vigilant for the stigmata of malnourishment presenting in the preoperative patient. Typical signs and symptoms include the following:

■ depression and apathy,

■ immuno-suppression,

■ reduced renal excretion of sodium and water,

■ hypothermia,

■ loss of shivering reflex,

■ cardiac and ventilatory impairment,

■ impaired gut integrity,

■ generalised oedema of non-cardiac origin.

Beyond a weight loss of about 45% original BW (i.e. 65% baseline weight) the changes associated with malnutrition become irreversible and death becomes inevitable. In males this point of no return corresponds to a BMI < 14, and in females a BMI < 12. A patient in acute catabolic critical illness can lose between 1% and 2% of lean body mass per day. Thus an unremitting acute catabolic state can bring a patient to the nutritional point of no return in approximately 20 days, where death will occur simply due to the affects of malnutrition quite apart from any other co-existent morbidities.

Level of nutritional support and appropriate substrate

Nutritional intervention ranges from simply encouraging a balanced oral diet, to full total nutrition either via the enteral or parenteral route.

Encourage oral feeding

Despite provision of hospital catering delivered to the bedside, many patients do not eat. This may be for a variety of reasons – the poor quality of the food, feeling nauseated and the presence of pain. These issues are easily corrected by the provision of high quality catering, treatment of relevant symptoms and proper supervision at meal times.

Food supplementation
So-called 'modular' feeds are incomplete, being composed of a single macronutrient, e.g. carbohydrate. They are only indicated to 'supplement' not replace normal dietary intake.

Promote digestion
So-called 'elemental' or 'pre-digested' feeds contain protein in the form of oligo-peptides or amino acids. Their use is indicated in states of reduced absorption capacity such as short bowel syndrome or inflammatory bowel disease. One practical drawback of these feeds is their consequently high osmolarity.

Total nutritional support
Total enteral or parenteral nutrition involves the provision of a fully balanced diet in the form of a solution. A balanced diet has four basic components:

- water,
- electrolytes,
- macronutrients (metabolic substrates),
- micronutrients (catalysts and cofactors).

Water
This acts as the universal solvent for all biological reactions. Sufficient water should be provided in a balanced diet to account for both sensible and insensible loss. The issue of sensible loss and fluid repair is addressed in the chapter on fluid balance. Any nutritional regimen should account for insensible fluid loss – and the provision of 'maintenance' fluid.

Typical insensible water loss = 35 ml/kg BW in 24 h, i.e. about 2.5 l in the average man (these values refer to adults only, see Chapter 4).

Historically, by shear coincidence calorific requirements were also calculated to be 35 kcal/kg in 24 h. Thus, parenteral and enteral solutions were made up to an energy concentration of 1 kcal/ml solution. Precise daily calorific requirements remain an issue for debate, and the tendency in recent years has been to revise down the figure. Modern feeding solutions are thus now available that contain calories at lower concentration, thus avoiding the risk of overfeeding while at the same time providing for adequate fluid maintenance.

Electrolytes
In contrast to the provision of calories where the absolute amount and precise mixture remain an issue of unresolved debate (see below), the provision of electrolytes is well established. Any feeding regimen should provide the following basic electrolytes:

- sodium = 1–2 mmol/kg/day,
- chloride = 1–2 mmol/kg/day,
- potassium = 1–2 mmol/kg/day,
- calcium = 0.1 mmol/kg/day,
- magnesium = 0.1 mmol/kg/day.

Electrolytes function to maintain the functional distribution of water between the various intracellular and extracellular compartments, and to regulate membrane potentials in the excitable tissues namely muscle and nerves.

Macronutrients
Their function is to provide the two prime elements in nutritional support, namely:

- nitrogen,
- calories (in the form of free energy substrates).

Nitrogen: Analogous to the concept of insensible fluid loss is the concept of nitrogen flux. Nitrogen flux arises from the cell turnover and wastage that occurs in maintaining tissue viability. Nitrogen is the end product of protein breakdown and is excreted in the urine. Thus, just as analysis of carbon dioxide (and oxygen) in exhaled breath can be used to calculate calorific requirement, so analysis of nitrogen excreted in the urine can be used to calculate nitrogen losses and replacement.

14

Urinary nitrogen loss is calculated as follows:

nitrogen g/24 h = urinary urea (mmol/l)
$$\times \text{ urine volume (l in 24 h)}$$
$$\times 0.28 \times 6/5$$

This formula allows for the conversion of mmol of urea to grams of nitrogen and corrects for the fact that urea accounts for approximately five sixths of total urinary nitrogen loss.

As discussed in Chapter 13 on the APR, catabolism may be thought of as an evolutionary mechanism to aid survival by providing nutrients, particularly amino acids for the APR. The assumption that high protein feeding is thus beneficial in catabolic patients may be invalid. High versus low protein feeding is known to cause increased mortality in famine victims. Two issues may be important here. It is not only the requirement for *absolute* amounts of various amino that increase in catabolism, but also their *relative amounts.* For example, there are high demands for glutamine and arginine for the immune system; cysteine and glutathione for the anti-oxidant system. Standard nutritional regimens may thus fail on two counts, firstly in failing to provide adequate levels of conditionally essential amino acids, secondly in providing a toxic excess of non-useful amino acids.

Current recommendations for nitrogen intake in 24 h have been revised down from 0.3 to 0.2 g/kg/24 h, 1 g of urinary nitrogen equating to 30 g of skeletal muscle. Thus, the average man (70 kg) loses 14 g of nitrogen per day equivalent to 420 g of skeletal muscle. (To put that in perspective, an average beef steak weighs 400 g.)

Calorific provision: As previously stated there are three basic sources of high-energy substrate namely, fats, protein and carbohydrate. Fats and carbohydrate are stored in specialised storage tissues, whereas protein is stored as *functional* tissue, mobilisation of protein calories thus comes at a price – the loss of functional tissue, principally skeletal muscle.

Formulation of feeds aims to provide the entire calorific requirement as a combination of carbohydrate and fat calories, and thus facilitate 'protein sparing'. There are various advantages and disadvantages of each calorie source (see below) and the precise optimal ratio of fat to carbohydrate calories still remains a subject for active debate. Typically the ratio lies somewhere between 30% and 50% as fat calories, and 50% and 70% as carbohydrate calories. The provision of calories is linked to the amount of nitrogen provided in the feed, thus approximately 150 kcal of energy is provided per 1 g of nitrogen present. (Note 1 kcal = 4.2 kJ.)

The efficacy of 'protein sparing' feeding regimens in the acutely catabolic patient remains to be established.

Micronutrients

These facilitate the delivery of free energy indirectly by providing catalysts and cofactors to the pathways of intermediate metabolism, in simple terms they facilitate mobilisation of free energy stores. Their other major contribution is in the synthesis of important anti-oxidants.

Daily requirements for important micronutrients are listed in Table 14.1.

The composition of liquid enteral feeds

So-called 'polymeric' feeds contain both macro- and micronutrients, including whole protein yielding approximately 5 g of nitrogen per litre of feed. They are formulated to give an energy concentration of 1 kcal/ml, although some formulations provide energy concentrations of between 1.5 and 2.0 kcal/ml to allow for a restricted fluid intake. Almost all preparations are lactose and gluten free. Some feeds have added fibre to reduce constipation and facilitate gut motility. Paradoxically these feeds containing added fibre have been found useful in the management of diarrhoea – presumably by modulating gut flora and preventing opportunistic overgrowth. Two litres of feed administered over 24 h gives 2000 kcal and 10 g of nitrogen.

The composition of liquid parenteral feeds

Commercially available parenteral feeds contain a complete profile of macro- and micronutrients in solution. Most feeds are

Table 14.1 **Daily requirements for important micronutrients**

Copper	1.2 mg/day
Iodine	140 µg/day
Selenium	75 µg/day
Zinc	9.5 mg/day
Vitamin A (retinol)	Max. 8000 µg/day
Vitamin B1 (thiamine)	4000 µg/1000 kcal
Vitamin B2 (riboflavin)	1.2 mg/day
Vitamin B3 (niacin)	6.6 mg/1000 kcal
Vitamin B6	15 µg/g protein
Vitamin B12	1.5 µg/day
Folate	200 µg/day
Vitamin C	40 mg/day
Vitamin D	SUNLIGHT
Vitamin E	7 mg/day
Vitamin K	1 µg/kg/day

presented prepared in 2-l bags, each bag designed to give a patient's total fluid and nutritional requirement over 24 h. The various preparations available vary in two basic aspects.

Firstly, in relation to the nitrogen content of the feed, nitrogen content varies from 5 to 14 g of nitrogen per 2000 ml of feed. Very low nitrogen content feeds containing ~5 g/bag are designed for patients being phased into nutritional support who may be chronically undernourished and who are at risk of re-feeding syndrome (see below). Low nitrogen feeds containing ~8 g/bag are designed for use in chronic renal failure where nitrogen excretion may be compromised.

Secondly, in relation to osmolarity of the feeding solution, the majority of parenteral feeds are hyperosmolar with an osmolality ~1200 mosm/kg due to the high glucose concentration in solution required to provide the required concentration of calories. This hyperosmolality renders them highly irritant and necessitates their being administered through a central vein. A number of preparations are now available with osmolality ~800 mosm/kg which are suitable for administration through a peripheral vein, so-called 'peripheral feeds'. The reduction in osmolality in peripheral feeds is achieved by a combination of reducing the overall calorie concentration, and increasing the proportion of lipid to glucose calories in the preparation.

Nitrogen is supplied as a mixed solution of essential and non-essential amino acids. The precise composition of the mixture is based on egg protein, which is taken as the gold standard. It is composed, 51%, of essential amino acids.

Carbohydrate calories are supplied as glucose in hypertonic solutions. The energy value of glucose being rated at 4 kcal/g, and the maximum rate of administration at 5 g/kg/day. The two basic disadvantages of excess glucose calories are firstly the high osmolality of solution and consequent venous irritation, and secondly the high respiratory quotient and consequent carbon dioxide production.

Fat calories are supplied as 10–20% Intralipid® solution, l, which despite its isotonicity, is still intrinsically irritant. The energy value of lipid is rated at 9 kcal/g and the maximum rate of administration at 2 g/kg/day. The basic disadvantages of lipid calories are: firstly, the high oxygen consumption required for their oxidation; secondly, that the bodies capacity to handle lipid calories in acute illness becomes significantly restricted, and thirdly overload of lipid calories will lead to hepatic and reticulo-endothelial dysfunction.

Access for delivery of substrate

The debate about the relative merits of feeding via the enteral route versus feeding via the parenteral route continues. There is a clinical impression, supported by limited evidence from meta-analysis, that the enteral route is superior. However, in assessing the

14

available data there are four points that should be remembered:

- The administration of PN is often associated with underlying gut failure – itself a significant predictor of mortality.

- Examination of historical studies in PN feeding suggest there is a tendency to overfeed, hyperglycaemia being a common problem, recent studies suggest that 'tight' control of blood sugars between the range 6–12 mmol, is itself associated with improved outcome.

- Feeding via the enteral route is functionally 'self limiting' in that sick patients do not absorb well, thus the risks associates with overfeeding (probably more significant than the risks associated with underfeeding) are avoided.

- The theory that gut wall 'integrity' is preserved in enteral feeding has no support in comparative histological examination – the degree of villous atrophy, and level of bacterial translocation, being equal across both PN and EN groups.

Theoretical advantages and disadvantages of the parenteral route

Parenteral feeds may be administered centrally through a central vein (usually the internal jugular or subclavian) or may be administered peripherally through a forearm vein. The precise choice is dependent on the planned level and duration of nutritional support, and the osmolality of the feeding solution selected.

Advantages
- Guaranteed delivery of substrate.

- Indicated in 'gut failure'.

- Comfortable for the patient.

Disadvantages
- Risk of overfeeding.

- Risk of fluid overload.

- Risk of hyperglycaemia.

14

- Vein injury.

- Infection at line sites.

- Chemical interaction between feed components in solution, e.g. the conditionally essential amino acid glutamine is unstable in solution.

Theoretical advantages and disadvantages of the enteral route

Enteral feeds may be administered either gastrically or in cases of gastric stasis post-gastrically.

Access to the gastric route may be via a fine bore NG tube passed under X-ray guidance or via a percutaneous endoscopic gastrostomy (PEG) sited endoscopically. Access to the post-gastric route may be achieved via a needle-catheter jejunostomy sited at laparotomy, or via a percutaneous endoscopic lejunostomy (PEJ) sited endoscopically.

Advantages
- 'Self-limiting' gut regulation of absorption.

- Liver activation.

- Preservation of gut wall integrity.

- Simple and cheap.

Disadvantages
- Tube displacement.

- Aspiration.

- Poor absorption.

- Diarrhoea.

- Patient discomfort.

Key points in clinical practice

Studies suggest that nutritional intervention prior to surgical insult, improves outcome. In contrast, nutritional intervention following surgical insult is not associated with any demonstrable improvement in outcome, and may in fact worsen outcome through overfeeding.

However, studies also indicate that maintenance function, including wound healing, can become impaired when individuals loose as little as 5–10% baseline BW. In catabolic patients post-major surgery this level of starvation can be achieved in about 5 days, thus despite the lack of an evidence base, it would seem prudent to *cautiously* feed the surgical patient as soon as possible after surgery. The following practical pointers should be used to guide nutritional support:

- In the first few days following surgery calculated energy requirements are estimated at BMR + 30%. However, various issues around the stress response and reduced gut motility in the postoperative period, limit substrate absorption and assimilation. There is thus some logic in restricting calorific intake, certainly for the first 48 h postoperatively, to 50% of calculated requirements.

- It is rare for even very sick patients to require more than 2000 kcal/day.

- The enteral route is the preferred route of administration in respect to 'self-limiting' absorption, reducing the risk of fluid overload and overfeeding.

- There is no evidence to support the notion that enteral feeding immediately after the first 24 h post-bowel surgery increases the risk of dehiscence.

- Given the broad concepts of pre-optimisation (Chapter 4) and the difficulties of absorption and assimilation that occur once the stress response is invoked, it is imperative to 'feed up' nutritionally vulnerable patients *before* major surgery. This would seem particularly true for elderly patients undergoing major elective surgery. Scandinavian studies have shown that a glucose challenge of 400 g given immediately prior to surgery, either by the enteral or parenteral route will decrease post-surgical stress as measured by insulin resistance and nitrogen flux, reducing the postoperative length of stay by up to 20%. Although explanations remain speculative, it would seem that glucose is altering metabolic settings perhaps via insulin stimulated membrane pumping. The body seems to cope better with injury when metabolically active rather than down regulated, perhaps this is also the reason for the benefits of nutritional support having little to do with the reversal of nitrogen wasting.

- Studies indicate that maintaining tight control on blood sugar levels, between the range 6.0–12.0 mmol/l with insulin infusion, has a beneficial effect on outcome compared to patients where sugar levels are just allowed to drift.

- Regular monitoring of hepatic function and infection screening should be carried out throughout the period of nutritional support.

The re-feeding syndrome

As stated above, 25% of basal energy consumption is directed to maintenance of membrane pump activity. In states of substrate depletion, pump activity is depressed, with consequent ICF shifts – manifest clinically as tissue oedema.

The re-feeding syndrome is simply a clinical manifestation of sudden membrane pump re-activation and is characterised by massive shifts of fluid back into the extracellular compartments with the consequent risk of cardiovascular overload. Sudden shifts of potassium and phosphate back into cells lead to clinical hypokalaemia and hypophosphataemia with the risk of cardiac dysrhythmias and skeletal muscle dysfunction, respectively.

14

15

Myocardial ischaemia, acute circulatory failure, life support and cardiopulmonary resuscitation

Aims

The aims of this chapter are to

- describe aspects of the functional anatomy of the cardiovascular system (CVS) which are appropriate to perioperative care of the patient;

- describe relevant aspects of cardiovascular physiology, and relate structure to function;

- discuss the cardiovascular response to surgery and anaesthesia;

- describe the pathophysiology associated with cardiovascular disease;

- discuss the perioperative management of patients with common cardiovascular diseases;

- discuss the theory and practice of basic life support (BLS) and advanced life support (ALS).

Objectives

After reading this chapter, you should be able to

- understand the physiological stresses placed on the body by surgery and anaesthesia;

- identify patients who are at greater risk of perioperative cardiovascular problems, such as those with left-ventricular failure, hypertension, chest pain and myocardial ischaemia;

- request and interpret appropriate investigations for such patients;

- rationalise treatment according to clinical indication;

- use your theoretical knowledge to confidently employ basic and ALS algorithms.

Introduction

Cardiovascular disease is the major cause of mortality and morbidity in Western countries.

Advances in general medicine and perioperative care have resulted in perioperative physicians encountering an increasingly elderly population (the number of surgical patients over the age of 65 is projected to increase by 100% by 2020), who are undergoing ever more invasive surgery. The multiple cardiovascular stresses associated with long, complex surgery and anaesthesia may reveal previously undiagnosed myocardial disease, or may substantially worsen pre-existing poor cardiac function.

In the US, approximately 30 million individuals a year undergo non-cardiac surgery, 10 millions of which have cardiac disease or major cardiac risk factors. In the UK, 20,000 deaths occur annually within 30 days of surgery, 40% of which have a cardiovascular aetiology. For every death, it is estimated that 5–20 patients suffer cardiovascular complications in the perioperative period, particularly if they have pre-existing cardiac disease. For example, the incidence of perioperative myocardial infarction (MI) is increased 10–50-fold in patients who have had previous coronary episodes; perioperative MI reduces 2-year survival from 95% to 23%.

Many researchers have attempted to stratify the risk of adverse cardiovascular outcomes in patients according to their preoperative condition and the type of non-cardiac surgery they are due to undergo (e.g. Goldman cardiac risk index, New York Heart Association classification). Some scoring systems have a better predictive value than others, but none are highly sensitive or specific. However, several factors may be identified that together suggest a patient is at risk of adverse cardiovascular events in the perioperative period. These are classified into patient-specific, surgery-specific and 'miscellaneous' factors (Table 15.1).

Rather than assessing the above risk factors in detail, the purpose of the first part of this chapter is to provide an anatomical and pathophysiological basis for the reader to understand the aetiology of perioperative cardiovascular disease, its consequences and the rationale for acute and chronic medical interventions.

15

Table 15.1 **The risk of perioperative cardiovascular complications in relation to patient-specific, surgery-specific and 'miscellaneous' risk factors**

| | Factor | Risk of perioperative cardiovascular complications | | |
		Low risk	Medium risk	High risk
Preoperative patient-specific risk factors	IHD	Abnormal ECG (LVH, LBBB, ST segment and T-wave abnormalities)	MI > 6 months ago Stable angina	Recent MI Unstable angina
	Cardiac failure	Poor exercise tolerance	Compensated – optimised by medical treatment	Decompensated (e.g. pulmonary/ systemic oedema)
	Cardiac dysrhythmia	Abnormal rhythm (e.g. AF)	Bi/tri fascicular block Temporary pacing	Paroxysmal VT, complete degree heart block, SVT with rapid ventricular rate
	Valvular heart disease			Severe AS, MS or MR leading to ventricular hypertrophy, cardiac failure or dysrhythmia
	Non-cardiac	Advanced age Cancer Anaemia Previous CVA	Diabetes Coagulopathy COPD Smoking	
Surgery-specific risk factors		Endoscopy Eye surgery Surface and breast surgery	CEA Maxillo-facial Orthopaedics Urology Non-emergency abdominal or thoracic	Emergency abdominal, cardiothoracic or trauma surgery Major vascular surgery Prolonged procedures requiring significant fluid transfusion
'Miscellaneous' risk factors		Out-of-hours operating	Non-availability of ITU or HDU care Grade of doctor	Inadequate monitoring facilities Poor medical knowledge Poor application of medical knowledge

Low risk = less than 1% rate of perioperative cardiac-related death or MI; medium risk = 1–5%; high risk = more than 5%; CEA = carotid end arterectomy; CVA = cerebrovascular accident; AS = aortic stenosis; MS = mitral stenosis; MR = mitral regurgitation.

15

Myocardial ischaemia

Ischaemia describes the loss of an adequate supply of oxygenated blood leading to cell hypoxia and consequent cell injury. Infarction occurs when ischaemia is severe enough to cause tissue death. In any organ of the body, ischaemia generally occurs when oxygen demand exceeds oxygen supply. The heart is no exception. Therefore, an understanding of the determinants of myocardial oxygen supply and myocardial oxygen demand is essential, in order to be able to diagnose the cause of myocardial ischaemia as well as to guide corrective treatment.

Ischaemia produces reversible increases in myocardial intracellular concentrations of hydrogen ions, potassium ions and lactate. Cellular necrosis ensues within 30 min, unless ischaemia resolves, resulting in the measurable release of cardiac enzymes, creatine kinase (CK) (MB subtype), lactate dehydrogenase and proteins (troponin I, myoglobin). Necrosis impairs both electrical conduction and myocardial contraction, leading to cardiac arrest, dysrhythmia and ventricular failure.

Myocardial oxygen supply

The arterial blood supply of the heart is derived mainly from the left and the right coronary arteries (LCA and RCA)(see Figs 15.1 and 15.2). There may be considerable population variation in terms of coronary artery 'dominance', i.e. the relative percentage of blood supplied to the heart by the LCA and RCA. The RCA originates from the anterior aortic sinus, passes between the pulmonary trunk and the right auricle, runs along the atrio-ventricular (AV) groove and descends across the anterior surface of the heart to the inferior surface, where it anastomoses with branches of the LCA. The RCA supplies blood to the sino-atrial (SA) node, the right atrium (RA), right ventricle (RV), and in the majority of the population (90%) the AV node. Therefore, ischaemia or infarction resulting from the loss of RCA blood flow will have three main

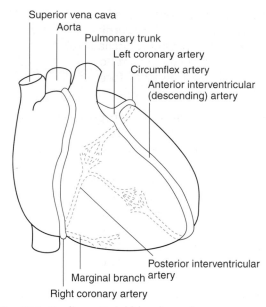

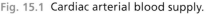

Fig. 15.1 Cardiac arterial blood supply.

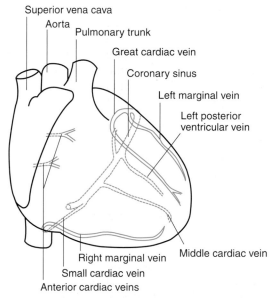

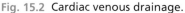

Fig. 15.2 Cardiac venous drainage.

clinical effects:

- right heart failure, caused by RA and RV damage (the central venous pressure (CVP) will be high);

- dysrhythmia, caused by SA or AV node damage (particularly, supra-ventricular dysrhythmias and various degrees of AV nodal block);

15

■ ECG changes. Dysrhythmia may be seen. ST depression (sub-endocardial ischaemia) or elevation (transmural ischaemia) may be seen in those leads that 'look' at the right lateral and inferior surfaces of the heart, i.e. leads II, III and aVF.

The LCA arises from the left posterior aortic sinus, passes the pulmonary trunk laterally and runs in the left AV groove, where it divides into the left anterior descending (LAD) or interventricular artery and the left circumflex (LCx) artery. The LAD descends anteriorly in the interventricular groove to the apex, where it anastomoses with the posterior interventricular artery (a branch of the RCA); it supplies the RV, left ventricle (LV) and interventricular septum. The LCx artery follows the AV groove to the posterior surface of the heart, where it anastomoses with the RCA; it supplies the left atrium (LA) and LV. It should be noted that although the LCA and RCA anastomose with each other, their interface is insufficient to prevent myocardial ischaemia during complete obstruction of one or other of the vessels. Ischaemia or infarction resulting from the loss of LCA blood flow will have two main clinical effects:

■ left heart failure, caused by LA and LV damage (with or without mitral valve incompetence), resulting in pulmonary oedema and reduced systemic tissue perfusion (cardiogenic shock)

■ ECG changes. Ischaemic changes may be seen in those leads that 'look' at the posterior (V_1), anterior (V_2, V_3), septal (V_3, V_4) and left lateral (aVL, V_5, V_6) surfaces of the heart. Main stem LCA blockage is, therefore, likely to produce ischaemic changes in V_1–V_6, LAD blockage in V_2–V_5 and LCx blockage in V_1 and V_6.

Coronary arterioles penetrate the myocardium in order to distribute blood transmurally. The ventricular endocardium, however, to a depth of 1 mm is supplied by oxygen derived directly by diffusion from intraventricular blood.

The venous drainage of the heart occurs predominantly (65%) via the great, middle and small cardiac veins to the coronary sinus, which empties into the RA; 30% occurs via the anterior cardiac veins and 5% via the Thebesian veins (which drain directly into the RA).

Physiologically, myocardial oxygen supply is calculated as the product of the coronary blood flow (CoBF) and the oxygen content of the coronary blood:

myocardial oxygen delivery (MDO$_2$) (ml/min)
$$= CoBF \times arterial\ oxygen\ content$$

arterial oxygen content
$$= O_2\ bound\ to\ Hb + O_2\ dissolved\ in\ plasma$$
$$= (Hb\ (g/L) \times SpO_2/100 \times 1.34)$$
$$+ (10 \times PaO_2 \times 0.0225)$$

The oxygen extraction ratio (OER) describes the proportion of arterial O_2 content that is removed during the passage of blood through tissues. It is calculated according to the equation:

$$OER = (arterial\ O_2\ content - venous\ O_2$$
$$content)/arterial\ O_2\ content$$

It is usually equivalent to 20–30%. However, the myocardial OER is nearer 65%, mainly due to the metabolic requirements of restoring transmembranal electrical potentials in cardiac tissues. The physiological consequence of an increased OER is that increased metabolic demands (e.g. during exercise) must be met by increasing oxygen supply rather than by increasing tissue oxygen extraction. Anaerobic respiration accounts for less than 1% of myocardial energy production (although this ratio can increase to 10% during ischaemia).

Effectively, therefore, there are three main determinants of MDO$_2$ – CoBF, Hb and arterial oxygen saturation.

Coronary blood flow

In the resting human, the cardiac output (CO) is approximately 5 l/min:

$$CO = stroke\ volume\ (SV) \times heart\ rate\ (HR)$$

$$CO = 70\ ml \times 70\ bpm = 5\ l/min$$

CoBF is equivalent to 5% (or 250 ml/min) of this. In turn, the CoBF (Fig. 15.1) is dependent upon:

■ *The cardiac cycle.* LCA flow is markedly reduced during LV systole.

Laplace's law states that, for spheres, the transmural pressure is twice the wall tension

15

divided by the radius of the sphere:

transmural pressure

= (2 × wall tension)/radius of curvature

or,

P = 2T/R

Ventricles are biological spheres. The myocardial thickness (and, therefore, the wall tension in systole) of the LV is three times that of the RV; therefore, the transmural pressure in systole is six times greater in the LV than the RV, and is high enough to temporarily occlude blood flow in the LCA during systole.

■ *The systolic time* (ventricular depolarisation to the end of ventricular re-polarisation).

This is relatively fixed in duration (0.4 s), being dependent on electrochemical and electromechanical processes. An increase in HR is, therefore, achieved by shortening diastole, which in turn reduces coronary filling time, potentially leading to myocardial ischaemia. For this reason, perioperative tachycardia is potentially dangerous for patients with ischaemic heart disease (IHD), and should be treated according to its cause. Sinus tachycardia may result from pain, hypoxia, hypercarbia, hypovolaemia (amongst others). Non-sinus tachycardia may result from a primary cardiac dysrhythmia or due to perioperative ischaemia; medical intervention (including cardioversion and administration of amiodarone, as well as oxygen and pain relief) may be required to reduce the ventricular rate.

β-1 adrenoceptor-blocking drugs (e.g. atenolol) have a dual beneficiary effect on myocardial oxygen balance, and they significantly reduce cardiac complications after surgery. By reducing the ventricular rate, β-blockers simultaneously reduce myocardial oxygen demand (see below) and prolong LCA diastolic filling time.

■ *Coronary perfusion pressure* (CoPP).

This is the sum of the diastolic BP minus the LV end-diastolic pressure (LVEDP):

CoPP = diastolic BP − LVEDP

= 80 − 10 = 70 mmHg

The CoPP represents the LV transmural BP difference during diastole; fluids, including

blood, can only flow from a high-pressure area to a low-pressure area, and therefore any factor that reduces the diastolic BP in relation to the LVEDP, or raises the LVEDP relative to the diastolic BP will reduce the CoPP, and thus myocardial oxygen delivery, leading to ischaemia.

Diastolic BP depends on cardiac preload (see below) and the compliance of the systemic arterial circulation. Consequently, the diastolic BP may be reduced by haemorrhage and vasodilation (e.g. by drugs and hypercarbia).

The LVEDP reflects LV preload, and is linearly related to LV end-diastolic volume in patients with a compliant, non-diseased LV.

The LVEDP is elevated by hypervolaemia (increased preload) and reduced ventricular compliance and contractility (e.g. after MI, due to left-ventricular hypertrophy secondary to aortic stenosis (AS), or due to dysrhythmia).

The diastolic pressure time index (DPTI) is a useful derived value that indicates HR-dependent LCA flow, and represents myocardial O_2 supply:

DPTI = CoPP × diastolic time

This value can be compared to the tension time index (TTI), which is representative of myocardial O_2 demand, to derive an 'endocardial viability ratio':

TTI = systolic BP × systolic time

endocardial viability ratio = DPTI/TTI

Endocardial blood supply is critically dependent on LVEDP, increases in which produce compression ischaemia of the endocardium. The endocardial viability ratio reflects this, both the numerator and the denominator being in part dependent on changes in the LVEDP. Normally, the ratio approximates to 1 or more than 1; critical endocardial ischaemia occurs when the ratio falls below 0.7.

Patency of the coronary arteries

The Hagen–Poiseuille equation states that for laminar flow of fluid through a tube (Chapter 3):

$$\text{flow} = \frac{\text{pressure gradient} \times \text{radius}^4 \times \pi}{8 \times \text{fluid viscosity} \times \text{tube length}}$$

$$= \frac{Pr^4\pi}{8 \times l}$$

Flow is, therefore, related to the fourth power of the radius of the vessel (only approximately as the equation was originally intended to apply to homogenous fluids flowing through rigid vessels). Consequently, in small vessels, such as the coronary arteries, reductions in vessel radius may lead to significant reductions in blood flow. Percutaneous transluminal coronary angioplasty works by increasing the coronary arterial radius. Coronary artery bypass grafting circumvents coronary stenoses, using non-stenosed, wider-bore vessel grafts.

The CoBF is subject to autoregulation, such that intramyocardial vascular resistance (i.e. coronary radius), and therefore CoBF, is adjusted to match myocardial oxygen demand. Adenosine, liberated from ATP, is a potent vascular smooth muscle vasodilator. Nitric oxide, prostacyclin, thromboxane and endothelins, which are synthesised and released from the coronary endothelium, also regulate vascular tone. IHD is thought to result from endothelial damage caused by risk factors for IHD, such as smoking, hypertension, diabetes and hypercholesterolaemia, such that the release of vasodilatory nitric oxide is reduced, while release of vasoconstricting endothelins are increased. In addition, atheroma formation can lead to reductions in arterial radius through mechanical obstruction and by stimulation of thrombus formation. Exogenous nitrates are often beneficial in reducing myocardial ischaemia because they increase CoBF. Similarly, endothelin receptor antagonists may in future be used in the treatment of myocardial ischaemia.

Neurogenic control of CoBF is of less physiological importance. α-adrenoceptor stimulation causes arteriolar vasoconstriction, which is of clinical importance when using noradrenaline in ICU; the α-adrenoceptor effect is often countered by using β-adrenoceptor-stimulating drugs (e.g. dopamine) that cause coronary vasodilation. Vagal stimulation increases CoBF providing bradycardia is avoided.

Haemoglobin

Arterial oxygen content is directly related to blood Hb concentration, which means that, all other factors remaining equal, a fall in Hb from 14 to 7 g/dl halves myocardial oxygen delivery. In younger people with patent coronary arteries, such a fall is unlikely to cause myocardial ischaemia – indeed, 7 g/dl (rather than 10 g/dl) is now recognised as the lower limit for blood transfusion. However, in more elderly patients with coronary artery disease, CoBF is reduced. Myocardial oxygen delivery, therefore, is relatively more reliant on arterial oxygen content, such that the Hb concentration below which myocardial ischaemia occurs is elevated – the blood transfusion trigger may be 10 g/dl rather than 7 g/dl (or 100 g/l rather than 70 g/l).

Smokers often have polycythaemia, a physiological response to relative hypoxia (10–15% of the total body Hb may be carboxy-Hb in smokers). However, polycythaemia increases blood viscosity, which is inversely related to blood flow (Hagen–Poiseuille, see above), which may actually reduce myocardial oxygen delivery rather than improving it.

Arterial oxygen saturation

Perioperative hypoxia may have a number of causes (Chapter 16) including atelectasis, pneumonia, pulmonary embolism (PE) and ARDS, and may be severe enough to contribute to myocardial ischaemia. Treatment is aimed at the cause of hypoxia.

Myocardial oxygen demand

The heart is approximately 15% efficient in terms of useful energy expended. Basal metabolism and electrical activity account for about 20% of myocardial oxygen demand. A further 15% occurs as a result of volume work. The majority (60%) of myocardial oxygen demand is determined by pressure work. Myocardial work, as related to oxygen demand (along with HR and contractility), is related to tension, which is the product of pressure and volume (see above).

Volume work

Volume work occurs in response to myocardial distension, and is dependent on cardiac preload. Cardiac preload is defined as the end-diastolic filling pressure of the ventricle prior to contraction, and is dependent on the

15

venous return to the heart. Frank showed that in *individual cardiac muscle fibres* force of contraction was dependent on the initial length of the fibre (Fig. 15.3). Starling demonstrated the same effect in the intact myocardium. Frank–Starling's law of the heart, therefore, describes an intrinsic regulatory mechanism of myocardial contraction, and states that the force of myocardial contraction is proportional to initial muscle fibre length, up to a point. This is the Frank–Starling or ventricular function curve (Fig. 15.4).

The force of contraction may be represented by the CO or SV. The initial myocardial fibre length may be represented by the LVEDP or CVP.

Cardiac preload, and therefore myocardial oxygen demand, is increased by hypervolaemia, head-down positioning and increases in venous tone (e.g. when patients are cold, scared or in pain) and sudden increases in venous return (e.g. release of pneumoperitoneum, conversion from positive-pressure ventilation to spontaneous ventilation).

Cardiac preload, and therefore myocardial oxygen demand, is decreased by sitting the

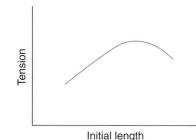

Fig. 15.3 Frank curve for isolated muscle fibre.

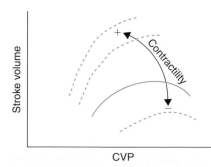

Fig. 15.4 The Frank–Starling (or ventricular function) curve for intact myocardium.

patient up and reducing venous tone (e.g. warming the patient, analgesia, use of spinal/epidural anaesthesia or nitrates). Pathological decreases in preload may occur with haemorrhage, pulmonary embolism (PE) and pericardial disease.

Pressure work

Pressure work describes the cardiac work required to overcome cardiac afterload. Cardiac afterload is defined as the resistance to flow that the LV must pump against, and is equivalent to the SVR, which is calculated as the mean arterial pressure (MAP) divided by the CO.

Ohm's law states that

volts = current × resistance   V = IR

which is analogous to

MAP = CO × SVR

therefore,

SVR = MAP/CO

Ohm's law may be rearranged as

$$I = \frac{V}{R} \quad \text{or} \quad flow = \frac{\text{change in pressure}}{\text{resistance}}$$

From the Hagen–Poiseuille equation:

$$flow = \frac{\Delta Pr^4 \pi}{8\eta L}$$

Combining the two equations:

$$\text{resistance (i.e. SVR)} \propto \frac{8\eta L}{\Delta Pr^4 \pi}$$

i.e. SVR is proportional to viscosity.
In turn:

$$\text{viscosity} = \frac{\text{tangential force}}{\text{cross-sectional area} \times \text{velocity gradient}}$$

From these equations, a number of factors that alter afterload (and therefore, the majority of myocardial oxygen demand) become apparent:

■ *MAP:* The MAP increases with age, as a result of arteriosclerotic change. MAP will

15

also be increased by endogenous (e.g. during physiological or psychological stress, via sympathetic nervous system (SNS) stimulation and the endocrine release of adrenaline and noradrenaline) or exogenous catecholamines (e.g. used in the treatment of cardiogenic shock or resuscitation).

- *CO:* The CO is the product of the SV and the HR:
  $$CO = SV \times HR$$

- *Increases in CO:* These occur when the HR and heart contractility increase, which may occur through intrinsic (Frank–Starling's law, Bowditch effect (contractility increases as HR increases)) or extrinsic mechanisms (SNS, endogenous/exogenous catecholamines).

- *Cross-sectional area of the left-ventricular outflow tract:* This is reduced by AS. All other elements remaining equal, a greater pressure gradient (i.e. increased cardiac work) must be produced in order for blood to be ejected in systole. In addition, AS leads to non-laminar flow in systole, which increases blood viscosity.

- *Cross-sectional area of the arteriolar tree:* Arterioles have the greatest comparative vascular wall tension, and therefore are the major determinants of SVR, which is increased by vasoconstriction and reduced by vasodilation.

- *Blood viscosity:* Blood viscosity may be increased after surgery due to dehydration, cold and the release of a number of acute phase proteins into the plasma. This effect may be countered by i.v. fluid haemodilution, anaemia and use of thrombo-prophylactic anticoagulants.

Perioperative prevention of myocardial ischaemia may, therefore, be achieved either by increasing myocardial oxygen supply or by reducing myocardial oxygen demand (Fig. 15.5). These are achieved by

- reducing SNS activity:
  - analgesia,
  - temperature regulation,
  - maintenance of normocapnea,
  - anxiolysis (talking to patients/pharmacological),
  - use of α-adrenoceptor- and β-adrenoceptor-blocking drugs;

- avoidance of hypoxia:
  - oxygen therapy,
  - cessation of smoking,
  - chest physiotherapy and mobilisation;

- continuing perioperative anti-hypertensive drugs;

- blood transfusion, as appropriate;

- reducing blood viscosity:
  - cessation of smoking,
  - mild haemodilution,
  - temperature regulation,
  - anti-thrombogenesis;

- surgical intervention prior to major surgery:
  - percutaneous transluminal angioplasty,
  - coronary artery bypass grafting,
  - aortic valve replacement.

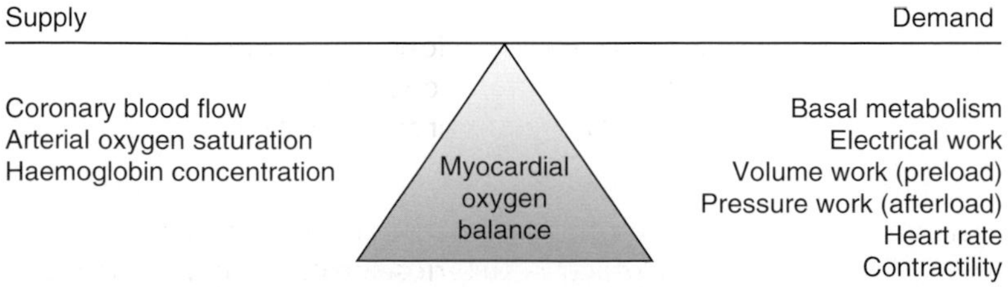

15

Supply		Demand
Coronary blood flow		Basal metabolism
Arterial oxygen saturation		Electrical work
Haemoglobin concentration	Myocardial oxygen balance	Volume work (preload)
		Pressure work (afterload)
		Heart rate
		Contractility

Fig. 15.5 Factors influencing myocardial oxygen supply and demand.

Ventricular failure

Heart failure is a common and debilitating disease. Approximately 1 person per 1000 per year develops the condition, although this figure rises to 10 per 1000 per year in the over 85s. Ventricular failure describes the inability of the heart to produce a blood flow that is sufficient to prevent systemic ischaemia, which occurs when systemic oxygen delivery (DO_2) fails to meet systemic oxygen demand. DO_2 is calculated as the product of the CO and the arterial oxygen content.

A number of terms are used to classify heart failure:

- *Left/right heart failure:* Left heart failure reduces systemic perfusion (forward failure), and produces dyspnoea due to pulmonary capillary congestion with oedema formation (backward failure). Right heart failure is associated with systemic venous congestion (raised CVP, hepatomegaly, ascites and leg oedema).

- *Congestive cardiac failure* describes simultaneous right and left heart failure, the former being caused by the latter.

- *High output cardiac failure* is associated with increased preload and increased cardiac work.

- *Cardiogenic shock* is a severe form of cardiac failure, and describes systemic shock (i.e. systolic BP <80 mmHg, with systemic ischaemia) that results from acute left-ventricular failure, such as occurs after acute MI.

Failure occurs for four reasons:

1. *Myocardial contractility is decreased:* Frank–Starling's curve is moved to the right (Fig. 15.4). Thus, the force of contraction is reduced relative to the same initial fibre length, or, for the same force of contraction the initial fibre length is increased. Reduced myocardial contractility occurs due to myocardial ischaemia, dysrhythmia, myocarditis and cardiomyopathy (e.g. perioperative sepsis, acidosis, chronic alcoholism).

2. *Increased cardiac work*: Increased wall tension increases myocardial work and oxygen demand. This results from the increased volume work resulting from increases in cardiac preload (which may occur due to hypervolaemia, anaemia, ventriculo-septal defect (after acute MI) and aortic/mitral valve regurgitation). Increased pressure work results from increases in cardiac afterload, which may occur due to systemic hypertension, AS and PE (right heart failure).

3. *Pericardial disease*, for example constrictive pericarditis or cardiac tamponade (e.g. after MI, or cardiac surgery).

4. *Reduced myocardial compliance* (e.g. fat infiltration, hypertrophic obstructive cardiomyopathy (HOCM), myocardial fibrosis after MI). 'Stiffer' ventricles develop smaller increases in volume (or end-diastolic fibre length) associated with a given increase in pressure than more compliant ventricles.

A number of compensatory physiological mechanisms occur:

- LVEDP rises, leading to ventricular hypertrophy.

- Ventricular compliance falls. Myocardial contractility initially increases (Frank–Starling's law) up to a point, whereupon contractility is reduced in response to increases in the LVEDV. SV therefore falls, and CO is maintained by increases in HR.

- Ventricular hypertrophy increases myocardial oxygen demand, at a time when CoBF is reduced (diseased coronary arteries, increased muscle mass, increased LVEDP, tachycardia).

- Reduced renal perfusion activates the renin–angiotensin–aldosterone system, resulting in sodium and water retention (which in turn increase preload).

15

A vicious cycle develops:

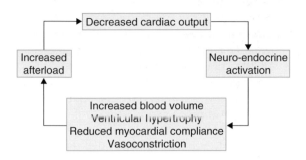

The perioperative management of acute heart failure (see chart below) is aimed at treating the underlying cause, increasing myocardial contractility and improving systemic perfusion.

Chronic medical treatment includes the use of a number of drugs that may have implications for perioperative management. Nevertheless, these therapies should be continued throughout the perioperative course. ACE inhibitors can cause hypotension in dehydrated patients and blood dyscrasias. Diuretics can cause electrolyte disturbances (hypokalaemia, hyponatraemia, hypercalcaemia), blood dyscrasias and hyperglycaemia. β-blockers (bisoprolol and carvedilol) can cause bradycardia, heart block, peripheral limb ischaemia, bronchospasm and confusion. Digoxin can cause confusion, dysrhythmias and heart block, and thrombocytopaenia.

Cardiac dysrhythmias

Cardiac dysrhythmias are defined as aberrations of normal sinus rhythm. The conducting system of the heart is shown diagrammatically as given in the diagram in p. 216.

Note: there is a 0.1-s delay in electrical transmission across the AV node, in order to

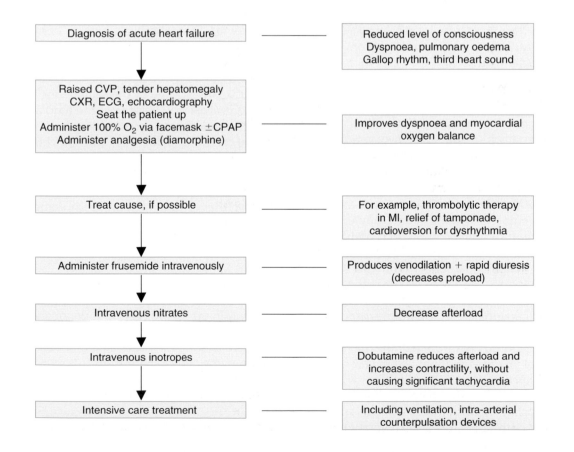

15

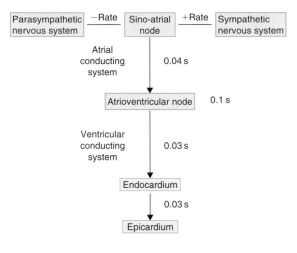

allow the completion of ventricular diastole, before systole.

Dysrhythmias are sub-classified according to their form and severity.

Disorders of electrical impulse generation

Disorders of electrical impulse generation are sub-classified into supra-ventricular (i.e. those arising from the SA node, atrial or AV node) and ventricular (i.e. those arising from the ventricular tissue):

■ *Supra-ventricular dysrhythmias:* These occur frequently, but are rarely dangerous. The SA node is particularly susceptible, especially if the patient is hypoxaemic or hypercapnoeic. Sinus bradycardia frequently follows vagal stimulation (e.g. during ocular, biliary, gynaecological, carotid and bronchial surgery), and may be prevented or treated with atropine. Atrial premature contractions (APCs) are commonly associated with hypokalaemia and hypomagnesaemia. Atrial fibrillation (AF) is associated with IHD, mitral valve disease, acute hypovolaemia, PE and cardiomyopathies. DC cardioversion may be required if the patient is hypotensive, with a high ventricular rate (i.e. the majority of atrial impulses result in ventricular conduction and contraction); less acute cases merit medical therapy aimed at reducing AV conduction, e.g. digoxin, amiodarone, β-blockers and verapamil.

■ *Ventricular dysrhythmias:* These occur for a variety of reasons. 'Opportunist' ectopics may occur, if the sinus rate slows excessively, but these are usually easily over-ridden by simply increasing the HR with atropine. Multifocal ectopics occurring in the otherwise normal patient may be caused by hypoxia, hypercapnia, anxiety, pain or the administration of exogenous catecholamines. In rare circumstances (more frequently in patients with IHD), these factors may lead to ventricular tachycardia (VT) or fibrillation. DC cardioversion may be required as a matter of urgency (see below). Medical treatment with β-blockers, lidocaine or amiodarone may be indicated.

Disorders of electrical impulse conduction

These are sub-classified according to whether they occur due to slowed or blocked conduction pathways (e.g. complete heart block), or due to aberrant conduction pathways (e.g. Wolff–Parkinson White syndrome). Complete heart block is associated with hypotension, ventricular dysrhythmias and sudden death. There is complete dissociation of P-waves and QRS complexes on the ECG; bradycardia at the radial pulse and cannon waves may be seen in the jugular pulse (caused by atrial contraction against a closed tricuspid valve). Complete heart block is more common in the elderly and may occur after MI, cardiac surgery and administration of β-blockers or digoxin. Treatment involves oxygen therapy and increasing the ventricular rate with isoprenaline until temporary myocardial pacing wires can be inserted.

Perioperative ECG monitoring

It is only in the last 30 years that perioperative ECG monitoring has become routine. Patients with pre-existing cardiac disease and ECG changes obviously benefit from ECG monitoring, but what changes and abnormalities can be detected from its use in the previously fit patient? First, it is necessary to consider apparatus and lead placement (Fig. 15.6).

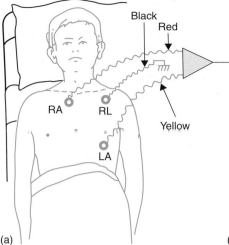

(a)

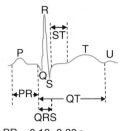

PR   0.12–0.20 s
QRS 0.07–0.10 normal ECG
QT   0.33–0.43

Junctional rhythm

(b) Ventricular bigemini

Fig. 15.6 ECG monitoring in the perioperative period: (a) the CM5-lead placement and (b) common types of rhythm disturbance.

Apparatus and lead placement

The conventional 12-lead ECG is obtained using an electrocardiograph from which a printed record is obtained for analysis. For 'real-time' perioperative ECG monitoring, an oscilloscope is used on which the electrical signal from the heart is directly displayed. Most units also employ 'memory' devices which enable abnormalities to be stored and separately displayed using a 'freeze' and 'cascade' facility. For permanent records, a separate printer is necessary, although these are not routinely available.

It would obviously be inconvenient to place electrodes on every patient to allow a full 12-lead record to be obtained. Indeed, most monitors are only equipped for 'bipolar' electrodes (3-lead systems) and not those necessary for the augmented or chest leads obtainable from the 12-lead ECG. Electrical filters are used to cut out spurious noise and movement artefact. Although the signal obtained is clearer, there is an unfortunate tendency for it to be degraded, and as a result, the ECG (particularly the ST segment) changes are more difficult to interpret. Switching the filters off is possible in some units by changing from the 'monitoring' to the 'diagnostic' mode.

With only three leads available, it is important that lead placement is optimised to produce the most useful information. The bipolar leads involve measurement and display of the difference in electrical potential (from the heart) between two points on the body surface. Conventionally, the three limb leads utilised are, I, II and III. 'I' measures the difference in potential between right arm and left arm, 'II', right arm and left leg and 'III', left arm and left leg. The three leads include two that are 'active', and one that is 'inactive' (earth). The former two may be placed to record leads I, II or III, the inactive lead being placed anywhere on the body surface. However, the information that primarily needs to be obtained relates to dysrhythmia and ischaemia detection.

While lead II is useful for the diagnosis of supra-ventricular dysrhythmias, none of the three bipolar leads is really suitable for detection of ischaemia. With regard to the conventional 12-lead ECG, it has been found that about 90% of detectable ischaemic changes are present in lead V5. Although this cannot be measured directly with a 3-lead ECG, a modified V5 (CM5) system can be employed. This involves placing the *red* active lead (usually designated the 'right arm') on an electrode over the upper right of the sternum, and the other (the 'left arm') *yellow* electrode placed in the usual V5 position (sixth intercostal space at the anterior axillary line under and lateral to the left nipple). The inactive *black* lead is usually placed on the

15

217

left shoulder (Fig 15.6). This CM5 configuration not only produces a modified V5 record for ischaemia detection, but also is excellent for dysrhythmia monitoring as it is aligned in the same direction as lead II. One also notes, in practice, that the amplitude of the signal is greater in this position (as one electrode is over the LV), allowing for the gain (and also the noise) of the ECG amplifier to be reduced.

Valvular heart disease

The perioperative management of patients with valvular heart disease is often poorly understood by junior physicians; it is, however, relatively straightforward.

Several general principles apply:

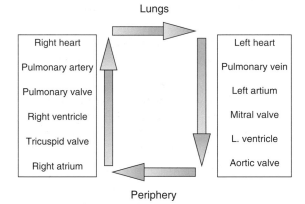

Lungs

Right heart	Left heart
Pulmonary artery	Pulmonary vein
Pulmonary valve	Left artium
Right ventricle	Mitral valve
Tricuspid valve	L. ventricle
Right atrium	Aortic valve

Periphery

Murmurs are caused by turbulent blood flow. They may occur in normal hearts. Left-sided murmurs (aortic and mitral) are heard more loudly than right-sided murmurs (tricuspid and pulmonary), because a greater muscle mass produces more turbulent blood flow. Ventricular systolic murmurs (best heard with the diaphragm of a stethoscope) are louder than diastolic murmurs (best heard with the bell of a stethoscope) for the same reason. Murmurs are best heard over the valve in which they occur. Radiation of a murmur depends on which direction the blood is flowing through the valve. Valvular heart disease may occur in any one (or more) of the four heart valves, and may be either stenotic or regurgitant in nature.

Stenotic murmurs

These are produced by disease that reduces the cross-sectional area and pliability of the valve (e.g. rheumatic fever). The murmurs occur early during the systolic phase of the upstream heart chamber – this is the atrium for the mitral and tricuspid valves, and the ventricle for the pulmonary and aortic valves. The murmur of mitral stenosis (MS) is therefore best heard over the mitral valve, and occurs during ventricular diastole (i.e. when the LA is contracting), producing a low-pitched mid-diastolic murmur. The murmur of AS is best heard over the aortic valve, and occurs during ventricular systole, producing an ejection systolic murmur. The heart chamber upstream of the affected valve hypertrophies. Left-sided stenotic disease results in a fixed CO; the MAP, therefore, depends on the SVR – hypotension may thus be caused by vasodilation (epidurals, nitrates), hypertension by vasoconstriction (cold, pain).

Regurgitant murmurs

These are produced by disease (e.g. rheumatic heart disease, MI, infective endocarditis) that damages the muscular annulus of the valve, such that it fails to close properly when the upstream chamber relaxes. Murmurs occur when blood flows in the opposite direction to normal, depending on the pressure gradient generated across the valve. The murmur of mitral regurgitation (MR) occurs during left-atrial diastole and throughout LV systole producing a pansystolic murmur. The murmur of aortic regurgitation (a sign of aortic dissection) occurs during LV diastole, but only when the aortic pressure exceeds the LVEDP (i.e. an early diastolic murmur). The chamber upstream of the affected valve hypertrophies:

- Left-sided valve disease is associated with systemic embolisation phenomena (e.g. embolic stroke), particularly if associated with dysrhythmia.

- Right-sided valve disease is associated with pulmonary disease, e.g. PE and abscess formation.

15

■ Aortic valve disease may cause coronary ischaemia by decreasing CoBF through occlusion of the coronary artery annuli.

■ Mitral valve disease is associated with dysrhythmias, particularly AF.

■ All patients with valvular heart disease require prophylactic antibiotics before undergoing surgical procedures that may produce bacteraemia (see Chapter 11).

The aims of perioperative management of patients with valvular heart disease are three-fold:

1. Keep the circulation moving in the correct direction. This involves maintaining preload (e.g. fluid therapy) and reducing afterload (e.g. analgesia).

2. Keep the patient in sinus rhythm, avoiding bradycardia and tachycardia. This reduces cardiac work, and makes contraction both more efficient and more effective. Bradycardia worsens regurgitation. Tachycardia reduces left-ventricular filling time, and may worsen stenotic disease. Treatment may involve oxygen administration, anti-dysrhythmic drugs, correction of electrolyte imbalance, cardiac pacing or cardioversion.

3. Maintain myocardial contractility, by avoiding cardiac depressors (e.g. excessive administration of anaesthetic agents) and cardiac stressors, which increase myocardial oxygen consumption in poorly perfused, hypertrophic myocardium. Therapies include analgesia and β-adrenoceptor blockade.

Basic life support and advanced life support

Cardiopulmonary arrest has a poor outcome, with a hospital discharge survival rate of around 15% (although initial resuscitation in hospital may be effective in a third of cases). In view of this figure, there has been intense ethical debate concerning whether or in what circumstances cardiopulmonary resuscitation (CPR) should be attempted. In general, CPR should always be undertaken unless the patient has expressly refused CPR in advance, or if the prognosis is so poor that CPR would be futile (in this instance, the decision should still be relayed to the patient, if possible). Survival is most likely when the event is witnessed, when help is summoned, when the heart arrests in fibrillation, and when ALS and defibrillation occur at an early stage.

Basic life support

BLS means the maintenance of an airway and the support of breathing and the circulation (ABC) without the use of equipment other than a simple airway device or protective shield. In the perioperative hospital setting, BLS continues until support staff are in attendance. The BLS algorithm, as modified for use by hospital doctors, is shown in Fig. 15.7.

Airway maintenance is described in Chapter 8. Three manoeuvres are employed in BLS:

1. *head tilt*, where the head is extended on the neck, is achieved by advancing one hand, placed on the occiput of a supine patient, in a caudal direction, such that the chin becomes elevated;

2. *chin lift* augments the effect of head tilt, and is achieved by placing two fingertips under the point of the chin to lift it forwards;

3. *Guedel airways* are presented in a range of sizes. In general, green Guedel airways are used for adult women, orange for adult males, and red for large adult males. They are interposed between the pharynx and tongue, in order to clear the airway.

Suction equipment should be available on all wards, and should be used rather than a 'finger sweep' to clear the airway of debris (e.g. vomit, blood). Dentures should be removed. Gloves should be worn at all times.

Breaths should be delivered to a tidal volume of 700–1000 ml (10 ml/kg, i.e. one large compression of a standard

15

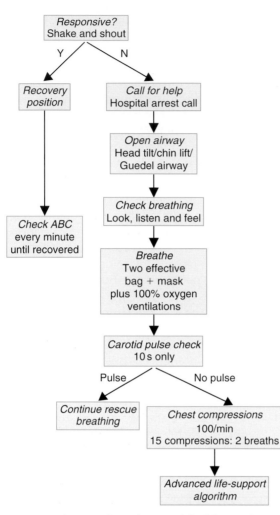

Fig. 15.7 The BLS algorithm, modified for use by hospital doctors.

2-l self-inflation bag, connected to 100% oxygen), over a 2-s duration (in order to allow the expansion of collapsed bronchioles); 2–4 s of expiration should be allowed between each breath, although the exact timing is not critical.

Chest compressions
The correct site for chest compression is in the centre of the lower half of the sternum. The heel of one palm should be placed two fingerbreadths cephalad to the xiphisternum. The other palm should be placed over the lower hand, and the fingers interlocked. With the arms straight and the elbows locked, firm pressure should be applied to the patient's chest, in order to depress the sternum by about 4–5 cm. Chest compressions should continue at a rate of 100/min, as a compromise between the optimisation of coronary perfusion and the minimisation of rescuer fatigue. CoPP rises throughout a cycle of chest compressions, and is higher after 15 than 5 consecutive compressions. Rescue breathing is associated with a rapid reduction in perfusion, and therefore a ratio of 15 compressions to two breaths is recommended for all resuscitations. The compression phase and the release phase should take a similar length of time. Even when performed optimally, chest compressions do not achieve more than 30% of the normal cerebral perfusion.

Two theories have been proposed to explain the efficacy of chest compression. The 'heart pump' theory describes the idea that ventricular output is achieved by compressing the ventricles between the sternum and thoracic vertebrae. This theory was somewhat discredited in the 1970s, firstly, because echo-cardiography demonstrated valvular incompetence during compression, and secondly, because coughing alone was shown to produce a life-sustaining circulation. The 'thoracic pump' theory proposes that chest compression increases intrathoracic pressure, propelling blood out of the chest; forward flow occurs because the vena cavae are compressed during chest compression while the arteries remain patent. During chest compression release, the intrathoracic pressure is only minimally positive/negative, allowing venous return from the relatively higher pressured head and abdomen.

Advanced life support
ALS describes the use of advanced airway management skills combined with defibrillation and use of vasopressor and anti-dysrhythmic drugs in order to restore a spontaneous circulation. ALS improves patient outcome compared to BLS. Note that successful patient outcomes equate to the patient leaving hospital without disability, and not merely the restoration of a (vasopressor-supported) CO.

Advanced airway techniques

These are described in more detail in Chapter 8. Endotracheal intubation (ETI) and ventilation with 100% inspired oxygen remains the gold standard of airway management. However, the use of both the laryngeal mask airway (LMA) and the Combitube® has grown in popularity. Both of these airway devices are advocated by the European Resuscitation Council and the UK Resuscitation Council as effective methods of airway control. Both have the added advantage of ease of insertion by relatively untrained personnel.

The Combitube® is an oesophageal obturator device, designed to provide a secure airway after 'blind' insertion. A schematic diagram is shown in Fig. 15.8 with all pictures (Figs 15.8–15.11) courtesy of http://www.akh-wien.ac.at/combitube/combit2.html.

The Combitube® is inserted with gentle downward pressure applied in a curved direction, such that the tip of the tube passes along the hard and soft palates to the laryngo-pharynx, until resistance is felt (Fig. 15.9).

The oesophageal balloon (blue) is inflated with 40–85 ml of air; this balloon seals the mouth and nose. The distal cuff is then inflated with 5–15 ml of air. Bag-mask ventilation is started via the blue, oesophageal lumen. If the tip of the Combitube lies in the oesophagus (as is most likely after blind insertion), the trachea is ventilated via the side holes of the oesophageal lumen, and air is

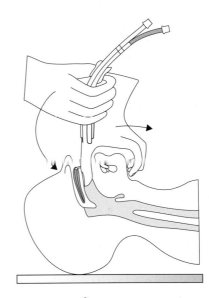

Fig. 15.9 Combitube® insertion.

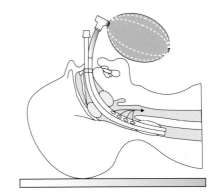

Fig. 15.10 Combitube correctly placed in the oesophagus with tracheal ventilation via the side holes.

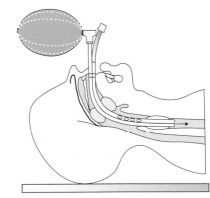

Fig. 15.11 Combitube placed in the trachea. Ventilation takes place 'conventionally' via the tracheal lumen.

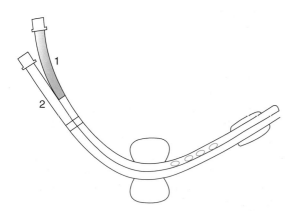

Fig. 15.8 Schematic diagram of a Combitube®.

15

prevented from entering the stomach by the 'tracheal' balloon (Fig. 15.10).

Air entry should be heard in both lungs and not over the stomach: if the reverse happens, then the tip of the tube is in the trachea, and bag-mask ventilation should be reconnected to the clear tracheal lumen (Fig. 15.11).

If ventilation is not possible via either lumen, the Combitube® should be withdrawn by 2–3 cm before re-attempting ventilation. Subsequent conversion to ETI is recommended.

Chest compressions

As described above, CoPP falls if chest compressions are interrupted. Chest compressions should, therefore, continue at a rate of 100/min, stopping only for pulse checks and defibrillation. Ventilation may be continued *during* compressions if a LMA or Combitube are used. Synchronous chest compression and endotracheal ventilation can result in rapid rises in airway pressure, increasing the risk of barotrauma. The maintenance of a small amount of continuous positive airways pressure between breaths and during compressions may be beneficial.

Defibrillation

Electrical defibrillation provides the definitive treatment for ventricular fibrillation (VF). Fibrillation describes unco-ordinated spontaneous depolarisation, which results in the loss of any effective CO. This leads to the cessation of coronary flow, and progressive myocardial and cerebral ischaemia. BLS slows the rate of ischaemia. However, as ischaemia becomes more profound the amplitude of VF decreases until asystole occurs. Defibrillation offers the best chance of successful recovery of spontaneous cardiac activity and is most effective the sooner it is applied after the onset of fibrillation; the chances of successful defibrillation decline by 7–10%/min of fibrillation. Only rarely does fibrillation spontaneously revert to a survivable rhythm, and drug therapy is ineffective at preventing or stopping fibrillation. A pre-cordial thump may occasionally abolish fibrillation, if delivered within 30 s of commencement.

Application of a potential difference across a capacitor results in the storage of charge, which may be subsequently released through the defibrillator paddles (Fig. 15.12).

The stored energy (in joules) is equivalent to the voltage applied and the coulombs of charge stored:

energy stored (J)
= potential difference (V) × charge (C)
charge (C) = current (A) × time applied (s)

The energy delivered is equivalent to half this amount:

$$\text{energy delivered (J)} = \frac{V \times C}{2}$$

In practise, a potential difference of 8000 V is developed across the capacitor. A current

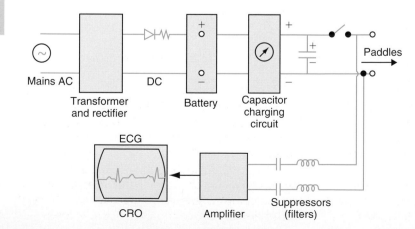

Fig. 15.12 Defibrillator circuit.

pulse of 30 A applied for less than 0.002 of a second delivers defibrillation energy of about 200 J. However, it is the actual current flow, rather than the energy of the delivered shock, that determines the success of defibrillation. The magnitude of current flow is a function of the energy delivered and trans-thoracic impedance. The trans-thoracic impedance describes the overall opposition to current flow, and is the sum of reactance (opposition to current flow in the capacitor) and resistance (i.e. opposition to current flow in the patient). Resistance is decreased by

- a thin, small body habitus;

- previous delivery of shocks;

- reduced intrathoracic volume (therefore, disconnect ventilation before shocks to reduce lung size);

- correct size of defibrillator paddles and correct paddle placement;

- firm pressure applied to the defibrillator paddles;

- use of conductive electrode gel between the patient and the defibrillator paddles.

There has been much interest in the potential use of alternating current (AC) defibrillators. In AC circuits, current and voltage do not reach steady state, varying sinusoidally, out of phase. The delivered waveform is bipolar, and has been shown to more effectively convert VF, and at lower energies (thereby reducing potential myocardial damage).

Delivery of a sufficient amount of current depolarises a significant proportion of the myocardium. This is followed by a short phase of myocardial stunning, which (hopefully) precedes spontaneous recovery of normal pacemaker function.

Management of dysrhythmias

VF is the commonest initial rhythm that leads to cardiac arrest. It is particularly common in patients with IHD and may be seen in up to 80–90% of patients who die suddenly outside hospital. It is recognised by a random waveform on the ECG, irregular in both frequency and amplitude. The amplitude decreases as time progresses.

Ventricular asystole describes complete ventricular standstill, with suppression of all myocardial pacemakers. It accounts for 10% of out-of-hospital arrests. In hospital, patients are more likely to develop asystole from the outset as a result of electrolyte and acid–base disturbances, anoxia and drug administration (e.g. β-blockade) superimposed on pre-existing myocardial disease. No ventricular activity is seen on the ECG.

Similarly, pulseless electrical activity (PEA, formally known as electromechanical dissociation (EMD)) is more likely to occur in inpatients than the figure quoted for out-of-hospital arrests (5%). Asystole and PEA account for 25% of in-hospital arrests, and are associated with a much worse prognosis than VF. PEA describes cardiac arrest despite normal myocardial electrical activity. PEA results from two main causes:

- Failure of excitation–contraction coupling:
  - hypo/hyperkalaemia or other electrolyte disturbances,
  - hypoxia,
  - hypothermia,
  - toxic/therapeutic disorders (drugs);
- mechanical obstruction to venous return or CO:
  - hypovolaemia,
  - tension pneumothorax,
  - tamponade,
  - thrombo-embolism (i.e. PE).

These causes may be remembered as 'four Hs' and 'four Ts'.

In order to rationalise and simplify matters, both the European Resuscitation Council and the UK Resuscitation Council have introduced a combined peri-arrest algorithm for VF, asystole and PEA. This is shown in Fig. 15.13.

Defibrillation may also be required for perioperative broad complex (ventricular) or narrow complex (supra-ventricular) tachycardias, particularly if the systolic BP is

15

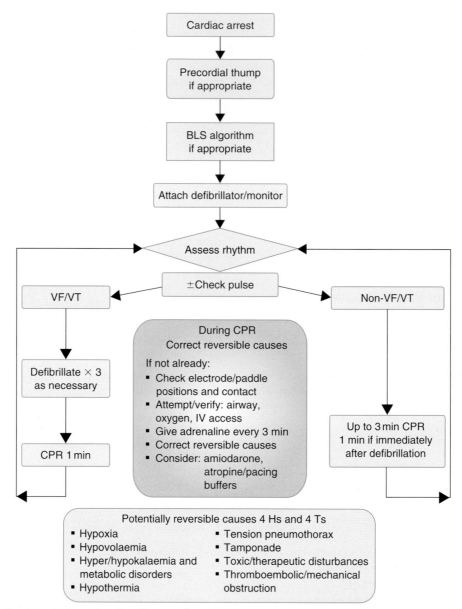

Fig. 15.13 Combined algorithm for VF, asystole and PEA.

less than 90 mmHg, the ventricular rate is more than 150 bpm (250/min for SVT), or if there is associated chest pain, heart failure or loss of consciousness. The most recent (2002) algorithms for broad and narrow complex tachycardia are shown in Figs 15.14 and 15.15. AF is managed differently from SVT (see Fig. 15.16).

Synchronised DC cardioversion is attempted in order to restore sinus rhythm. A DC current

(of lower energy than that used for defibrillation i.e. 50–100 J) is delivered to a sedated patient, such that the current pulse is synchronised to occur with the R-wave of the ECG; if delivery occurs during ventricular re-polarisation, VF may result (R- on T-phenomenon).

The management guidelines for perioperative bradycardia are shown in Fig. 15.17.

15

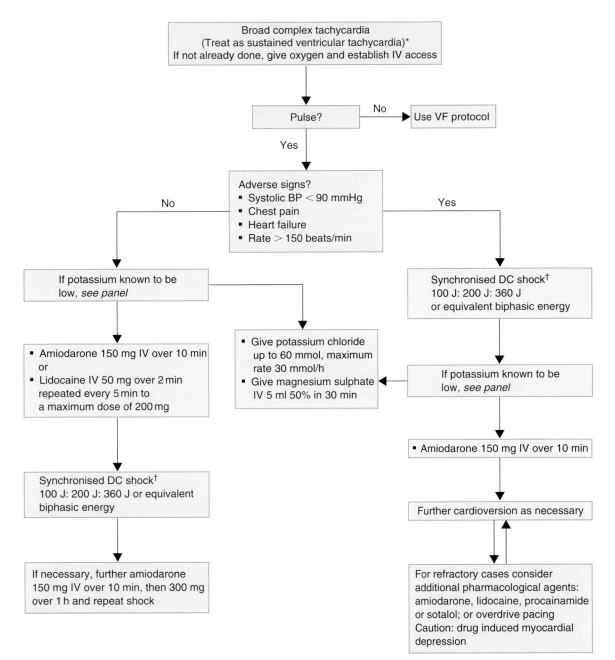

Fig. 15.14 Algorithm for broad complex tachycardia. Doses throughout are based on a adult of average body weight. *For paroxysms of *tosades de pointes,* use magnesium as above or overdrive pacing (expert help strongly recommended). †DC shock is always given under sedation/general anaesthesia.

An expert should institute transvenous pacing under fluoroscopic guidance. Successful transvenous pacing requires that the electrodes are in contact with the right-ventricular endocardium (CXR and impedance studies check this), that a sufficient threshold current is being applied to the endocardium (see ECG and check pulse to confirm electromechanical capture) and that the pacing rate is higher than the

15

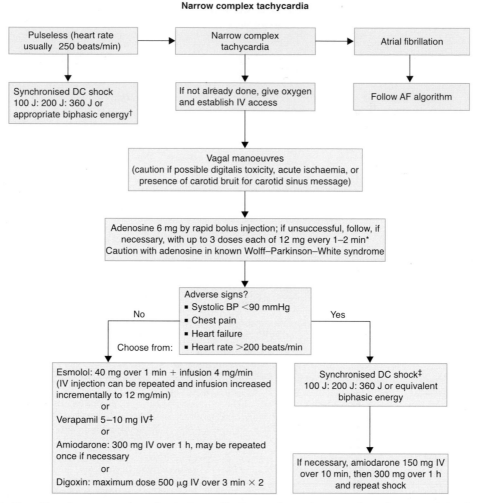

Narrow complex tachycardia

Fig. 15.15 Algorithm for narrow complex tachycardia. Doses throughout are based on an adult of average body weight. A starting dose of 6 mg adenosine is currently outside the UK license for this agent. *Theophyline and related compounds block the effect of adenosine. Patients on dipyridamole, carbamazepine, or with denervated hearts have a marked exaggerated effect which may be hazardous. †DC shock is always given under sedation/general anaesthesia. ‡Not to be used in patients receiving β-blockers.

15

spontaneous ventricular rate (again, check for electromechanical capture – the pulse rate should equate to the pacing rate).

Drugs used in cardiopulmonary resuscitation

As stated, successful defibrillation provides the best chance of survival from cardiac arrest. However, a number of drugs may be used that

■ make the chances of defibrillation success more likely,

■ reduce cerebral ischaemia until circulation is re-established,

■ reduce the likelihood of cardiac dysrhythmia.

These include (but are not limited to) oxygen, adrenaline, atropine, lidocaine, calcium, sodium bicarbonate and amiodarone. When attempted, i.v. access should be secured using a short, wide-bore (14–16G) cannula. The i.v. access may be difficult during CPR, if the patient is fat or peripherally vasoconstricted

Atrial Fibrillation

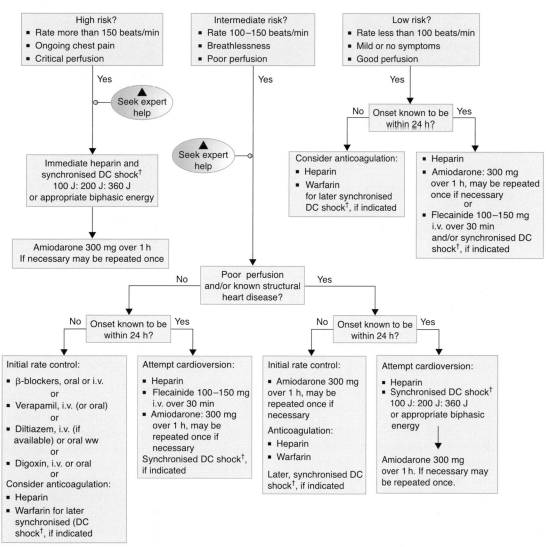

Fig. 15.16 Algorithm for AF. Doses throughout are based on adult of average body weight. †DC shock is always given under sedation/general anaesthetic. ‡Not to be used in patients receiving β-blockers.

by hypothermia or hypovolaemia. In this instance, endotracheal administration of some drugs (adrenaline, atropine and lidocaine) may be attempted, until central venous access is obtained. In practice, intra-cardiac injections are only administered on television. The i.v. administered drugs should be flushed into the (poor) circulation using at least 20 ml saline.

Adrenaline

Adrenaline is currently the only drug recommended for the management of VF,

asystole and PEA. Its beneficial effects are exerted via agonist effects at α- and β-adrenoceptors (Chapter 3):

- *α-agonism:* Peripheral vasoconstriction occurs primarily through $α_2$-agonism ($α_1$-mediated vasoconstriction is less apparent during hypoxia). Venous return is increased, which improves the SV per chest compression, increasing cerebral and CoBF (diastolic BP is increased).

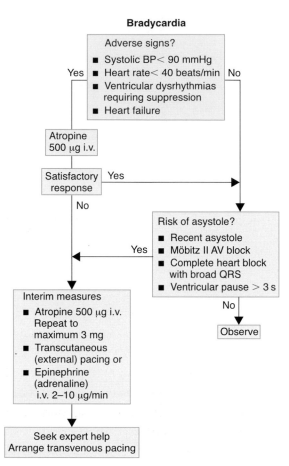

Fig.15.17 Management guidelines for perioperative bradycardia. Includes rate inappropriately slow for haemodynamic state. If appropriate, give oxygen and establish i.v. access.

- *β-agonism:* β-agonism increases the likelihood of successful defibrillation. However, β-agonism increases the HR, which increases myocardial oxygen demand; this is partially offset by β-mediated coronary artery vasodilation. (*Note:* α₂-agonists are coronary vasoconstrictors.)

Atropine

Atropine is an antagonist at muscarinic parasympathetic nerve synapses (Chapter 3). This affects increased sinus node rate and automaticity and augments AV node conduction. Perioperative bradycardia may be caused by excessive parasympathetic tone (particularly if the SNS is antagonised by, e.g. β-blocking drugs), which may be countered by atropine.

Lidocaine

Lidocaine is an amide local anaesthetic agent that renders excitable membranes less likely to depolarise by inhibiting sodium ion influx (Chapter 10). Phase 4 pacemaker tissue depolarisation is less likely, which reduces the automaticity of the heart. In addition, the fibrillatory threshold is increased, less conduction is likely to occur through re-entrant electrical pathways, and there is decreased disparity in conduction times between live and dying myocardium.

Calcium

Calcium plays a vital role in cardiac excitation–contraction coupling. However, its use is now limited to proven cases of hypocalcaemia or hyperkalaemia; indiscriminate use may be associated with coronary and cerebral artery spasm, and myocardial necrosis.

Sodium bicarbonate

Sodium bicarbonate is of questionable benefit during CPR. Its administration increases the $PaCO_2$ (at a time when ventilation may be inadequate), which may worsen any acidosis, reducing the fibrillatory threshold and exacerbating cerebral oedema. However, severe metabolic acidosis (pH < 7) is associated with a very poor outcome; careful titration of sodium bicarbonate, aimed at restoring plasma bicarbonate levels (in a setting of adequate ventilation), may increase the fibrillatory threshold and potentiate the effects of catecholamines.

Amiodarone

Amiodarone is a potent anti-dysrhythmic drug with a complex pharmacological profile, best used to prevent the development of potentially lethal dysrhythmias. It increases the refractoriness of all cardiac tissue, blocking sodium and calcium channels, and having anti-adrenergic and anti-fibrillatory effects. Myocardial contractility is mildly reduced, but this is offset by coronary vasodilation.

16

Oxygen and oxygen toxicity

Aims

The aims of this chapter are to

- discuss the crucial role of oxygen and oxygen delivery to tissues in promoting the availability of energy for cellular oxygen function by allowing aerobic metabolism;

- discuss the means by which oxygen is delivered and its dependence on the haematopoetic, cardiovascular and respiratory systems;

- emphasise that oxygen delivery must be always matched to demand in a cell, organ or the whole body;

- discuss the effects of reduced oxygen delivery to cells and the effect on organ function;

- outline the causes of reduced oxygen delivery in the perioperative period;

- describe means of overcoming oxygen delivery problems in the context of the perioperative period.

Objectives

After reading this chapter, you should

- have a sound understanding of the crucial role of oxygen for cellular and organ function from which to base sound therapeutic interventions in the perioperative period;

- be able to diagnose and treat the common causes of decreased oxygen delivery in the perioperative period;

- be able to decide on which type of oxygen therapy and ventilation is needed in a particular patient.

16

Introduction

Oxygen is essential to life due to its function as the final electron and H^+ acceptor in the

mitochondrial cytochrome chain, whereby ATP is produced as the cellular energy source. Without 'aerobic' metabolism, ATP production is not only reduced 20-fold but lactic acid is produced in excess, causing intracellular acidosis and eventually death. The reserves of ATP are small, so a constant supply of oxygen is necessary for living cells. Many disease states lead to failure to deliver oxygen to tissues, which often is the ultimate cause of death (Chapter 14).

The alveolar air equation

This is one of the fundamental equations in physiology. It can look very complicated, but the underlying concept is simple to understand. Breathing atmospheric air, the amount of 'space' left for oxygen in the alveolus is dependent on the tension of nitrogen, water vapour and carbon dioxide. The former two are fixed quantities and do not change, i.e. there is normally no net movement of nitrogen or water vapour in or out of the alveolus. The space available for oxygen is thus only dependent on the amount of oxygen in the air and the amount of carbon dioxide in the alveolus. If carbon dioxide tension rises (e.g. due to respiratory depression), oxygen tension falls and vice versa. The 'space' available for oxygen is thus the inspired oxygen tension minus the tension of carbon dioxide. However, there is a subtle adjustment to this equation because, normally, more oxygen is taken up than carbon dioxide is produced (the respiratory exchange ratio or respiratory quotient, R). This has the effect of diluting the oxygen tension still further as is seen in the equation:

$$PAO_2 = (PIO_2 - PaCO_2)/R$$

PIO_2 refers to the inspired O_2 tension ($FIO_2 \times$ barometric pressure, BP). Thus, working in kPa (mmHg), at an FIO_2 of 0.21, and a BP of 100 (760), with water vapour pressure in the lungs of 6 (47), reducing this to 94 (713), PIO_2 is equal to about 20 (149). R refers to the respiratory exchange ratio, i.e.

the amount of CO_2 produced divided by the amount of O_2 consumed (in ml/min). This ratio is normally 0.8. Thus, if the PIO_2 is 20 (149) and $PaCO_2$ is 5.5 (40):

$$PAO_2 = (19 - 5.2)/0.8 \quad (PAO_2 = (149 - 40)/0.8$$
$$= 13.2\,kPa \quad (99\,mmHg)$$

The difference between the calculated alveolar PAO_2 and the actual arterial PaO_2 gives the 'A–a' gradient, (A–a) dO_2. This is a useful estimate of the amount of venous admixture or shunted blood passing through the lungs without coming into contact with alveolar air. An increase in the gradient suggests an increased admixture. The alveolar air equation also emphasises the deleterious effect on PaO_2 of a rise in $PaCO_2$, and why an increase in FIO_2 goes some way in compensation.

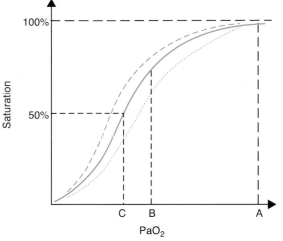

Fig. 16.1 The Hb dissociation curve: (·····), R-shift due to increase in CO_2, H^+, temperature and 2,3,DPG* (increased p50), (———), L-shift due to decrease in CO_2, H^+, temperature and 2,3,DPG (decreased p50). * 2,3,DPG is formed from 1,3,DPG in the glycolytic pathway. It binds preferentially to the reduced form of Hb, thereby aiding O_2 release to the tissues. A: Normal arterial point $PaO_2 = 13\,kPa$ (97 mmHg), $SaO_2 = 98\%$; B: Normal venous point $PvO_2 = 5.3\,kPa$ (40 mmHg), $SaO_2 = 75\%$; C: p50, i.e. tension at which Hb is 50% saturated. Normally $= 3.6\,kPa$ (27 mmHg).

Blood oxygen content and dissociation curve

Hb is employed as a specialised oxygen-carrying system. Simple solution of oxygen in plasma, at ambient pressure and concentration, is insufficient for cellular oxygen demand. (Since only 3 ml of O_2 is carried per litre of plasma, thus for a normal O_2 demand of 250 ml/min to be met from plasma, dissolved oxygen would require a cardiac output of at least 80 l/min!) The relation between the partial pressure of oxygen in blood and Hb saturation is a sigmoid curve, with the steepest portion occurring in the range 2.6–9.3 kPa (20–70 mmHg) as seen in Fig. 16.1.

One gram of Hb can carry 1.34 ml of oxygen, when fully saturated. Thus, with an Hb of 150 g/l, an arterial oxygen tension (PaO_2) of 13.3 kPa (100 mmHg) and a saturation (SaO_2) of 98%:

arterial oxygen content
$$= 150 \times 1.34 \times 0.98$$
$$= \text{(ignoring that dissolved in plasma)}$$
$$= 200\,ml/l \text{ of blood}$$

Hypoxia and oxygen delivery to tissues

Oxygen delivery

Oxygen carried in blood leaving the lungs has to reach the cells to allow aerobic metabolism to take place. The concept of tissue 'oxygen delivery' or 'availability' is an important one because it gives a good idea of the factors determining tissue oxygenation:

overall oxygen delivery
$$= \text{arterial oxygen content} \times \text{cardiac output}$$

Normally, cardiac output (Q) is about 5 l/min and oxygen content 200 ml/l. Thus:

oxygen delivery $= 5 \times 200$
$$= 1000\,ml/min$$

Note the three variables which affect oxygen availability: Hb, SaO_2 and Q. At an oxygen

16

231

consumption of 250 ml/min, this leaves 750 ml of oxygen returning to the lung in the venous blood. This oxygen extraction ratio (OER) of 25% (250/1000) is found in normal volunteers at rest. In cases where oxygen delivery is deficient or demand excessive OER may go up to a maximum of 50%. Thus, if each one of the variables is halved, oxygen delivery is reduced to 1/8 of normal, i.e. to 125 ml/min. This results in anaerobic metabolism, lactic acid production and cellular acidosis. Uncorrected, this leads inexorably to organ failure and death.

Note: Since normal alveolar ventilation is 5 l/m (minute volume around 7 l) and each litre of air also contains about 200 ml of oxygen, then *1000 ml/min* of oxygen is delivered to the alveoli by the respiratory system. This underpins the close matching of ventilation to perfusion (V/Q) and oxygen delivery to consumption. If oxygen demand goes up, not only must oxygen delivery to the tissues increase but also the delivery of oxygen to the alveoli. When assessing adequacy of ventilation, the oxygen requirements of the body must also be taken into account. An oxygen delivery of 1000 ml/min may not be sufficient, if oxygen demand has doubled or tripled.

Types of hypoxia

Anoxic or hypoxic
This is due to a fall in the partial pressure of the inspired gas (PIO_2) such as at altitude, or if inspired oxygen is reduced in accidental misconnection of pipes under anaesthesia. This results in a fall in PAO_2. An increase in $PaCO_2$ or in the alveolar to arterial gradient for oxygen ($(A–a)dO_2$) lowers PaO_2 directly.

Anaemic
This is due to failure of oxygen carriage, as a result of low Hb, with normal cardiac output and saturation, or to alteration in the oxygen-carrying capacity of Hb as a result of combination with carbon monoxide. The latter binds more strongly with Hb than does oxygen with the result that the tissues receive an inadequate oxygen supply.

Ischaemic or stagnant
This results from inadequate blood perfusion to tissues due to myocardial failure, sepsis, raised SVR or arterial embolism.

Histotoxic
Here, the oxygen delivery to the tissue is normal, but mitochondrial oxygen utilisation is defective, such as in cyanide poisoning.

Oxygen cascade from environment to cell

Oxygen therapy is ultimately designed to ensure adequate mitochondrial oxygen tensions. The points at which failure to achieve this may occur are outlined in Table 16.1.

Matching of ventilation to whole body oxygen consumption

As oxygen is taken up from alveolus to capillary, the partial pressure in the alveolus (PAO_2) declines unless oxygen is constantly added by ventilation. At a normal oxygen consumption of 250 ml/min with alveolar ventilation of 5 l/min, the PAO_2 is 13.2 kPa (99 mmHg). If oxygen consumption doubles, as a result of raised temperature, requirement of a healing wound, excessive muscular activity or shivering, then the same alveolar ventilation only results in a PAO_2 of (say) 8 kPa (60 mmHg). Although the healthy patient may be able to double or triple alveolar ventilation to compensate for the increased demand, postoperative or sick patients may not. Increasing the inspired oxygen fraction (FIO_2) to 0.4 compensates partially (see later).

Matching of ventilation and perfusion in the lung

Ventilation (V) and perfusion (Q) must be closely matched so that oxygen delivery by

16

Table 16.1 **Causes and classification of hypoxia**

System level	Defect	Classification
Inspired gas	Low inspired oxygen tension (PIO_2) Low barometric pressure (pB)	Hypoxic
Inspired gas to alveolar gas	Low alveolar ventilation Raised oxygen consumption	Hypoxic
Alveolar gas to arterial blood	Venous admixture or shunt V/Q inequality (>1) Impaired diffusion	Hypoxic
Arterial blood to cell	Low or inadequate blood flow	Ischaemic
Arterial blood to cell	Low Hb Carbon monoxide poisoning	Anaemic
Cell	Metabolic poisons Increased metabolism	Histotoxic Ischaemic

ventilation to the lungs (1000 ml/min) matches oxygen uptake and transport from the lungs to the tissues (1000 ml/min). Although we can look at the lung as a whole, it is obviously important that each alveolus and its perfusing blood supply are also closely matched for V and Q in a ratio of 1:1. In health, due to the effect of gravity, the alveoli at the base of the lung tend to be relatively overperfused (V/Q – 0.8:1), while those at the apex, which do not receive such a good blood supply, are relatively overventilated (V/Q – 2:1). Overall, the figure is close to 0.9:1.

If ventilation to an alveolus is restricted (due to secretions, oedema or bronchospasm leading to atelectasis) and its perfusion is maintained, then the V/Q ratio would fall from around 1:1 to say 0.2:1. Oxygen uptake exceeds supply so that blood leaving the alveolus is not properly oxygenated. This hypoxic blood meets arterialised blood from normal alveoli and results in an overall reduction of PaO_2. This is called 'venous admixture' and is correctable to an extent by increasing the FIO_2. This has the effect of increasing the actual amount of oxygen reaching the alveolus by increasing the

concentration. If ventilation to an alveolus is obstructed completely, no amount of additional oxygen will help and the patient has a true 'shunt'. This may be due to complete atelectasis or an extra-pulmonary shunt as in congenital heart disease.

Causes of compromised oxygen delivery in the postoperative period

In the perioperative period, oxygen delivery is often compromised by the following factors.

Reduced oxygen delivery to the alveoli

1. The patient's respiratory drive is depressed as a result of opioid analgesics and residual quantities of other CNS depressants.

2. When controlled ventilation is instituted during balanced anaesthesia, there is often a tendency to reduce the patient's arterial carbon dioxide tension ($PaCO_2$). This,

16

233

together with the effect of residual CNS depressants, leads to hypoventilation in the immediate postoperative period until $PaCO_2$ has been restored to normality. As a result, oxygen delivery to the alveoli may be insufficient to maintain oxygenation unless its concentration in the inspired gas is increased.

3. The capacity to ventilate the lungs and to cough may also be impaired due to residual effects of long-acting neuromuscular blockers and to pain.

Reduced oxygen delivery from the alveoli to the tissues

1. Inadequate fluid administration may lead to occult hypovolaemia and lowered cardiac output and thus oxygen delivery. In addition, the oxygen-carrying capacity of blood may be decreased due to red cell loss.

2. The cardiac output may also be significantly reduced due to heart disease or to depressant drugs. Regional perfusion is impaired as well.

Increased tissue demand for oxygen

1. Wound healing following tissue injury (due to trauma or surgery) increases the metabolic demand for oxygen.

2. A pyrexial patient has an increased metabolic rate and demand for oxygen.

3. A fall in the patient's temperature intra-operatively due to

    □ a cold operating theatre,

    □ administration of inadequately warmed fluids and blood,

    □ lack of warming and humidification of inspired gases,

    □ loss of the patient's normal mechanisms of heat conservation under anaesthesia,

    □ exposure of large areas of bowel.

As soon as the operation is complete, the patient restores body temperature to normal by shivering, resulting in big increases in

oxygen demand. All these causes can be minimised or eliminated altogether and the patient left with a normal temperature at the end of surgery.

These are some of the important reasons why oxygen therapy is indicated postoperatively.

Therapeutic implications

In assessing the patient's respiratory status perioperatively, it must always be done in the context of the intricate relationship between the haematopoietic, cardiovascular and respiratory systems. Although simply increasing the FIO_2 counteracts the deleterious effects of atelectasis in the short term, no effort should be spared in assisting the patient to re-expand the collapsed alveoli. Atelectasis predisposes to infection and effectively reduces lung volume and respiratory reserve. Thus, especially following upper abdominal surgery, and particularly if the patient is a heavy smoker or has COPD, breathing exercises and physiotherapy are encouraged to prevent this serious complication.

Oxygen administration

From the above, it can be seen that raising the FIO_2 is a primary form of treatment for many of the conditions causing hypoxia. It is symptomatic and not curative. The effect that increased FIO_2 has on PAO_2 even when $PaCO_2$ is raised (due to the causes mentioned previously) can be determined from the 'alveolar air equation' as we saw earlier, i.e.

$PAO_2 = (PIO_2 - PaCO_2)/R$

Working in kPa (mmHg), at an FIO_2 of 0.4, with a $PaCO_2$ of 8 (60), PIO_2 is equal to about 37 (280):

$PAO_2 = (37 - 8)/0.8$ $(PAO_2 = (280 - 60)/0.8$
$\qquad = 27\,kPa\ (205\,mmHg)$

Thus, the raised FIO_2 more than compensates for the raised $PaCO_2$ and the PAO_2 is still

16

above the normal range, thus ensuring adequate Hb saturation.

Devices for oxygen therapy

Devices for delivering oxygen (raising the FIO_2) include masks, nasal prongs, tents and hyperbaric chambers.

Two types are in common use and are shown in Fig. 16.2.

Low-flow devices

These are simple, cheap devices such as the Mary Catterall (MC), Hudson mask and nasal prongs (Fig. 16.2a). A fixed flow of oxygen (2–4 l/min) enters the mask (or nasopharynx) so that the patient inspires an oxygen–air mixture. The flow of oxygen is less than the airflow during inspiration so the final oxygen concentration is determined, not only by the oxygen flow rate into the mask but also by

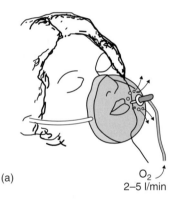

(a)

O_2
2–5 l/min

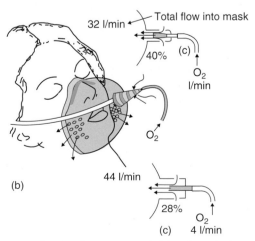

(b)

32 l/min ← Total flow into mask

40% (c)

O_2
l/min

O_2

44 l/min

28%

(c)   4 l/min

O_2

Fig. 16.2 Types of oxygen mask (a) MC or Hudson and (b) Vickers Ventimask.

the patient's minute volume. If the latter declines, the fractional concentration of inspired oxygen (FIO_2) increases. In those patients who are dependent on hypoxic drive with chronic CO_2 retention, too high an initial FIO_2 may be achieved, leading to hyperoxia, hypoventilation and a further rise in FIO_2 as the minute volume falls. The ensuing increase in $PaCO_2$ may be sufficient to render the patient unconscious. For this reason, low-flow devices are reserved for those patients in whom a precise knowledge of inspired oxygen concentration is unnecessary, e.g. postoperative recovery. In the average adult, a flow of 4 l/min into the mask results in an FIO_2 of approximately 0.4.

Air entrainment devices

In patients dependent on hypoxic drive to ventilation, a more precise concentration of oxygen is needed to prevent hyperoxia and respiratory depression. This mask (e.g. Vickers Ventimask) uses a 'constant pressure jet mixing' mechanism (Fig. 16.2b). This ensures entrainment of a large flow (30–40 l/min) of room air through side holes by a small but constant flow of oxygen (3–8 l/min). Low flows of oxygen entrain air to a concentration of about 24%, while higher flows allow the oxygen concentration to reach over 50% (Fig. 16.2c). However, as the oxygen 'enriched' air always exceeds the patients' maximum inspiratory flow and minute volume a known, fixed FIO_2 can be delivered (usually 0.24, 0.28 or 0.35).

Oxygen toxicity

Although essential to life, prolonged increases in PIO_2 above normal may result in toxicity. This is particularly seen in the premature neonate as retinopathy of prematurity, and in the older patient as pulmonary oxygen toxicity.

Pulmonary oxygen toxicity

Oxygen radicals are utilised by the body's defence systems, particularly the polymorphs,

16

235

for killing harmful micro-organisms. This involves the production of free superoxide radicals (O_2 + electron), which are then broken down to hydrogen peroxide by superoxide dismutases, and thence by catalases to oxygen and water. There is evidence that excess oxygen pressures increase superoxide formation and decrease its breakdown by inhibition of superoxide dismutase.

Excess free radicals are normally rendered harmless by scavenging compounds that contain −SH (sulphydryl) groups. The latter are also affected by high oxygen concentrations that leave the free radicals to able to attack cell membrane phospholipids producing lipid peroxidation. This occurs primarily in the lung, presumably as it faces the highest partial pressures. Capillary endothelial damage results, and this leads to ISF accumulation and reduced compliance with consequent pulmonary failure. PIO_2 should always be kept below about 40 kPa (300 mmHg, FIO_2 0.4) to reduce the likelihood of this occurring.

16

17

Acute respiratory failure

17

Aims

The aims of this chapter are to discuss the

- physiological background, causation and types of acute respiratory failure, especially those likely to occur in the perioperative period;

- management of acute respiratory failure, the role of oxygen therapy (Chapter 16) and indications for respiratory support and admission to HDU and ICU.

Objectives

After reading this chapter, you should be able to

- make a differential diagnosis of acute respiratory failure occurring in the perioperative period;

- manage a patient with acute respiratory failure using appropriate methods of oxygen therapy and ventilatory support;

- know when to call for a second opinion and referral to HDU and ICU.

Definition

Acute respiratory failure exists when the patient's breathing apparatus fails in its ability to maintain arterial blood gases (ABGs) within the normal range breathing room air. By definition, acute respiratory failure is present when the blood gases demonstrate:

- an arterial oxygen tension (PaO_2) of <8 kPa (60 mmHg) with normal or low $PaCO_2$ (Type I or hypoxaemic respiratory failure) or

- an arterial carbon dioxide tension ($PaCO_2$) of >6.7 kPa usually accompanied by a fall in pH (<7.3, $H^+ > 45$ nmol/l) in addition to hypoxaemia (Type II or ventilatory respiratory failure).

Hypoxaemia on its own does not always mean respiratory failure, e.g. if the subject is at altitude or has a right to left shunt due to congenital heart disease.

In this chapter we are concerned only with acute respiratory failure, one of the most dramatic and life-threatening emergencies that the house officer and SHO may have to deal with in the hospital setting. Chronic obstructive pulmonary disease (COPD) is the fourth leading cause of death and one-third of patients, who have acute respiratory failure in COPD die.

Pathophysiology

The following section should be read in conjunction with the chapter on oxygen therapy (Chapter 16). There are four parts of the respiratory system that may be involved in the causation of a respiratory emergency, i.e. the

- respiratory centre in the central nervous system (CNS);

- respiratory apparatus (e.g. chest wall and lungs);

- respiratory muscles including the diaphragm, the main respiratory pump; here the effect of muscle fatigue is of crucial importance;

- gas exchanging units in the lung, i.e. the respiratory bronchioles and the alveoli.

It is chastening to remember that in assessing patients with acute respiratory failure, most attention is usually paid to what is happening at the alveolar level, i.e. the blood gases rather than problems elsewhere. The reason for this is the difficulty in measuring parameters such as phrenic nerve function or respiratory muscle fatigue in the clinical (versus experimental) setting.

For example, in COPD there are alterations in ventilation (V) and perfusion (Q) in the lung such that there is localised destruction of alveoli without reduction in ventilation leading to high V/Q ratios or increased dead space. In other areas, there is reduction in ventilation due to destruction or collapse of respiratory bronchioles and relatively normal alveoli leading to low V/Q ratios or shunt. Both co-exist in COPD. This leads potentially to hypercarbia and hypoxaemia.

A prominent defect in COPD is loss of elastic support for respiratory bronchioles that make them prone to collapse on expiration causing the typical vibration and wheeze. Increased lung volumes at the end of expiration compensate for this in an attempt to pull the bronchioles open. Loss of elasticity also results in failure to exhale all the gas so the next breath begins before the previous one has finished. Airway trapping occurs and this causes a shift in the position of the alveoli on the volume pressure curve to a less compliant position. Since respiratory work is equal to pressure times volume, more work is needed to generate a tidal volume as well as to bring the airway pressure back to normal to

allow gas to enter the lung for the next inspiration. As the lung becomes more distended due to air trapping, the diaphragm becomes flattened, decreasing its mechanical advantage (it normally acts like a piston), the blood vessels become crimped and the ribs more horizontal. This again diminishes their efficiency. It is no surprise that the respiratory muscles may become fatigued due to increased work and diminished blood supply.

In acute respiratory failure resulting from COPD, there will be a worsening of hypercarbia, which is primarily related to an increased frequency of ventilation together with a fall in tidal volume. In other words, minute volume may not be diminished. In addition, the pattern of respiration changes to one of decreased inspiratory time and variability.

Examples of conditions causing acute respiratory failure are shown in Table 17.1.

Table 17.1 **Causes of respiratory failure**

Site	Type	Examples
Respiratory centre (CNS)	II	Depressant drugs, opioids; traumatic and ischaemic lesions Loss of respiratory sensitivity to CO_2
Spinal cord and peripheral nerves	II	Spinal injury, Guillain-Barré, poliomyelitis
Neuromuscular junction	II	Myasthenia, neuromuscular-blocking drugs
Muscle	II	Myopathies, respiratory muscle fatigue in COPD
Pleura and thoracic cage	II	Flail chest, pneumothorax, haemothorax deformities, trauma (e.g. rib fractures), loss of optimal shape due to chronic lung hyperinflation
Airways	II	Extrathoracic: foreign bodies, croup Intrathoracic: asthma, bronchiolitis, chronic bronchitis
Gaseous exchange, e.g. alveolus	II	Emphysema, pulmonary oedema, ARDS, pneumonia
Lung vasculature	I	Pulmonary oedema, embolus, ARDS

For ARDS see later.

17

Clinical picture

The clinical picture varies with the cause but any of those mentioned in Table 17.1 leads to deterioration in the patient's respiratory gas exchange. The subsequent changes that occur in blood gases, particularly carbon dioxide, cause medullary chemoreceptor and other compensatory mechanisms to be activated. The patient becomes aware of the necessity to breathe, and as the precipitating cause progresses, exhibits overt signs of distress, i.e. dyspnoea. Eventually, blood gases can no longer be kept in the normal range and acute respiratory failure supervenes.

Acute respiratory failure resulting from CNS depression as a result of drugs (e.g. anaesthetic agents) or injury does not produce overt signs of respiratory distress. Accurate diagnosis is dependent on a high index of suspicion and is confirmed by ABG analysis.

Clinical signs and symptoms

Generally, the onset of acute respiratory failure is heralded by the patient becomes increasingly anxious and preoccupied with the necessity to concentrate every effort on ventilation. The eyes are closed and the accessory muscles of ventilation are fully used. Hypoxia and hypercarbia produce characteristic effects on the CNS and cardiovascular system (CVS), e.g.:

- Hypoxia:
    - CNS – uncooperative, confused, drunken-like state;
    - CVS – Bradycardia, variable BP, cyanosis.
- Hypercarbia:
    - CNS – tremor and overt flap;
    - CVS – raised pulse rate, peripheral vasodilation with pink peripheries, BP changes are variable.

Diagnosis

Diagnosis depends on history, clinical examination and special investigations, such as chest X-ray (CXR), peak expiratory flow rate (PEFR) and ABG analysis. It is important to establish the causative site (Table 17.1).

For example, the history gives a clue to pre-existing disease, such as chronic bronchitis and asthma, or may distinguish between acute epiglottitis (sudden onset) and laryngo-tracheo-bronchitis (slower onset over 24 h), when the clinical signs are equivocal. On clinical examination, expiratory wheeze suggests intrathoracic airway obstruction while inspiratory wheeze suggests that it is extrathoracic. CXR reveals parenchymal causes such as pneumonia, airway obstruction due to foreign bodies (ipsilateral hyperinflation of lung), pleural and thoracic cage causes, such as effusion, pneumothorax and fractured ribs. Raised bicarbonate levels in the blood gases suggest chronic pre-existing disease, and a combination of hypoxia, hypocarbia and an initial metabolic alkalosis followed by acidosis is a common accompaniment of ARDS.

Treatment

Whatever the cause, three important principles of treatment apply.

Establish an airway

This applies particularly to the unconscious patient, e.g. due to overdose, general anaesthesia, CNS trauma and so on. The patient is placed on the side with the head-down, and lower jaw pulled forward to prevent the tongue falling back and obstructing the upper airway. At this stage, it may become obvious that the obstruction is due primarily to foreign bodies or vomit, so this must be cleared, if possible (Chapter 8).

Indications for artificial airways
1. *Oropharyngeal:* This is useful where it is expected that the patient will soon recover consciousness, e.g. postoperatively, or where there is lack of expertise in endotracheal intubation (ETI). A laryngeal mask may be used as an alternative in this situation.

2. *Endotracheal tube (ETT):* If unconsciousness is expected to last for more than a matter of minutes, as in drug overdose, then an ETT must be used both to ensure and to protect the airway (e.g. from aspiration of gastric contents). If ventilation is depressed or inadequate due to trauma or disease, then intermittent positive pressure ventilation (IPPV) will be required.

3. *Cricothyrotomy and tracheostomy:* Obstruction above the cords due to disease or infection may make intubation impossible. Cricothyrotomy or tracheostomy is then necessary to restore the airway.

4. *Bronchoscopy* may also be required for bronchial toilet, removing viscid mucous and obtaining specimens for microscopy and culture.

Administer oxygen to ensure adequate tissue oxygenation

It is of paramount importance to maintain a PaO_2 sufficient to give an arterial Hb saturation of at least 90% (i.e. 8–9 kPa or 60–70 mmHg). Hyperoxia should be avoided, particularly in the bronchitic, who retains carbon dioxide and is dependent on hypoxic ventilatory drive (Chapter 16).

Maintain alveolar ventilation and treat underlying cause

These two are inextricably linked. The causes of acute respiratory failure are many and varied as are the requisite therapies. If treatment of the underlying cause is not successful (e.g. steroids, bronchodilators in asthma, physiotherapy, antibiotics, mucolytics, bronchodilators in acute or chronic bronchitis), then the carbon dioxide tension will begin to rise inexorably, possibly necessitating IPPV. There is no place for respiratory stimulants, except perhaps narcotic antagonists in opioid overdose. Note: Infection is a cause of exacerbation of acute respiratory failure in COPD in <50% of cases. Other causes, such as heart failure, dysrhythmias and pneumothorax must be excluded and treated where necessary.

In acute respiratory failure due to COPD, muscle fatigue is a major contributory factor to continuing hypoxia and hypercarbia. Non-invasive methods of ventilation (e.g. nasal mask) as well as ETI and IPPV may be needed.

17

Special problems encountered which may require high-dependency or intensive care unit support

Despite the fact that there are many causes of acute respiratory failure, anaesthetists and intensivists are faced with a relatively small number of problems, which occur frequently.

Acute severe asthma

This is an attack of asthma that has not been controlled by the patient's usual medication. Patients with severe asthma have

- inability to complete a sentence in one breath;
- respiratory rate ≥25 breaths/min;
- tachycardia ≥110 bpm;
- PEFR <50% of predicted normal or best.

Life-threatening features are

- a silent chest, cyanosis or feeble respiratory effort;
- exhaustion, confusion or coma;
- bradycardia or hypotension;
- PEFR <30% of predicted normal or best (approximately 150 l/min in adults).

This usually occurs in the perioperative period in a patient with a pre-existing asthma history.

Management

- Additional oxygen therapy (Chapter 16) should be administered immediately.

- The patient should be transferred to a high-dependency area (Chapter 12) for monitoring of ECG, non-invasive BP, respiratory rate, PEFR, SpO_2 and baseline ABGs.

17

■ Bronchodilators should be begun immediately. Nebulised salbutamol 2.5–5 mg in 2–4 ml saline, 2–4 hourly, is the treatment of choice. Aminophylline 5–6 mg/kg over 20 min followed by 0.5 mg/kg/h may be given provided the patient has not been on the drug before. Levels should be monitored. Ipratropium 0.5 mg in 2 ml saline may be useful in patients with COPD and asthma.

■ Steroids should be begun immediately in a dose of 100 mg i.v. stat followed by 100 mg 6 hourly.

■ Antibiotics should be administered as appropriate and chest physiotherapy instituted.

If the patient's clinical condition worsens as evidenced by obvious fatigue, reduction in PEFR and worsening ABG (especially, a rise in $PaCO_2$), then more senior help should be requested.

By the time the patient with an acute severe asthmatic attack reaches the ICU, the intensivist is faced with one of the most difficult management problems. The patient is often exhausted, tachycardic, hypoxic, hypercarbic, acidotic and dehydrated, yet needs intubation and ventilation to restore reasonable blood gases. Attempting to intubate the patient 'awake', may precipitate complete obstruction and cardiovascular collapse. Following intubation, ventilation is usually extremely difficult necessitating high inflation pressures, which can only be lowered by prolonging inspiration, and yet air trapping requires that expiration is also prolonged. This conundrum requires considerable compromise with ventilator settings and can often only be accommodated by accepting relatively high $PaCO_2$ levels.

The chronic obstructive pulmonary disease patient, who may require ventilation

In a previous section, it was mentioned that the COPD patient, who presents in acute respiratory failure might proceed, despite optimal therapy (see above, Management guidelines under Acute severe asthma), to the point where nasal mask and non-invasive ventilation or ETI and IPPV is required. In such cases, it is paramount that the patient is assessed as to the suitability of this form of treatment. This involves a thorough history from the patient (or relatives) with particular regard to

■ previous hospital admissions, with lung function tests and blood gases;

■ previous requirements for IPPV or tracheostomy;

■ exercise tolerance.

Only guidelines can be given, but in cases where the patient has had frequent previous admissions with IPPV treatment, progressive lung damage can be anticipated so that further periods of IPPV may be unwarranted. This is also applicable to cases where the patient is housebound and/or breathless at rest. However, recent studies suggest that the patient with acute respiratory failure due to COPD has as good a chance of weaning from IPPV as a patient with an acute attack of asthma.

Adult respiratory distress syndrome

In recent years, it has become evident that the lung can be injured primarily (as in aspiration pneumonitis) as well as by a secondary process in severe illness or trauma. Generally speaking, it is the vascular and alveolar endothelium that is affected. Damage from any of the causes below results in loss of membrane integrity and thus increased permeability to fluid and protein. This leaks into the interstitial space and lymphatics, producing an exudative 'non-cardiogenic pulmonary oedema', with a characteristic 'fluffy' appearance on CXR. It is distinguished from 'cardiogenic pulmonary oedema', by demonstration of a normal or low pulmonary capillary wedge pressure (PCWP), and from oedema due to a low colloid oncotic pressure by demonstration of a serum albumin of >30 g/l. A pronounced decrease in functional residual capacity (FRC) and compliance occurs, with a resulting increased work of breathing and dyspnoea. This together with the associated endothelial damage results in an imbalance of ventilation and perfusion, with hypoxia and increase in dead space. A pronounced inflammatory and fibrotic stage may supervene and lead to permanent lung damage.

ARDS may result from

- ischaemia (following major trauma and hypotension);

- complement and neutrophil activation (as in sepsis, or prolonged hypovolaemia);

- disseminated intravascular coagulation (DIC) with vascular microthrombosis and ischaemia;

- fat embolus syndrome;

- acid aspiration causes primarily alveolar epithelial damage, but vascular endothelial damage follows leading to ARDS;

- inhalation injury, e.g. noxious fumes.

The symptoms are those of severe acute respiratory failure with dyspnoea being prominent. The 'clinical' condition of the patient may not immediately give cause for concern, e.g. in early 'fat embolism'. However, sampling of the ABGs reveals profound hypoxaemia ($PaO_2 < 5\,kPa$ or $35\,mmHg$) and secondary hyperventilation with a low $PaCO_2$ ($<4\,kPa$ or $30\,mmHg$). If left untreated, CO_2 retention and metabolic acidosis develop. The profound hypoxia is often unresponsive to additional oxygen by mask, in which case ETI with IPPV and positive-end expiratory pressure (PEEP) are required. The latter works by increasing FRC by backward distending pressure thus reducing V/Q mismatch and improving compliance at the same time.

17

18

Gastrointestinal system

Aims

The aims of this chapter are to

- describe aspects of the functional anatomy and physiology of the gastrointestinal (GI), hepatic and renal systems, which are appropriate to perioperative care of the patient;

- describe the pathophysiology of common perioperative GI, hepatic and renal problems;

- provide a rational for the treatment of those problems.

Objectives

After reading this chapter, you should be able to

- understand the causation of abnormal GI function in the perioperative patient;

- recognise abnormal GI function in the perioperative patient;

- investigate abnormalities and interpret the results of investigations;

- integrate the importance of renal function as an indicator of clinical status.

Introduction

Diseases of the GI tract (GIT) system constitute a considerable proportion of the general surgical workload. Symptomatic GIT problems (such as nausea and vomiting, constipation and diarrhoea) account for a significant amount of perioperative morbidity. In addition, patients may present for surgery with co-existent hepatic and renal problems, which may in themselves complicate perioperative management, or which may be made worse by the pathophysiological response to surgery and anaesthesia.

Postoperative nausea and vomiting

Introduction

Postoperative nausea and vomiting (PONV), the incidence of which has remained unchanged for several decades at 30%, only rarely causes significant morbidity, but is nevertheless distressing for the patient. As well as delaying oral intake and hospital discharge it increases the perioperative risk of haemorrhage, wound dehiscence, myocardial ischaemia and aspiration pneumonia. Prolonged or excessive vomiting can result in hypochloraemic metabolic alkalosis, with dehydration and hypokalaemia (due to aldosterone secretion in response to dehydration).

Mechanism

Physiologically, a number of triggers activate the vomiting centre in the reticular formation of the medulla (see Fig. 18.1). The vomiting centre integrates and co-ordinates afferent information, and stimulates efferent impulses in cranial nerves V, VII, IX, X and XII (to the upper GIT) and spinal nerves (to the diaphragm and abdominal muscles). Increased salivation (waterbrash) preceeds deeper breathing and closure of the glottis; breath is then held in mid-inspiration, as the abdominal muscles contract and the oesophageal sphincters relax, creating a pressure gradient that expels the gastric contents outwards.

Factors associated with an increased incidence of postoperative nausea and vomiting

Patient factors

- Children are more prone than adults.

- Female sex, particularly in the second half of the menstrual cycle – incidence decreases after the menopause.

- Obesity.

- Previous PONV.

- History of motion sickness.

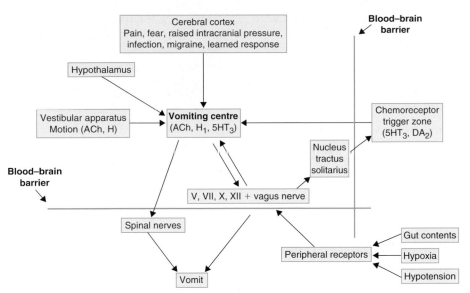

Fig. 18.1 Pathophysiology of vomiting. The chemoreceptor trigger zone (CTZ) is situated on the systemic side of the blood–brain barrier, on the floor of the fourth ventricle, adjacent to the area postrema. Neurotransmitters involved: ACh: acetylcholine, H_1: histamine, $5HT_3$: serotonin, DA_2: dopamine.

- Pain and distress.

- Preoperative full stomach.

- Early postoperative eating and drinking.

- Learned behaviour – those who expect to vomit are more likely to do so.

Surgical factors
- Type of surgery – gynaecological, genital, eye, middle ear and abdominal surgery are more closely associated with PONV.

- Intra-operative factors – haemorrhage and hypotension, hypoxia, use of nitrous oxide and neostigmine during anaesthesia.

- Postoperative factors – use of opioid and anticholinergic drugs, hypoxia and hypotension, excessive early movement.

PONV usually resolves within 4 h after surgery. Treatment involves avoidance of triggers, and administration of fluids, oxygen, non-opioid pain relief and anti-emetics. Anti-emetics may be prescribed in combination, and used prophylactically for high-risk patients.

Anti-emetics
Given the number of neurotransmitters involved in the vomiting pathway, a number of drugs that competitively inhibit neurotransmitter action have anti-emetic properties. Anti-emetics may be classified as follows:

- *Antihistamines,* e.g. cyclizine (50 mg p.o./ i.m./slow i.v. tds). These are effective anti-emetics that act by histamine-1 (H_1)-receptor antagonism. They are mildly sedative.

- *Serotonin ($5HT_3$-receptor) antagonists,* such as ondansetron (4 mg i.v. bd), are highly effective anti-emetics, but expensive, which limit their use to high-risk patients and children (who are prone to the anti-dopaminergic side-effects of other drugs). Propofol has anti-serotoninergic properties; patients anaesthetised with propofol infusions have a lower incidence of PONV, than those anaesthetised using anaesthetic gas mixtures.

- *Anti-dopaminergic agents.* These include substituted benzamides (metoclopramide), butyrophenones (haloperidol), benzimidazole derivatives (domperidone) and phenothiazines (prochlorperazine). Oculogyric crisis (muscle rigidity and involuntary jaw and eye movements) is

18

a rare side-effect, and may be treated with procyclidine.

■ *Anticholinergic drugs* (e.g. hyoscine and atropine) are rarely used, because they cause sedation, confusion, dry mouth and blurred vision.

■ *Miscellaneous* – cannabinoids, benzodiazepines, steroids, ginger and acupressure are anti-emetic, but are more commonly used in chemotherapy than after surgical operations.

Gastroduodenal ulceration

Peptic ulcer disease is relatively common in the population, causing discomfort to the patient and increasing their risk of upper GI haemorrhage. Ulcers that bleed are likely to re-bleed. Ulcers may occur at single or multiple sites. A number of perioperative factors may worsen existing ulceration, or cause new ulceration. These include:

■ *Shock:* The splanchnic circulation is prone to ischaemia during shock; e.g. as little as 30 s of absolute ischaemia may lead to necrosis of small intestine villi. Splanchnic hypoperfusion may be caused by hypovolaemia and hypotension, manual obstruction and splanchnic vasoconstrictors (e.g. noradrenaline).

■ *Sepsis and multi-organ failure* (MOF).

■ *Burns* (Curling's ulcers).

■ *Head injury* (Cushing's ulcers).

■ *Polytrauma*.

■ *Surgery:* Ulceration may occur along suture margins after gastroduodenal surgery.

■ *Drugs:* Non-steroidal anti-inflammatory drugs (NSAIDs), particularly in tablet form, may cause ulceration, particularly if the patient is otherwise nil-by-mouth, and dehydrated.

Any subsequent bleeding may be made worse by vomiting, coagulopathy and respiratory failure. High-risk patients (in addition to addressing the underlying cause) should be given prophylactic anti-ulcer therapy, which may include one (or a combination) of the following drugs:

■ Histamine-2 (H_2)-receptor antagonists (e.g. ranitidine), which reduce acid secretion by competing with histamine at the H_2-receptor on the gastric parietal cell.

■ Proton-pump inhibitors (e.g. omeprazole, lansoprazole), which inhibit H^+/K^+ adenosine bisphosphatase, the enzyme responsible for gastric acid secretion.

■ Sucralfate is a complex of aluminium hydroxide and sulphated sucrose. It has no antacid effect, but effects ulcer protection through stimulation of mucus production, mucosal blood flow and local prostaglandin production (i.e. by cytoprotection).

■ Antacids (solutions of bases, containing, e.g. magnesium and aluminium) are rarely used, because they cause constipation and diarrhoea, and must be given regularly.

■ Msstil (a prostaglandin E_1-analogue) is a rarely used 'antacid' with cytoprotective actions usually used alongside NSAIDs (Chapter 10).

Antacids, H_2-antagonists and proton-pump inhibitors may also be given (in combination with metoclopramide) preoperatively to patients who are at risk of gastro-oesophageal reflux, in order to alkalinise any stomach material that might potentially be aspirated into the lungs.

Perioperative drug administration in 'nil-by-mouth' patients

Patients are invariably placed 'nil-by-mouth' before operations, in order to avoid the risk of aspiration of gastric contents on induction of anaesthesia. Unfortunately, 'nil-by-mouth' is often *too* rigidly adhered to by ward staff, such that patients fail to receive essential preoperative medications. Even in patients starved for 6 h, the stomach may contain

200–300 ml of fluid, resulting from continuous gastric secretions. The risk associated with increasing this volume by 10 ml or so of water (in order to swallow pills) is, therefore, negligible in comparison to the increased perioperative risks of, e.g. omitting preoperative anticonvulsant therapy or premedicant drugs prescribed by anaesthetists. In other instances, oral drugs may have a short plasma half-life; their omission may not affect anaesthesia, but can lead to a postoperative worsening of symptoms (e.g. L-dopa in Parkinson's disease, oral morphine in chronic pain patients).

A selection of drugs, which should be omitted preoperatively (check with the anaesthetist first) are as follows (Chapter 4):

■ Aspirin and warfarin in operations likely to be bloody (e.g. transurethral resection of prostate). In many operations, aspirin can be continued.

■ Longer-acting oral hypoglycaemic agents, particularly chlorpropamide, glibenclamide and gliclazide.

■ Monoamine oxidase inhibitors (MAOIs) (tranylcypromine, phenelzine and isocarboxazid).

■ Oral contraceptive pill (debatable).

Diarrhoea and constipation

Both problems occur commonly in the perioperative period. Normally, patients' bowel habits vary widely, and therefore diarrhoea and constipation are in part defined subjectively. However, abnormal changes in bowel habit in the perioperative period may be painful or embarrassing for the patient, and require attention.

Diarrhoea

This is usually defined as the passage of more than 300 ml per 24 h of loose stool. In many cases, the cause may be idiopathic. Table 18.1 details the more common identifiable causes of perioperative diarrhoea and their treatment. The most effective anti-diarrhoeal is codeine phosphate (30 mg 6 hourly p.o. or i.m.).

Constipation

Stools may be described as infrequent, incomplete or unduly hard. A number of causes may be identified:

■ *Lack of oral intake and reduced mobility:* Preoperative starvation may reduce bowel motility. Gradual return to normal life often improves bowel function.

■ *Postoperative ileus:* This results from intra-operative handling of the bowel, and usually resolves within a matter of days. Prolonged ileus is associated with subacute splanchnic ischaemia, acid–base disturbances and electrolyte imbalances (e.g. hypercalcaemia, hypokalaemia and dehydration). Correction of the underlying abnormality improves motility, as may use of osmotic laxatives (e.g. lactulose).

■ *Pain:* Anorectal surgery may be associated with pain on attempted passage of stool, together with fear of defaecation. Non-opioid analgesics and stool softeners and lubricants (e.g. glycerol suppositories) are indicated.

■ *Analgesics:* Opioid analgesics reduce bowel motility (and are effective anti-diarrhoeal agents). Their withdrawal improves motility, which may be further enhanced by the use of GI stimulants (e.g. senna and metoclopramide).

■ *Miscellaneous:* Neurological disorders, such as paraplegia, multiple sclerosis and senility and epidural anaesthesia are associated with interrupted autonomic nervous control of defaecation, and may require use of enemas or manual disimpaction. Surgical obstruction (e.g. sigmoid volvulus and hernia) may require surgery.

Alcohol abuse

The pathophysiology associated with acute or chronic alcohol consumption contributes to approximately 20% of male and 10% of female admissions to hospital, in the UK. Alcohol is a systemic poison that can damage all organs, as well as harming personal and

18

Table 18.1 **The causes of perioperative diarrhoea and their treatment**

Cause	Treatment
After GI surgery	
Mesenteric ischaemia	Fluids, oxygen, splanchnic vasodilator drugs, surgery
Dumping phenomena	Resolve over time
Short bowel syndrome	
Drug-induced	
Laxatives, including bowel preparations	Withdraw drugs
Antacids	Anti-diarrhoeals should be used with caution
Many others	
Miscellaneous	
Old age	
Overflow diarrhoea in the constipated	Treat constipation
Electrolyte disturbances	Correct
Endocrine causes	
Nasogastric feeding	Alter composition
Infective	
Viral/bacterial cross-contamination of food	Hygiene
Altered bowel flora secondary to antibiotic use	Avoid indiscriminate use of broad-spectrum antibiotics
Clostridium difficile infection	Vancomycin

interpersonal interactions. Patients may be acutely intoxicated, chronically dependent or withdrawing from the effects of alcohol.

Acute intoxication

The degree of physiological derangement depends on the plasma concentration, a reflection of the time course and amount of alcohol imbibed. Patients may present after trauma caused by the impaired sensorium (slowed reaction times, reduced inhibition) associated with alcohol. Patients may be unco-operative, and have a depressed level of consciousness, making assessment of head injury or concurrent drug intake difficult. Sedative drugs should be avoided.

Cardiac dysrhythmias, particularly atrial fibrillation (AF) and ventricular ectopics may occur. Ventricular dysrhythmias have been reported. Tachycardia is common. Peripheral vasodilation occurs, and patients may become rapidly hypothermic.

Coma preceeds respiratory arrest, and is associated with high levels of plasma alcohol (>400 mg/dl – equivalent to 15 units consumed rapidly). Alcoholic coma has a 5% mortality. It should be noted that acute intoxication can result in hypoglycaemia, causing convulsions and coma. Comatose patients are at increased risk of aspiration of stomach contents, peripheral mononeuropathy (especially, ulnar and radial) and rhabdomyolysis.

Alcohol inhibits anti-diuretic hormone secretion. The volume of urine passed while intoxicated therefore exceeds the volume of alcoholic drink consumed, and the patient becomes dehydrated.

Alcohol depresses gastric motility; therefore, patients should always be considered to have a full stomach, and be placed in the recovery position if they have a reduced level of consciousness. Alcohol may cause gastritis and pancreatitis, both of which can produce upper abdominal pain, radiating to the back. Acute pancreatitis is fatal in up to 40% of cases.

Retching and vomiting may cause Mallory–Weiss tears of the lower oesophagus (and, therefore, upper GI haemorrhage). Excessive vomiting may also lead to metabolic alkalosis, due to the loss of stomach H^+ ions (Chapter 8), although this may be balanced by ketoacidosis (ketone production occurs when concurrent fasting leads to fat being used as an energy source). Alkalosis may cause hypokalaemia, which worsens cardiac dysrhythmias and may produce seizures. Hypokalaemia and hypomagnesaemia are also caused by direct renal toxicity.

The metabolism of alcohol displays zero-order kinetics, being oxidised at a constant rate of about 1 unit/h. The fall in plasma concentration is, therefore, dependent on time, rather than plasma concentration.

Acutely intoxicated patients should be managed in the recovery position, or sitting up, with oxygen administered by facemask. They should be monitored continuously using ECG, oxygen saturation probes and nursing presence. Non-emergency surgery should be avoided, until the patient is sober. Full blood count, amylase, blood alcohol level and ABGs should be measured on admission. Blood glucose levels should be monitored hourly, until the patient resumes oral intake; i.v. fluids and H_2-receptor antagonists may be administered. The patient should be advised about sensible alcohol intake when recovered, and invited to speak to a specialist in alcohol abuse.

Chronic alcoholism

Chronic alcoholism may be defined as a physical and psychological dependence on alcohol. Behaviour patterns evolve that are based around drinking, and the patient is unable to function normally without alcohol. In addition, alcohol cessation produces withdrawal phenomena. Alcoholism has a number of systemic effects:

- Neurological:
  - Convulsions, particularly 7–48 h after withdrawal, that may lead to intracerebral haemorrhage.
  - Confusion.
  - Withdrawal phenomena – tremor, anxiety, hallucinations (delirium tremens), perioperative.
  - Confusion (Chapter 19).
  - Intracerebral and subarachnoid haemorrhage.
- Cardiovascular:
  - Dysrhythmia.
  - Hypertension.
  - IHD.
  - Dilated cardiomyopathy.
- Malnutrition:
  - Vitamin B deficiency – peripheral neuropathy.
  - Thiamine (vitamin B_1) deficiency is associated with Wernicke's encephalopathy (nystagmus, ataxia and deranged mental function), Korsakoff's psychosis (retrograde and anterograde amnesia, with confabulation), cerebellar degeneration and amblyopia (red/green blindness and blurred sight).
  - Folate (B_{12}) deficiency is associated with megaloblastic anaemia and amblyopia.
  - Direct bone marrow suppression may result in neutropaenia and thrombocytopaenia.
- Hepatic:
  - Fatty liver and hypertriglyceridaemia.
  - Alcoholic hepatitis. This is usually a progression from fatty liver, and is associated with abdominal pain, jaundice and fever. Liver function tests (LFTs) are deranged.
  - Cirrhosis. Fibrotic change in the liver may result from prolonged excessive alcohol exposure. Fibrosis results from recurrent attacks of hepatitis, together with direct toxic effects of the alcohol metabolite acetaldehyde.
  - Oesophageal varices may occur, which are prone to haemorrhage

18

(catastrophically, if the patient is also coagulopathic).

- Liver failure, with hypoglycaemia, coagulopathy and encephalopathy may occur, if the cirrhotic liver decompensates.

- Hypo-albuminaemia may result from liver disease or malnutrition, and is associated with ascites and congestive cardiac failure. Drug distribution of highly plasma-protein-bound drugs is affected.

- Infection, due to malnutrition, neutropaenia and poor social conditions (housing, sanitation, relationships).

History and examination may reveal little unless the patient has advanced disease. Drug abuse and tobacco use may co-exist. Routine investigations may be deranged, as described above. It is important to investigate the patient for coagulopathy (clotting tests and platelet concentration) and cardiomyopathy (ECG and echocardiography). Fresh-frozen plasma (FFP) and parenteral vitamin K may be required preoperatively. High concentration vitamin preparations (Pabrinex – vitamins B and C) should be given to patients both preoperatively and postoperatively; i.v. infusions of chlormethiazole, midazolam or even alcohol may be used prophylactically to avoid withdrawal phenomena, but these should only be administered to constantly monitored patients.

Evidence is beginning to accumulate that abstention of alcohol for a period of 1 month or so prior to major surgery, even in moderate drinkers, significantly reduces perioperative complications. The addition of disulfiram (an inhibitor of alcohol dehydrogenase and used to discourage alcohol consumption in alcoholics) may be necessary to ensure compliance with the regime in some patients.

Hepatic disease

Anatomy and physiology
The liver is the largest organ in the body, weighing between 1.2 and 1.5 kg. It is situated in the right upper abdominal quadrant, and is pyramidal in shape, the apex reaching xiphisternum. The liver is divided into two lobes (the right being six times the size of the left in adults) by the falciform ligament, and subdivided into lobules (50–100,000 in number), within which blood flows from a number of peripheral hepatic arterioles to a central hepatic vein through sinusoids, past hepatocytes (65% of liver cells) and non-parenchymal cells (35% – a third of which are Kuppfer cells (hepatic macrophages)). In fact, functionally, the liver may be divided into acini, in which blood flows from a central hepatic arteriole and terminal portal venule to a number of peripheral hepatic veins (see Fig. 18.2). Bile drains from each hepatocyte via several canaliculi to a collecting duct (that associates with the hepatic arteriole), emptying into larger ducts and finally the common bile duct.

Three functional zones may be identified in each acinus:

- Zone 1 lies nearest the hepatic arteriole, and is, therefore, supplied with well-oxygenated blood. Hepatocytes in this zone are responsible for protein anabolism and catabolism, which involve high-energy chemical reactions.

- Zone 2 is an intermediary zone.

- Zone 3 lies nearest the hepatic venule, and is most prone to ischaemic damage. Hepatocytes here contain high levels of cytochrome P450, and this is the area where phase I drug biotransformation (see below) takes place.

Afferent blood flow to the liver is derived from two sources, the hepatic artery (which supplies 35% of the blood (500 ml/min) and 65% of the oxygen) and the portal vein (which supplies 65% of the blood (1000 ml/min) and 35% of the oxygen – having already passed through the splanchnic circulation). The sources mix before entering the peripheral part of the hepatic sinusoids. Hepatic arteriolar tone lowers the distal arteriolar perfusion pressure to below that of

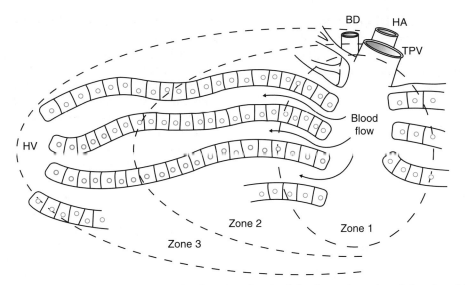

Fig. 18.2 Schematic diagram of an acinus – the functional unit of the liver. The acinus is bordered by the triad of terminal portal venule (TBV), bile ductile (BD) and hepatic arteriole (HA). Flow is unidirectional within the acinus from the triad to the hepatic venule (HV) and ultimately hepatic veins.

the portal venous pressure to avoid hepatic portal backwash.

20–25% (1500 ml/min) of the cardiac output flows through the liver (100 ml/100g/min); the liver may contain up to 15% of the total blood volume at any one time, 80% of which can be expelled within 20s after sympathetic nerve stimulation, adding 7–10% to the circulating blood volume.

The arterial supply is autoregulated in the physiological pressure range, while the hepatic portal system reacts as a passive vascular bed, with a linear pressure/flow relationship. Factors that reduce splanchnic perfusion pressure (such as hypoxia and noradrenaline) may therefore significantly reduce hepatic blood flow. Similarly, factors which reduce hepatic oxygen supply may be significantly reduced by factors that reduce either hepatic arterial flow (e.g. haemorrhage) or arterial oxygenation (e.g. respiratory disease). Acidosis increases flow in both vessels. Alkalosis decreases flow in both vessels. A degree of compensation may occur for changes in portal and arterial flow: if portal venous flow falls, hepatic artery flow increases; if portal venous flow increases, hepatic artery flow falls. General anaesthetic agents and regional

Table 18.2 Perioperative factors which decrease or increase hepatic blood flow

Decrease	Increase
Abdominal surgery	Supine posture
Anaesthesia	Food
▪ Positive-pressure ventilation	Acute hepatitis
▪ Hypoxia hypercarbia	Enzyme-inducing drugs
▪ Volatile anaesthetic agents	Acidosis
▪ Anaesthetic agents (i.v.)	
▪ Ganglion-blocking drugs	
▪ Thoracic epidurals	
H$_2$-receptor anatagonists	
Vasopressin	

anaesthesia decrease liver blood flow by about 25%; manipulation of intra-abdominal viscera during surgery, however, may reduce blood flow by up to 70%. Table 18.2 summarises the perioperative factors that increase or decrease hepatic blood flow.

Functions of the liver

The liver performs a variety of essential functions related to molecular anabolism, catabolism, detoxification and excretion. Of greatest importance are

- carbohydrate, fat and protein metabolism;

- bile formation;

- detoxification and biotransformation;

- synthesis of pro- and anticoagulant factors;

- haematological and immune function;

- acid–base regulation;

- storage of vitamins and minerals.

Carbohydrate, fat and protein metabolism

The liver helps maintain the blood glucose level within relatively narrow limits, the absolute level determining whether the liver stores or produces glucose. After food, approximately 25–50% of the glucose load is absorbed by the liver, and converted to glycogen or triglyceride. Insulin almost completely suppresses hepatic glucose production, and stimulates glycogen deposition through the activation of glycogen synthetase. Inhibition of glycogenolysis and stimulation of glycogen synthesis also occurs through a depression of hepatic vagal activity, in response to high glucose concentrations in the portal vein.

The liver is the only organ that can make glucose. When fasting, insulin levels fall and glucagon levels rise, which stimulates gluconeogenesis through activation of the glucose-6-phosphatase enzyme. Gluconeogenesis may also be achieved after sympathetic nervous stimulation and release of catecholamines. Lactate, pyruvate, glycerol and gluconeogenic amino acids may be used as substrates for gluconeogenesis.

Dietary fat, which reaches the liver via lymph and portal blood, is converted to glycerol and fatty acids by hepatic lipases. Glycerol is then oxidised, via carbohydrate enzyme pathways. Fatty acids are oxidised to acetyl coenzyme A, and either enter carbohydrate enzyme pathways, or form ketone bodies. The liver is the only organ that can form ketone bodies, which are in turn oxidised by other tissues as an energy source (producing carbon dioxide, water, heat and energy).

The liver is the major site of dietary amino acid metabolism, and is involved in catabolising amino acids to form substrates for carbohydrate and fat metabolism, in addition to synthesising a large number of bioactive proteins (e.g. clotting factors, transport proteins, albumin, antibodies). Nitrogen, a waste product of protein catabolism, is converted into urea, a small molecule that is freely excreted by the kidneys.

Bile formation

Bile consists of water, bile salts and pigments (bilirubin, biliverdin), cholesterol, fatty acids and inorganic salts. The liver produces about 750 ml/day. Bile salts are sodium and potassium salts of bile acids (derivatives of cholesterol) conjugated with taurine or glycine; their physicochemical composition facilitates lipid micelle formation in the gut, by reducing surface tension. Bile pigments are end products of haem catabolism; about 300 mg a day are produced.

In addition, bile increases colonic motility, aids excretion of lipophilic and protein-bound drugs, toxins and heavy metals, enhances gut mucosal immunity and reduces endotoxin absorption from the gut.

Detoxification and biotransformation

The liver plays a central role in detoxification and biotransformation for several reasons:

- It receives a high arterial blood flow, and is, therefore, theoretically exposed to the entire blood volume every four circulations.

- It receives blood from the portal tract. Therefore, anything absorbed by the GIT has to pass through the liver before reaching the systemic circulation.

- The transit time through the liver is slow – a function of the size of the liver, despite its high blood flow.

- The presence of Kuppfer cells (liver macrophages).

18

■ There is functional organisation of enzyme subgroups according to cellular oxygen tension.

The 'hepatic extraction ratio' (HER) describes the amount of a substrate that is removed from a volume of blood by one passage through the liver. The majority of a drug with a high HER (e.g. GTN and propranolol) is, therefore, removed by passage through the liver (Chapter 3).

The liver catabolises insulin, inactivates steroid hormones, converts thyroxine to triiodothyronine and hydroxylates cholecalciferol. The liver also is the main site for production of pseudo-cholinesterase, which metabolises important drugs used in the perioperative period, such as suxamethonium and mivacurium.

Synthesis of pro- and anticoagulant factors
The liver is the site of synthesis of

■ all pro-coagulant factors, except factor VIII;

■ the anticoagulant factors anti-thrombin III and protein C;

■ the fibrinolytic factors plasminogen and α-2 anti-plasmin.

In addition, the liver stores vitamin K, and catabolises activated clotting factors and circulating fibrinolytic stimulators.

Haematological and immune function
After 2 months of age, the liver effectively has no haematopoetic function. However, the liver can produce erythropoetin in uraemic patients. In addition, the liver synthesises transferrin and is an important storage site for vitamin B_{12} and folate.

Kuppfer cells, which comprise 70% of the body's reticulo-endothelial system, act as biological filters that clear the portal blood of particulate and cellular debris, as well as acting as initiators of an immune response in response to exogenous material, particularly endotoxins. Kuppfer cells also have important antiviral and anti-tumour functions.

In addition, the liver synthesises and secretes IgA, and produces bile, which prevents adhesion of pathological bacteria to gut mucosal surfaces.

Acid–base regulation
In alkalosis, H^+ ions released from ammonia (during the synthesis of urea) neutralise excess HCO_3. The liver also converts lactate to glucose and carbon dioxide (Chapter 8).

Storage of vitamins and minerals
The liver stores the fat-soluble vitamins A, D, E and K, and also acts as a reservoir of vitamin B_{12} and iron.

Liver failure
Like the kidneys, the liver has a high physiological reserve – a significant proportion of its maximal physiological capability can be damaged before pathological decompensation occurs.

Perioperative liver failure may occur for a number of reasons (Table 18.3).

The clinical effects of hepatic failure may be predicted from an understanding of the normal physiological functions of the liver. Therefore, in failure, the following occur (Table 18.4):

■ *Hypoglycaemia*. Occurs due to failure of gluconeogenesis and reduced catabolism of insulin.

■ *Hypo-albuminaemia*: This has two main consequences: a reduction in plasma oncotic pressure (leading to ascites, high-output cardiac failure and pleural effusion), and a reduction in plasma protein transport (which increases the free plasma concentration of highly plasma protein-bound drugs, such as phenytoin and diazepam – increased levels of which can have adverse side-effects).

■ *Coagulopathy*: Occurs due to decreased production of pro-coagulants, reduced vitamin K absorption and storage, synthesis of abnormal clotting factors (e.g. dysfibrinogen), decreased clearance of activated clotting factors, excessive fibrinolysis and reduced clearance of endogenous heparin.

18

18

Table 18.3 Common causes of perioperative liver failure

Prehepatic causes

Ischaemic hepatic necrosis
- Prolonged hypotension
- Splanchnic vasoconstrictors (e.g. noradrenaline)
- MOF

Surgery

Hyperthermia

Hepatic causes

Infective hepatitis
- Hepatitis viruses B, C, D
- Cytomegalovirus

Drug-induced hepatitis
- Halothane
- Paracetamol
- NSAIDs
- Phenytoin

Acute fatty liver of pregnancy

Alcohol

Hepatic venous obstruction (Budd–Chiari syndrome)

Cirrhosis (with acute episodes of failure)

Posthepatic causes

Cholangitis

Biliary obstruction

Cholestasis
- Pregnancy
- ITU patients
- Parenteral nutrition

Table 18.4 Summary of pathological consequences of acute hepatic failure

Hypoglycaemia

Hypo-albuminaemia

Coagulopathy

Jaundice

Encephalopathy

Immuno-compromise

Metabolic derangement

Impaired drug metabolism

- *Encephalopathy.* This is generally attributed to the accumulation of toxic substances (including ammonia, gamma-amino butyric acid (GABA) and endogenous benzodiazepine receptor ligands), that produce direct cerebral depression, as well as cerebral oedema. As encephalopathy worsens, the patient becomes more drowsy and unrousable, develops clonus and has reduced reactivity to painful stimuli.

- *Jaundice.* Occurs due to failure of bilirubin transport (hypo-albuminaemia) and hepatic conjugation. Bilirubin (amongst other toxins) is nephrotoxic, and renal failure is common after hepatic failure.

- *Immuno-compromise:* Severe infections, particularly with Gram-positive and -negative aerobes originating from the gut and urinary tract, are common.

- *Metabolic disturbances:* Dilutional hyponatraemia and hypokalaemia occur. The latter may also occur due to co-existent metabolic alkalosis.

- *Impaired drug metabolism:* Drugs with a high HER (>60%) produce high peak drug concentrations in hepatic failure; their dose, rather than their frequency of administration, should be reduced.

Drugs with a low HER of <30% (e.g. diazepam) are relatively unaffected by hepatic failure; their frequency of administration, rather than their dose, should be reduced.

A number of investigations may be performed perioperatively in order to assess the degree of liver dysfunction. These are summarised in Table 18.5.

In the perioperative period, surgery is usually deferred in patients with acute hepatic failure, due to the very high mortality risk, although surgery may include life-saving procedures (e.g. sclerotherapy for varices) or transplantation.

Table 18.5 **Summary of investigative findings likely in liver disease**

Parameter	Result
Full blood count	Anaemia ■ Macrocytic – B12 and folate depletion ■ Microcytic – iron depletion, malnutrition Thrombocytopaenia – due to portal hypertension and hypersplenism
Urea and electrolytes	Urea decreased, may be increased if renal failure also present Hypo/hypernatraemia Hypokalaemia, hypomagnesaemia, hypophosphataemia Hypoglycaemia
ABGs	Respiratory alkalosis (in encephalopathy), metabolic alkalosis, metabolic acidosis (after paracetamol overdose)
LFTs	Bilirubin >35 mmol/l produces clinically noticeable jaundice; >90 mmol/l increases chance of perioperative renal failure + mortality Hypo-albuminaemia (often <30 g/dl) Alanine transaminase (ALT) and aspartate aminotransferase (AST) >40 mmol/l (though these may be normal if severe hepato-cellular loss has occurred, because their synthesis is reduced) Alkaline phosphatase (ALP) – particularly after biliary obstruction Gamma glutamyl transpeptidase (GGT) – particularly after alcohol intake
Coagulation function	The International Normalised Ratio (INR) is a sensitive test of liver synthetic function, elevations indicating a reduction in liver function
Blood cultures	A variety of GI and urinary G+/− aerobes. Serology is sent for HBV, HCV and CMV
Electrocardiogram	Ischaemia and dysrhythmias may occur
CXR	Pleural effusions, pulmonary oedema
Abdominal girth measurements	Increases as ascites collects
Electroencephalography (EEG)	To diagnose hepatic encephalopathy in unconscious or sedated patients
Intracranial pressure (ICP) monitoring	ICP increases with cerebral oedema, although the correlation is poor
Computerised tomography and ultrasound scanning	To visualise ascites, pleural effusions, biliary tree obstruction
Endoscopy	To assess oesophageal varices
Liver biopsy	To assess hepato-cellular or parenchymal liver disease Hazardous, if patient is coagulopathic

18

Similarly, patients with chronic liver disease have significant perioperative mortality, which may be in excess of 75% at 1 month, if there is co-existent encephalopathy, renal or respiratory failure, or coagulopathy. Preoperative care is multidisciplinary. Coagulopathy should be treated with FFP and vitamin K (and platelet transfusion, cryoprecipitate and vasopressin, as required). Ascites may need to be drained to avoid diaphragmatic splinting when the patient lies supine. Patients with severe hypo-albuminaemia (i.e. <15 g/dl) may benefit from i.v. albumin infusions. A sliding scale insulin/glucose/potassium infusion should be started. Patients will require an intensive care bed postoperatively.

Intra-operative care is aimed at maintaining fluid and electrolyte homeostasis (use of appropriate i.v. fluids and diuretics, monitoring renal function/urine output, maintaining blood glucose level) and avoiding/treating coagulopathy. Universal precautions should be taken.

Postoperatively, opioids are minimised because most constrict the sphincter of Oddi (causing reduced biliary flow) and are CNS depressants. NSAIDs are also avoided because of their nephrotoxic side-effects. Regional analgesia (in the absence of coagulopathy), pethidine and paracetamol may be used for pain relief. Renal, coagulant and cerebral function are closely monitored. Hypotension and hypoxia should be avoided. High protein nutritional regimes are avoided to reduce the incidence of encephalopathy. Postoperative jaundice may be associated with haemolysis after extensive surgery, heart failure (with hepatic congestion), drug reactions (erythromycin, phenothiazines), sepsis and Gilbert's syndrome (benign unconjugated hyperbilirubinaemia).

Acute renal failure

Introduction

Acute renal failure (ARF) may be defined clinically by a rising serum creatinine, increasing at a rate exceeding 40 μmol/day coupled with either a urine output of < 0.5 ml/kg/h (oliguric renal failure) or a urine output exceeding 2.0 ml/kg/h (polyuric renal failure).

Episodes of ARF will occur in some 1–2% of all hospital admissions and 20% of all intensive care admissions. The onset of ARF significantly contributes to subsequent mortality by up to 30%. Most importantly given the potential negative impact of ARF, it is estimated that up to 50% of the episodes of ARF occurring within the hospital setting are iatrogenic in origin and therefore essentially preventable. The commonest cause of ARF is acute tubular necrosis (ATN) occurring as a result of systemic hypoperfusion (shock).

Functions of the kidney

In health, the kidneys perform two primary functions. These are the excretion of the end products of nitrogen metabolism (urea) together with the conservation of substrates of nitrogen-based synthesis (amino acids) and glucose; and the control of the electrolyte and hydrogen ion content of body fluids. These processes are achieved through the formation of an hypertonic urine. Urine is essentially an ultrafiltrate of blood, which is subsequently modified by absorption and secretion.

Conceptually, nephron function can be divided into two physiological phases, one passive and one active. The first stage is the formation of an ultrafiltrate by the glomerulus. This is essentially a passive function for the kidney as energy is provided in a potential form in the pressure head delivered by the heart. The integrity of this filtration function is usually estimated by measuring *creatinine clearance*. In clinical practice, the production of urine is taken to be synonymous with a functioning kidney, reflecting in turn blood flow to the renal parenchyma. Both of these assumptions are in point of fact invalid. Even a dead kidney can produce a 'dilute' urine isotonic with the plasma through passive ultrafiltration conditional only on mean arterial pressure and the patency of the ultrafiltration pores in the glomerular basement membrane.

18

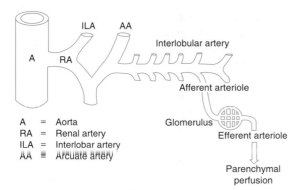

A = Aorta
RA = Renal artery
ILA = Interlobar artery
AA = Arcuate artery

Fig. 18.3 The renal circulation.

Further, the arrangement of the renal circulation is such that its two basic functions, glomerular function and renal parenchymal perfusion occur in series, not in parallel (Fig. 18.3). The practical import of this arrangement is that in conditions of adequate systemic arterial pressure, there is adequate blood flow to maintain both filtration and renal perfusion.

However, in states of reduced systemic arterial pressure (shock), glomerular filtration (GF) pressure is maintained by vasoconstriction in the efferent arterioles creating a backpressure and thus maintaining primary urine production. However, this efferent vasoconstriction has the unwanted side-effect of shutting down perfusion to the renal parenchyma distal to the glomerulus. Thus, contrary to popular belief, urine output and renal blood flow are not necessarily synonymous.

Of greater import in the assessment of kidney function is the second (active) stage in urine formation. This second stage involves the subsequent modification of the primary urine, involving the creation of ion fluxes against concentration gradients (thus requiring the consumption of energy), and ultimately leading to a urine hypertonic with respect to the plasma. The measurement of urine *osmolality* and its value in relation to plasma osmolality give some indication of the integrity of this active principle (Chapter 6):

normal plasma osmolality = 300 mosmol/kg

normal urine osmolality range
= 600–1000 mosmol/kg

normal urine to plasma osmolality ratio
= 2:1 to 3:1

The osmolality ratio is a particularly useful index of renal function in that being an active principle, it is very sensitive to changes in oxygen delivery to the renal parenchyma. Thus changes in the ratio are a useful *early* sign of renal dysfunction *preceding* any overt changes in urine volume.

Prevention of acute renal failure

Given the reportedly high incidence of iatrogenic episodes of ARF, the primary management of ARF should be preventative. Through all episodes of major surgery or postoperative critical care particular attention should be paid to the maintenance of adequate BP and levels of hydration. In addition, it is important to avoid drugs with potential renal toxicity such as the amino glycoside antibiotics, and the NSAIDs. It is important to remember that even the new generation NSAIDs the so-called 'Cox 2-specific' drugs although demonstrating a reduced incidence of GI bleeding, still maintain the same profile of renal toxicity (Chapter 10). It goes without saying that particular diligence should be paid in patients who present with a pre-existing degree of renal dysfunction as evidenced by an elevated serum creatinine on admission.

Treatment of established acute renal failure

Of paramount importance when dealing with any organ damaged by ischaemia is the restoration of balance between oxygen supply and demand. The first step in this process has to be the re-establishment of an adequate perfusion pressure and circulating blood volume.

The options for pharmacological support are less well defined. Having established a perfusion pressure, by convention the next step is to provide a renal vasodilator to optimise oxygen delivery to the renal parenchyma. Historically dopamine remains

18

259

the mainstay of treatment, the rational basis for its use being the existence of vasodilatory dopaminergic receptors in the renal vascular bed, in common with other splanchnic organs. However, recent data suggests that the diuresis seen during dopamine administration is actually due to its natriuretic rather than vasodilatory effects.

Dopexamine hydrochloride an N-substituted analogue of dopamine, with activity at both dopaminergic and β2-receptors but lacking any intrinsic α-effect (unlike dopamine) is another drug with potential renal vasodilator effects. It also has the additional property, useful in some cases of ARF, of modulating serum potassium levels via β-mediated intracellular translocation. Its efficacy in ARF remains to be substantiated in randomised controlled trials.

18

19

Central nervous system

Aims

The aims of this chapter are to

- describe aspects of the functional anatomy and physiology of the central nervous system (CNS), which are appropriate to perioperative care of the patient;

- describe the pathophysiology of common perioperative problems related to the (CNS)

- outline the investigation and treatment of such problems.

19

Objectives

After reading this chapter you should be able to

- recognise, investigate and manage abnormal neurological functioning in the perioperative patient;

- understand the psychological stress of surgery for patients.

Introduction

An altered state of consciousness may be one of the first clinical indicators of CNS pathology in the perioperative period. Preoperatively, patients with CNS disorders may present for surgery to correct the disorder or its sequelae, or for surgery unconnected to the condition.

They may be taking a variety of long-term medications, a number of which may have side-effects that affect their perioperative care. A number of neurological diseases are a function of aging (e.g. cerebrovascular disease and dementia) and are likely to increase along with the average age of the population. Intra-operatively, anaesthesia has a major impact on the CNS rendering patients temporarily and reversibly unconscious during general anaesthesia, and temporarily paralysed in the case of regional anaesthesia. Postoperatively, a number of factors may combine to cause temporary or permanent neurological damage, in addition to aggravating preoperative conditions. In addition, the psychological stress of illness and surgery can trigger or worsen neuro-psychiatric disease. A functional understanding both of the anatomy and physiology of the central and peripheral nervous systems, and how they are affected by systemic dysfunction, allows the physician to rapidly diagnose, investigate and treat neurological pathology, which may prevent further deterioration.

Functional anatomy and physiology

The nervous system may be divided as given in the diagram below.

The functional anatomy and physiology of the *autonomic nervous system* is described in Chapter 3.

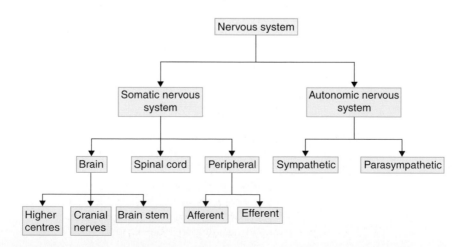

Brain

The brain is classically divided into forebrain, midbrain and hindbrain as shown in the diagram below.

The forebrain

The forebrain is divided into

- Cerebral cortex, comprising two hemispheres (left and right), which are subdivided into several lobes. The frontal lobes (anterior) which contain motor cortices and areas for memory and intellectual function.

- Parietal lobes (superolateral) which contain sensory cortices and sensory integrative areas.

- Temporal lobes (lateral) which contain the auditory cortices and integrative pathways and the limbic system (mood and memory).

- Occipital lobes (posterior) which contain the visual cortices and integrative pathways.

- Basal ganglia – grey matter within the cerebral hemispheres which integrates information about fine motor control.

- Diencephalon – consisting of the

  - *hypothalamus* (on the floor of the third ventricle, posterior to the optic chiasm) which controls autonomic nervous system activity, temperature regulation, thirst, hunger, sexual activity and the release of hormones from the posterior pituitary (to which it is attached by the hypothalamo-hypophyseal stalk);

  - *pituitary gland* (sits in the pituitary fossa of the sphenoid bone), which secretes growth hormone, prolactin, ACTH, thyroxine release hormone and LH/FSH from its anterior lobe, and stores and releases vasopressin and oxytocin from its posterior lobe);

  - *thalamus*, which integrates sensory pathways.

The midbrain

The midbrain communicates with the cerebellum, cranial nuclei III and IV and the pineal gland (and is, therefore, possibly concerned with the sleep/wake cycle).

The hindbrain

The hindbrain consists of the

- *cerebellum*, which lies in the posterior cranial fossa and regulates posture, co-ordination and muscle tone;

- *pons*, which lies between the midbrain and medulla, communicates with cerebellum, and contains the pontine nuclei and cranial nerve nuclei V, VI, VII and VIII;

- *medulla*, which is the most inferior part of the brain and is continuous with the spinal cord. It communicates with the cerebellum and contains cranial nerve nuclei IX, X, XI, XII, respiratory and cardiovascular centres, ascending sensory nerve fibres and descending motor fibres.

The midbrain, pons and medulla are collectively referred to as the brain stem and

19

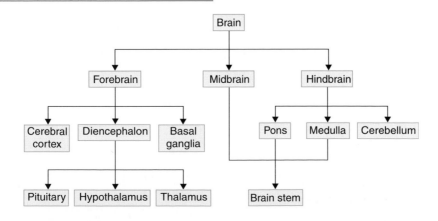

19

are grossly responsible for the control of vegetative functions – breathing, cardiovascular homeostasis, gastrointestinal function and balance.

Spinal cord

The spinal cord is continuous with the medulla and exits the base of the skull at the foramen magnum. It descends through the vertebral canal bordered anteriorly by the vertebral bodies and intervertebral discs, laterally by the pedicles, laminae and transverse processes of the vertebrae and posteriorly by the spinous processes of the lamina, before terminating inferiorly to form the conus medullaris (approximately at L1 or 2 in adults). Thirty-one pairs of spinal nerves are given off along this course (8 cervical, 12 thoracic, 5 lumbar, 5 sacral, 1 coccygeal).

Figure 19.1 shows a cross-section through the spinal cord and shows the position and function of the ascending and descending spinal tracts.

The blood supply of the spinal cord is derived from three sources:

- anterior spinal artery, which is derived from the vertebral arteries, descends in the anterior median fissure and supplies the anterior two thirds of the cord;

- posterior spinal arteries, which are derived from the vertebral arteries and supply the posterior third of the cord;

- radicular branches, which are derived from local arteries, such as the intercostal arteries.

Meninges and cerebrospinal fluid

The meninges consist of three layers of tissue that surround the brain, spinal cord and nerve roots. The inner layer, the pia mater, is closely adherent to the brain surface and is vascular. The arachnoid mater overlies the pia, but does not follow the pia mater into the brain sulci and clefts. The thick, fibrous dura mater is composed of two layers: an outer layer which is adherent to the periosteum of the skull/vertebrae, and an inner layer, which forms the falx cerebri and cerebelli, and tentorium cerebelli. In the brain, the inner and outer layers are adherent apart from transmitting the venous sinuses. In the spinal cord, the inner and outer layers are separated by the extradural space, which contains fat,

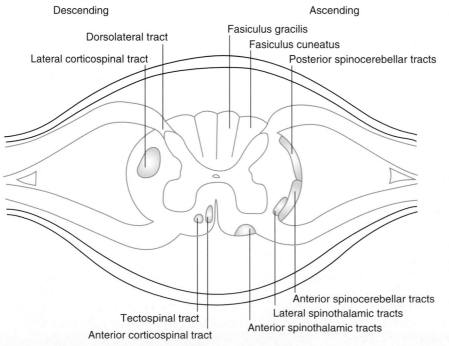

Fig. 19.1 Cross-section through the spinal cord and shows the position and function of the ascending and descending spinal tracts.

blood vessels and connective tissue, and is the space which is targeted for epidural anaesthesia (local anaesthetic remains contained in this space, and bathes the spinal nerve roots that exit the space laterally).

The space between the pia mater and arachnoid mater contains cerebrospinal fluid (CSF), a filtrate of plasma secreted by the choroid plexus in the third, fourth and lateral ventricles (CSF containing spaces that communicate bilaterally on the brain's inner surface). The CSF circulates around the surfaces of the brain and spinal cord, providing shock absorption and structural support to the soft nervous tissue, before being reabsorbed by the arachnoid villi to the cerebrovenous sinuses. CSF reabsorption is reduced if the central venous pressure (CVP) is raised. The volume of CSF is approximately 150 ml, which is replaced about three times a day.

Cerebral circulation

The cerebral circulation is derived bilaterally from the internal carotid arteries (65%) and the vertebral arteries (35%) forming the circle of Willis. Venous drainage passes posteriorly to the left and right transverse sinuses, which drain into the internal jugular vein (IJV).

In adults, the cerebral blood flow (CBF) approximates to 15% of the cardiac output, or 750 ml/min. The CBF may be altered by several factors:

Cerebral perfusion pressure

The cerebral perfusion pressure (CPP) is autoregulated between a mean arterial pressure (MAP) of 60–150 mmHg (Fig. 19.2).

Autoregulation is the process whereby tissues regulate their own blood flow, the mechanisms for which are unclear, but may involve a reactive contractility of vascular smooth muscle (myogenic theory) and hyperlocalised metabolic vasoactivity (metabolic theory). The MAP at which autoregulation occurs may be reset upwards (i.e. a higher perioperative MAP may be required to maintain CPP, thus avoiding cerebral ischaemia, in chronically hypertensive patients. The CPP may also be critically

reduced by a raised intracerebral pressure (ICP):

$$CPP = MAP - ICP \quad \text{(or CVP, whichever value is higher)}$$

The Monroe–Kellie doctrine

This states that the cranial vault is effectively a rigid box and its contents (brain tissue, CSF and blood) are incompressible. Therefore, potential increases in volume in one component (e.g. blood following cerebral haemorrhage or brain tumour) can only take place at the expense of reduction in volume elsewhere (e.g. normal brain tissue compression and reduced CSF volume). This effect may limit a rise in ICP for a while, but eventually the limit is reached and any further increase in bleeding or tumour size leads to raised ICP and a subsequent fall in CPP. If severe, this causes brain injury due to ischaemia and compression. Generally, the more rapid the change the more likely the injury (e.g. following acute subrachnoid haemorrhage).

Arterial PO$_2$ and PCO$_2$

Hypoxia and hypercapnia, such as may occur in perioperative hypoventilation due to sedation, increase CBF. Hypocapnia decreases CBF (Fig. 19.2).

Anaesthesia

All volatile anaesthetic agents and ketamine increase CBF; i.v. anaesthetic agents and sedatives decrease CBF.

19

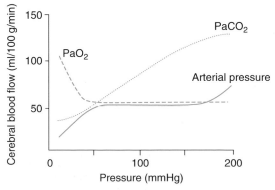

Fig. 19.2 Autoregulation of CBF with BP and changes resulting from alterations in PaCO$_2$.

19

Hypothermia

This decreases CBF but also decreases the cerebral metabolic rate for oxygen ($CMRO_2$), as do many sedatives. This is why mild hypothermia, sedation and avoidance of seizure activity may be cerebro-protective.

Investigation of neurological dysfunction

The most accurate assessment of CNS dysfunction remains the taking of a history and the performance of a thorough physical examination. Gross neurological disturbance is relatively easy to diagnose. However, fine aberrations may be more elusive to elicit, particularly if the patient is elderly, poorly communicative or had preoperative pathology. Evidence may well initially be provided by the patient's relatives, and the patient often requires formal assessment by a neurologist. Laboratory and radiological investigations may include the following tests.

X-ray

The use of X-rays has become superceded to a large extent by computerised tomography (CT) and magnetic resonance imaging (MRI) scanning. However, X-rays are still used to detect fractures of the cranial vault and vertebrae.

Computerised axial tomography

A thin beam of X-radiation is passed from a rotating source through the patient to a diametrically opposed fixed array of detectors, which measure the degree of X-ray absorption. Computers are used to integrate absorption information from the detectors, producing a two-dimensional display. By moving the patient through the scanner, axial 'cuts' (usually 5 mm apart) may be taken, producing a cross-sectional view of the patient. Scans are viewed as if looking up through the patient from feet to head. Bone appears white, soft tissue as a range of grey shades and air as black. The i.v. contrast agents are seen as whiteness on the scan, and may be used to demonstrate the presence of

intracranial haemorrhage. CT may also be of use in diagnosing cerebral oedema and infarction, trauma, tumour, arterio-venous malformations/aneurysms, abscesses and spinal cord compression.

Magnetic resonance imaging

Hydrogen protons align themselves along the axis of strong magnetic fields, such as that provided within an MRI scanner. If a radiofrequency pulse is beamed perpendicular to the magnetic field, the protons absorb energy and their spin is deflected. Withdrawal of the pulse results in realignment of the protons in the magnetic field, with a release of measurable radiofrequency energy. The rate at which hydrogen protons realign (and therefore, the differential rate of release of radiofrequency energy) depends on the physicochemical 'lattice' (i.e. the type of tissue) in which they are held. The proton density of tissue also varies. Computerised interpretation of this data produces a two- or three-dimensional image of the patient. MRI is particularly useful for assessing soft tissue damage (e.g. demyelination and spinal cord views), and avoids patient exposure to ionising radiation.

Positron emission tomography

This is a relatively new technique, and is not widely available. Radionuclides (positron-emitting isotopes, e.g. [11]carbon) are bound to compounds such as water or glucose and injected into patients. Positron release and interaction with electrons produces two photons that are emitted at 180° to each other and may be detected by fixed array detectors placed around the patient. The density of the labelled compound is determined by computer analysis, and is presented as a density image. Whereas CT and MRI provide information about structural damage, positron emission tomography (PET) scanning, which is mainly still a research tool, may in the future provide important information about functional damage (e.g. reduced oxygen extraction, reduced CBF in areas of cerebral ischaemia).

Electroencephalography

An array of electrodes attached to the scalp record micro-potentials, which are amplified, filtered and presented as a pen recorder display. The spontaneous electrical activity of the brain varies in amplitude, distribution and frequency, patterns of which may be characteristic of certain conditions, such as epilepsy, encephalopathy and coma.

Intracranial pressure monitoring

A transcranial ventricular catheter placed in the lateral ventricle is connected to a pressure transducer, which in turn is connected to a computerised recorder. Normal ICP is <10 mmHg, although small regular fluctuations may be seen. As the ICP rises past 20 mmHg (moderate elevation) towards 40 mmHg (severe), variable amplitude fluctuations occur, related to respiration, approximately every 30 s. Plateau waves occur when the ICP is raised above 50 mmHg for more than 5–10 min, and precede severe neurological deterioration. ICP monitoring is most often used perioperatively both to monitor the degree of cerebral oedema and assess the response to ICP lowering therapies.

Lumbar puncture

Occasionally, in the perioperative period, physicians may be required to perform a lumbar puncture in order to investigate possible meningitis, e.g. after ENT procedures or open skull fractures. Bacterial meningitis may be confirmed by the presence of turbid CSF, with a low glucose concentration (less than one-third blood glucose), high protein content (more than 0.5 g/l) and high WCC ($0.2–10 \times 10^9$ cells/l, mainly polymorphonuclear cells). Gram stain, culture and sensitivities confirm the infecting organism and suggest antibiotic strategy. The technique of lumbar puncture for spinal subarachnoid block is described in Chapter 10.

Electromyography/nerve conduction studies

These may be used to detect abnormalities of skeletal muscle, neuropraxia and peripheral neuropathies.

Newer techniques

Cerebral oximetry using two modified oximeter probes can be used to measure the regional saturation of oxygen (RSO_2) in the underlying brain, e.g. the watershed area of the brain if the probes are applied over the forehead (unilateral or bilateral). Real time changes in RSO_2 predict postoperative neuro-cognitive dysfunction and are increasingly employed during carotid endarterectomy (CEA), head injury and cardiac surgery. It is also possible to detect pulsation and flow in the middle cerebral artery using a transcranial doppler. This is again useful during CEA to assess the adequacy of collateral circulation during carotid clamping.

19

Perioperative management of CNS conditions

The following list highlights some of the perioperative considerations that should be taken into account when managing patients with neurological disease.

Epilepsy

Epilepsy affects about 1:200 of the population. The condition is associated with paroxysms of cerebral neuronal discharge, which may produce a variety of clinical symptoms that are classified according to the type of seizure produced. Generalised seizures are sub-classified into two:

- *Grand mal* – a tonic (sustained muscular contraction) phase precedes a clonic (jerking) phase, with loss of consciousness, and sometimes loss of urinary incontinence. Prodromal symptoms, such as headache, may precede the fit, and the patient may be aware that a fit is imminent (aura).

- *Petit mal* – or 'absence' seizures. These are rarely associated with loss of consciousness.

Partial, or focal seizures may occur with or without loss of consciousness. Temporal seizures classically present with auditory, visual or olfactory hallucinations and mood change. Jacksonian seizures spread from an extremity to involve the whole body.

While petit mal and focal seizures can be distressing to the patient, the focus of the perioperative care of epileptics is to avoid grand-mal seizures. Prolonged fitting has several effects: sustained muscular contraction can affect respiratory pattern (reducing respiratory capacity) at a time when cellular oxygen uptake is increased – the patient, therefore, becomes hypoxic. Fitting also increases the $CMRO_2$, and in conditions of systemic hypoxia this can render the brain more ischaemic (which in turn reduces the fitting threshold). At the same time, prolonged fitting can produce systemic hypoglycaemia; the brain has an absolute requirement for glucose as an energy source, and hypoglycaemia can further cerebral dysfunction and damage.

Prolonged muscular contraction has four other effects:

■ core temperature rises and with it, the $CMRO_2$, by 10%/°C above 37°C;

■ plasma potassium rises, which can cause serious heart dysrhythmias;

■ rhabdomyolysis occurs, which can precipitate renal failure;

■ metabolic acidosis occurs, which in turn can reduce the fitting threshold.

Loss of consciousness endangers the patient's airway. It should be noted that cerebral hypoxia can cause fitting even in non-epileptics.

Preoperatively, the physician should assess the type of seizures the patient experiences, their frequency, any triggering factors (e.g. preoperative starvation), when the last fit occurred and any anticonvulsant medications the patient might be taking. Clinical input should be sought from a neurologist, if the patient suffers frequent, grand-mal seizures, is on a complex treatment regime, or whose fits have previously proven refractory to medication. Anticonvulsant therapy should be continued on the day of surgery.

Anticonvulsants are associated with a number of side-effects. All are associated with drowsiness and confusion. Other drug side-effects include:

■ *carbamazepine* (for grand-mal epileptics) – anaemia, leucopaenia, thrombocytopaenia, hepatitis and cholestatic jaundice;

■ *sodium valproate* (all types of seizure) – impaired hepatic function, thrombocytopaenia;

■ *phenytoin* (tonic-clonic and partial seizures) – narrow therapeutic index (i.e. check plasma levels), hepatic dysfunction, peripheral neuropathy, blood dyscrasias, hypocalcaemia. Plasma levels may be raised by amiodarone, metronidazole, fluconazole, nifedipine and cimetidine, increasing the frequency of side-effects;

■ *ciprofloxacin and anti-psychotics* – anticonvulsant activity may be reduced;

■ *barbiturates* (grand-mal) – less used today, due to their side-effect profile, which includes liver enzyme induction, mental depression and anaemia;

■ *lamotrigine, gabapentin, ethosuximide, topiramate and vigabatrin* – all can cause blood dyscrasias.

Therefore:

■ Preoperatively, patients should have full blood count, urea and electrolytes and liver function tested.

■ Intra-operatively, it is important to avoid administering pro-convulsant anaesthetic agents (e.g. enflurane and ketamine) and hypocapnia.

■ Postoperatively, anticonvulsant therapy should be recommenced as soon as possible.

Advice may be required in the severe epileptic who must remain nil by mouth, and who will require conversion of their anticonvulsants to a parenteral (usually phenytoin) regime. Care should be taken to avoid hypocapnia (e.g. hyperventilation due to pain), dehydration, hypoglycaemia and sepsis.

Status epilepticus usually describes tonic–clonic seizures that are prolonged or so

19

frequent that the patient does not recover consciousness between fits. Although the condition usually occurs in epileptics that are poorly compliant with medication or have had their medication changed, it may also occur in head injured patients, after cerebral bleeds or alcohol withdrawal. The condition is a medical emergency, requiring prompt treatment:

General anaesthesia may be associated with increased frequencies of postoperative confusion; autonomic dysfunction is associated with intra-operative cardiovascular instability. Local or regional anaesthesia is well tolerated.

Postoperatively, anti-Parkinsonian medication should be recommenced as soon

19

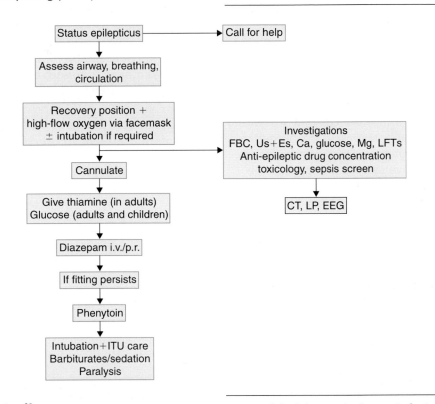

Parkinson's disease

This is a disorder of the extrapyramidal system with degeneration and loss of dopamine in the substantia niagra that gives rise to intention tremor, 'cogwheel' rigidity, hypokinesia and postural instability. The disease occurs in about 1:200 of the elderly. Preoperative assessment should consider the degree of tremor (which can make i.v. cannulation difficult) and autonomic impairment (e.g. salivation and postural hypotension), any ventilatory impairment (usually restrictive, due to a bent posture) and the effect of anti-parkinsonian medication. The medications themselves should be continued on the day of surgery (note that the half-life of L-dopa in particular is short).

as possible (alternatively, s.c. infusions of apomorphine can be given perioperatively after initial discontinuation of L-dopa therapy. This is particularly useful in severe cases or those in which it is difficult to continue oral therapy, e.g. GIT surgery). The patient should be encouraged to mobilise to avoid DVTs and respiratory complications. Dopamine antagonists, notably phenothiazines (used as postoperative tranquillisers for confused patients) and anti-emetics such as metoclopramide should be avoided. Postoperative sleep apnoea has been reported.

Multiple sclerosis

This is a chronic, progressive systemic disease (incidence 1:1000), characterised by relapsing and remitting episodes of axonal demyelination. Patients may present for any type of surgery, but may require orthopaedic procedures to ameliorate the effects of spastic contractions. Treatment is supportive but may involve steroid therapy. Patients may have restrictive respiratory defects. Spinal anaesthesia is generally avoided, due to concerns about exacerbating the condition. Postoperatively, care should be taken to mobilise the patient early.

Cerebral palsy, paraplegia and tetraplegia

Cerebral palsy (CP) includes a spectrum of non-progressive motor deficits that are caused by cerebral hypoxia, usually in the perinatal period. Improvements in physiotherapy and general supportive care have improved the life expectancy of severe sufferers. Patients with CP may present for a variety of corrective orthopaedic procedures. The condition may be associated with recurrent respiratory infections (restrictive lung defect and gastro-oesophageal reflux), poor nutrition (requiring gastrostomy feeding), poor mental function (although this is not always the case), bed sores, epilepsy and latex allergy (due to repeated medical procedures and long-term urinary catheterisation). Paraplegia describes paralysis of the lower limbs, and tetraplegia paralysis of all four limbs and the trunk.

Postoperative recovery from general anaesthesia may be slow in CP. Care should be taken with wounds, pressure areas and respiratory function, because the patient may not be able to sense a problem occurring, or may not be able to communicate. DVT prophylaxis is essential. Anticonvulsants should be recommenced as soon as possible after operation.

Myasthenia gravis

This is an autoimmune disease directed against acetylcholine receptors at the neuromuscular junction that produces muscular weakness and fatigability. It is more prevalent in females. Although it is a rare condition (1:25,000), it has several implications for perioperative management. Patients suffer repeated chest infections and may be taking immuno-suppressive therapy, including steroids. The conduct of general anaesthesia is made more difficult both by the preoperative administration of anticholinesterase inhibitors (e.g. pyridostigmine), and by the difficulties associated with intra-operative choice of paralysing agents, which can prolong the postoperative return of muscular function. Postoperatively, pyridostigmine should be restarted i.v. until oral intake resumes, and close monitoring of respiratory function, together with physiotherapy, is required to avoid the common complication of respiratory infection.

Intracerebral haemorrhage

Patients may present for surgery who have previously had a cerebrovascular accident (CVA). CVAs may also occur in the perioperative period. CVAs are caused by:

- cerebral infarction (80–85%) – which, in turn, may be caused by atheroma, embolism, arteritis or hypotension;

- cerebral haemorrhage (15–20%) – which may be caused by trauma, rupture of intracranial aneurysms and rupture of arterio-venous malformations. Hypertension and anticoagulant therapy may be contributory factors.

CVAs are more common after cardiac, carotid and neurosurgery. The clinical symptoms that develop acutely after a CVA depend on the site and degree of damage. Consciousness is usually impaired, at least temporarily. Infarction may occur of any intracerebral vessel, although the middle cerebral artery is most commonly affected. Ensuing cerebral damage may be limited by the re-establishment of blood flow and compensatory collateral flow. Haemorrhage due to trauma often originates from veins interposing the two-layered dura mater (see above), producing an extradural haematoma; this is often unilateral and produces a mass effect. Sub-dural haemorrhage occurs from blood vessels between the dura and arachnoid mater and occurs more commonly in the elderly and alcoholics; sub-durals may reach a considerable size before clinical signs or

19

symptoms are seen (confusion and sedation). Subarachnoid haemorrhage usually occurs from congenital aneurysms. The treatment of an acute CVA is supportive – initial resuscitation and investigation (CT scan, predisposing causes) is followed by chronic rehabilitation, involving physiotherapy and occupational therapy.

Patients requiring surgery who have previously had a CVA may present a variety of perioperative problems.

CVAs may be indicative of underlying pathology such as hypertension, atherosclerosis (and therefore, IHD and carotid disease), cardiac dysrhythmia, coagulation disorders or anticoagulant therapy and connective tissue disorders (e.g. polycystic kidney disease). Other problems include:

- *immobility*, due to hemiplegia, which predisposes to DVT and pressure sore formation;

- *increased likelihood of accidental trauma*, such as falls;

- *limb contracture formation*, which can complicate venous access;

- *restrictive respiratory defects* due to muscular wasting, which, together with immobility and bulbar palsy, may predispose the patient to postoperative chest infections;

- *chronic pain syndromes*, for which the patient may be prescribed anticonvulsants, antidepressants or opioids;

- *communication difficulties*, which can cause problems with complicity with treatment and provision of consent;

- *bulbar palsies*, which may predispose the patient to chest infections, as well as making enteral nutrition/swallowing and speech difficult;

- *facial weakness*, which affects speech and may predispose to corneal dryness and abrasion;

- *sensory inattention*, such that the patient is not aware of or does not complain of pain or pathology occurring in the limbs (e.g. wrist fractures may be missed after falls);

- *postoperative confusion* is common;

- *urinary and faecal incontinence*;

- *poor temperature homeostasis*.

Head injury and cerebral protection

Head injury is a common cause of mortality and morbidity, particularly in young males. Of all people who are admitted to hospital after sustaining a head injury (140/100,000 in the USA), 70% are released from hospital after 12–48 h with no intracerebral sequelae, 10% are dead on arrival, 10% have moderate head injury (Glasgow Coma Score (GCS), Chapter 20) of 8–14/15) and 10% (20/100,000) are classed as having a severe head injury (i.e. GCS < 8). Neurotrauma accounts for a third of all deaths from trauma. Head injury should be suspected in any major trauma, particularly falls and road traffic accidents. Trauma may be alcohol related, and alcohol may confuse the clinical presentation with respect to level of consciousness. Head injury may co-exist in trauma patients presenting for emergency cardiothoracic, abdominal or orthopaedic surgery. Two distinct phases of head injury are seen: an initial phase, in which brain damage is directly due to the trauma sustained (coup and contracoup injuries, rotational/shearing injuries), is followed by a more protracted phase during which secondary damage may occur, as a result of cerebral ischaemia caused by expanding haemorrhage, cerebral hypoxia or cerebral tissue oedema. Patients may initially be comatose or have reduced levels of consciousness or amnesia. Neurological function may recover in the short term, or may deteriorate as secondary brain injury occurs. Initial management requires resuscitation (airway, breathing, circulation, etc.) and investigation for intracerebral injury (clinical presentation and CT scan).

Cerebral ischaemia occurs when cerebral oxygen demand (i.e. the $CMRO_2$) exceeds cerebral oxygen supply. The cerebral damage that ensues depends on the duration, site and cause of ischaemia, together with co-existent patient factors (e.g. age and cerebral pathology). Damage results from ischaemia induced intracellular hypercalcaemia, free

19

radical production, lipid peroxidation, lactate production, changes in membrane permeability and transmembrane Na/K-ATPase activity, and neurotransmitter accumulation. In turn these factors lead to cerebral oedema, which further reduces CBF, worsening ischaemia. Cerebral oedema may be exacerbated by ingestion of toxins, encephalopathy, systemic acidosis and sepsis.

$CMRO_2$ represents the volume of oxygen consumed by the brain, and is represented by the equation:

$CMRO_2$ (ml/min)
= CBF (ml/min)
× arterio-venous O_2 content difference

CBF, as we have seen, is dependent in part on the cerebral perfusion pressure (although this relationship is less evident in the case of head trauma).

Cerebral oxygen supply is dependent on the CBF and arterial O_2 content:

$DO_{2(cerebral)}$ (ml/min)
= CBF (ml/min) × arterial O_2 content

Arterial O_2 content
= ([Hb] × O_2 saturation × 1.34 (Chapter 16)

It can be seen from these variables that a number of important factors contribute to cerebral oxygen supply and demand:

- *CBF*, which is reduced by a high intracranial pressure (cerebral oedema, intracranial haemorrhage), a low MAP (cardiac arrest or dysrhythmia, haemorrhage and hypotension) and hypocapnia (due to hyperventilation). CBF may be increased by correction of these factors.

- *Arterial O_2 content*, which is reduced by anaemia (e.g. due to haemorrhage or excessive haemodilution) and hypoxia (represented by a fall in arterial oxygen saturation, secondary, e.g. to chest injury, hypoventilation, chest infection).

- Oxygen extraction ratio (OER), reduced extraction occurs in damaged and hypoperfused brain areas.

- *CO*.

Indeed the above considerations are applicable to preventing ischaemia in any body tissue, and form the rationale behind the resuscitation strategies described by the advanced trauma and life support (ATLS) guidelines. Tissue ischaemia is prevented, therefore, by the restoration of tissue flow by adequately oxygenated blood, which is achieved by the use of respiratory and cardiac support, prevention of ongoing haemorrhage and fluid resuscitation (see Chapter 6).

'Cerebral protection' strategies aim to preserve cerebral function, and are an extension of the resuscitation methods described above. They are commonly employed after head injury, but are also used in the perioperative management of patients undergoing neurosurgery, cardiac surgery or carotid surgery, and following a cardiorespiratory arrest, CVA or severe poisoning. Protective techniques include:

- Improving cerebral oxygen supply (see above).

- Maintain MAP around 80–100 mmHg.

- Electively ventilate the patient, maintaining $PaCO_2$ between 4 and 4.5 kPa, and PaO_2 above 10 kPa.

- Maintain blood Hb concentration within the normal range (polycythaemia increases blood viscosity, reducing blood flow).

- Avoid coughing and straining on the endotracheal tube, keep head in neutral position to avoid kinking jugular veins, and avoid circumferential neck ligatures. All these manoeuvres avoid acute rises in the CVP.

- The patient is placed head-up by 20°, to reduce cerebral oedema and CVP.

- Surgical techniques may be required to decompress intracerebral haemorrhage.

- Reduce cerebral metabolism.

- Sedate the patient, preferably with an i.v. anaesthetic agent.

- Administer seizure prophylaxis (sedatives and phenytoin).

- Avoid hyperthermia by use of paracetamol and tepid sponging; moderate hypothermia (35°C) may be beneficial.

- Normalise blood electrolyte concentrations, particularly blood glucose.

- Avoid hyponatraemia (which may be caused by the syndrome of inappropriate anti-diuretic hormone release – SIADH).

- Treat acute rises in ICP.

- Monitor the at risk patient using direct intraventricular ICP measuring catheters

- Hyperventilate the patient to a $PaCO_2$ of 3.5–4 kPa.

- Mannitol (0.5–1 g/kg by i.v. infusion of 10–20% solution over 20–30 min) may reduce cerebral oedema and improve CBF. Mannitol and frusemide produce a diuresis and a degree of intravascular hypertonicity, which has a dehydrating osmotic effect on brain tissue.

- Nimodipine may reduce the incidence of cerebral vasospasm after intracerebral haemorrhage.

- Steroids may reduce isolated rather than global cerebral oedema.

- Use of free radical scavengers and glutamate antagonists are unproven.

Cranial diabetes insipidus is a common occurrence, and its presence should warn the physician to monitor the patient for acute rises in ICP. Disruption of the supraoptic nucleus/hypophyseal–hypothalamic tract axis results in reduction of ADH release, leading to hypo-osmolar polyuria, plasma hyperosmolality and hypotension. SIADH may also occur, but is associated with the intermediate phase of neural recovery.

Data concerning antibiotic prophylaxis after head injury is not convincing, even in the presence of a proven skull fracture, surgery or insertion of an ICP monitoring bolt. If antibiotics are to be used, penicillin is the drug of choice. Tetanus cover should be provided. Selective gut decontamination could be considered in a young multiple trauma victim. Physiotherapy should be instituted to avoid chest atelectasis and limb contracture formation. Conscientious pressure care and DVT prophylaxis are necessary. Cushing's gastric ulcer formation is particularly prevalent after head injury and prophylactic antacid and H_2 antagonist therapy should be started. Acute GI haemorrhage may ensue in 10–15% of treated severe head injuries and may be compounded by the idiopathic coagulopathy associated with head injury. Further, GI protection is afforded by early enteral nutrition. NG tubes should be passed with extreme caution, and not at all in suspected basal skull fracture. NG-tube-related sinusitis should be ruled out in patients with unexplained fever.

Brain death

Definition

'Brain death' may be the result of some of the pathologies described above, notably trauma and CVA. In the UK, 'brain death' is a legal definition that equates to the irreversible absence of brain stem function (i.e. midbrain, pontine and medullary death), such that circulation and respiration do not occur without artificial support. Even with support, cardiorespiratory function usually fails within 72 h. A brain stem dead person is legally dead, and the diagnosis has important implications for organ donation. Persistent vegetative state (PVS) describes a clinical condition that results from the death of the forebrain, but with intact brain stem function, in which case the patient is still legally alive. The legal position is described further in Chapter 5.

Diagnosis

Two medical practitioners make the diagnosis of death, independently. Several criteria must be fulfilled prior to testing:

- the patient must be deeply unconscious;

- the patient must have suffered an identifiable, irreversible cause for their coma;

- there should be no possibility of drug-induced paralysis or sedation;

- the patient should have no biochemical, endocrine or temperature abnormality.

19

273

The tests of brain stem death are as follows:

- *Cranial nerves*
  - absent pupillary reflex to light (III) and absent corneal reflex (V);
  - absent Doll's eye reflex (III, IV, VI) – the eyes do not remain fixed on a point when the head is turned;
  - absent response to facial painful stimulus (V, VII);
  - absent oculo-vestibular reflex (III, IV, VI, VIII) – no ocular deviation in either direction in response to cold water injected gently onto the eardrum (having ascertained that the external meatus is free of wax);
  - absent gag or cough reflex (IX, X).

- *Respiratory centres*
  - ventilator disconnection test.

The patient is pre-oxygenated with 100% O_2 and an arterial blood gas (ABG) sample is drawn, to check the $PaCO_2$. The ventilator is switched off and continuous oxygen mist be administered throughout the test to maintain $SpO_2 > 95\%$. The observer looks for any respiratory effort. The test finishes either if the patient becomes cardiovascularly unstable, or if a second ABG sample reveals that the $PaCO_2$ (which rises by approximately 0.5 kPa/min in apnoeic patients) has risen to more than 6.6 kPa.

Neuropraxias and nerve damage

Although relatively uncommon, intra-operative nerve damage is often (but not always) avoidable and can cause significant postoperative morbidity, as well as incurring expensive liability in medical negligence. Early postoperative recognition allows patient reassurance or explanation, and potentially curative treatment (removal of ligatures including bandages and orthopaedic splints). Investigation may involve electromyography (EMG) and nerve conduction studies, which provide the most conclusive results 2–3 weeks after the injury.

Nerve damage may occur in surgical patients undergoing general or regional anaesthesia. During the former, poor positioning of the patient or use of tourniquets can cause nerve compression and neural ischaemia (neurapraxia), while hypotension, hypothermia or extravasation of drugs can cause axonotmesis or neurotmesis. Neurapraxia tends to effect motor more than sensory loss (touch and proprioception); total recovery usually occurs within 6 weeks. Axonotmesis describes axonal damage and myelin loss, with complete motor and sensory loss; the nerve sheath remains intact, down which the nerve regenerates from the proximal site of damage, effecting some long-term recovery. Neurotmesis describes complete nerve transection, from which recovery is rare.

A number of sites are specifically vulnerable to degrees of nerve damage in the perioperative period:

- Ulnar nerve (C_7, C_8) at the elbow, producing a clawed hand and sensory loss in the little finger and ulnar half of the ring finger.

- Radial nerve (C_6, C_7, C_8) in the radial groove of the humerus, producing flexion deformities of the elbow and wrist and sensory loss over the lateral dorsal surface of the hand.

- Common peroneal nerve (L_4, L_5) (particularly after operations in lithotomy), resulting in weak dorsiflexion and eversion of the foot and foot drop, and sensory loss over the dorsal lateral surface of the foot.

- Supraorbital nerve, which may be damaged by facial pressure, resulting in loss of sensation to the scalp as far back as the vertex.

- Brachial plexus, particularly if the upper arm is abducted more than 90° (with the elbow flexed and pointing towards the head) causing plexial stretching, or if the patient undergoes surgery in the lateral position, causing plexial compression. The upper roots (C5, C6, C7) are more often affected than the lower roots (C8, T1), producing Erb's palsy and loss of sensation over the lateral aspect of the arm and forearm.

Recovery is protracted, occurring over a period of months.

Anterior spinal artery syndrome

This may occur after aortic aneurysm repair. It complicates 24% of emergency repairs, but only 1% of elective repairs, being more prevalent after thoracic than abdominal surgery. The anterior spinal artery supplies blood to the anterior 2/3 of the spinal cord (see above). Cord ischaemia, due to profound hypotension and aortic cross-clamping, results in paralysis with upper motor neurone signs below the level of ischaemia, in excess of sensory loss (pain and temperature are the most affected). Recovery is poor.

Perioperative confusion

Cognition is the mental process of perception, memory and information by which a person acquires knowledge, solves problems and plans for the future. Cognitive impairment may be apparent before surgery (e.g. dementia). Acute cognitive impairment may also present for the first time in the postoperative phase, commonly manifest by confusion and amnesia.

Precedent cognitive impairment

There are five important implications for the perioperative management of cognitively impaired patients who present for surgery:

1. *Cognitive impairment.* This may in part be caused by co-existent pathologies, including alcoholism and drug addiction (and withdrawal phenomena), mental illness, generalised vascular disease and hypertension, and advanced multiple sclerosis or parkinsonism. The majority of patients with dementia are elderly, with reduced physiological reserve.

2. *Physiological status.* The patient's physiological status may be poor. Demented patients, even with the best of community and medical support, are often undernourished and prone to infection (e.g. due to long-term catheterisation). Alcoholics are often undernourished and suffer from vitamin deficiency syndromes (e.g. Korsakoff's psychosis due to thiamine deficiency). Drug addicts may be alcoholic, undernourished, HIV positive and chronically infected with staphylococci (including infective endocarditis) and fungi.

3. *Medications.* Patients may be taking a number of neuro-psychiatric drugs that can interact with anaesthetic agents, or be neural depressants in their own right. Withdrawal phenomena can occur if the drugs are stopped in the perioperative period (particularly, for drugs with a short half-life). Alcohol is a neurodepressant. Alcohol withdrawal is associated with seizures, for which prophylactic benzodiazepines may be prescribed.

   - *Anti-psychotics.* These are prescribed for schizophrenia, and are commonly used to 'tranquillise' confused or agitated patients in the perioperative period (e.g. haloperidol). They have a variety of side-effects. 'Largactil' (chlorpromazine) derives its proprietary name from 'large spectrum of activity'. Patients taking anti-psychotics are prone to parkinsonism and tardive dyskinesia (anti-dopaminergic side-effects), hypothermia and hypotension, cardiac dysrhythmia, blood dyscrasias and CNS depression.

   - *Antidepressants.* These drugs are associated with anti-muscarinic side-effects, cardiac dysrhythmias and heart block, syncope and hyponatraemia (in the elderly), and withdrawal phenomena. Of particular concern are the MAOIs (tranylcypromine > phenelzine > isocarboxazid), which may precipitate a hypertensive crisis if sympathomimetic drugs (e.g. ephedrine and adrenaline) are co-administered. Chronic antidepressant use (especially of amitriptyline and dothiepin) may be seen in patients with chronic pain syndromes.

19

- *Hypnotics and anxiolytics.* These are commonly prescribed medications (e.g. benzodiazepines), to which patients may become physiologically and psychologically addicted. They are sedative, and are associated with withdrawal phenomena.

- *Anti-dementia drugs.* These are reversible acetylcholinesterase inhibitors, and, as such, may alter the degree of neuromuscular block when paralysing agents are given during anaesthesia (enhance depolarising block and antagonise non-depolarising block).

- *Drug addiction.* Illegal drugs are abused for their CNS effects, specifically alteration of mood and perception. Non-prescription polypharmacy is common (i.e. patients may take a variety of drugs simultaneously). Drug addiction and mental illness may be related through cause or effect. Cocaine, amphetamine and amphetamine-like substances (*Ecstasy*) are central stimulants; seizures may occur in chronic abusers for which prophylactic benzodiazepines may be prescribed (these may also be used specifically as hypnotics). Stimulant abusers may be prescribed anti-psychotics or antidepressants to control psychotic or bipolar mental illness. Opioids, barbiturates, benzodiazepines and cannabinoids are CNS depressants; acute intoxication reduces intra-operative anaesthesia and postoperative sedation requirements. However, chronic abuse of depressants may give rise to acute withdrawal symptoms, which are sympathomimetic in nature and require the administration of CNS depressants. Chronic opioid use may be seen in patients with chronic pain syndromes.

4. *Consent.* It may not be possible to obtain consent if the patients lacks legal capacity (see Chapter 5). Note that patients detained under the Mental Health Act, 1983 may still be able to consent or refuse medical treatment, if that treatment is not targeted at curing or alleviating their mental illness.

5. *Co-operation.* The patient may not be able to comply with simple commands, through lack of understanding. Confused patients, particularly those with impaired frontal lobe function, may be aggressive towards staff.

Postoperative cognitive impairment
This may occur in any age group after any operation, and in previously normal patients. It is more common in elderly patients (25% develop delirium) with precedent cognitive impairment, those who have undergone neurosurgery, cardiac or carotid surgery, or particularly long, invasive or complicated surgery.

Delirium is a global cognitive impairment with impaired levels of attention and consciousness that presents with irrational behaviour and agitation. Coma describes complete unawareness of self and surroundings, and lack of response to external stimuli. Conditions causing delirium may progress to coma, without intervention.

The cause of postoperative delirium is idiopathic in 40% of cases. However, potentially identifiable causes include:

- *Early (within hours)*

  - drugs – residual anaesthetic agents, ketamine;

  - pain and opioid analgesics;

  - hypoxia, hypercapnia, hypocapnia;

  - reduced CPP;

  - seizures;

  - hypotension, cardiac dysrhythmia, embolic events;

  - metabolic disturbance – hypoglycaemia, hypo/hypernatraemia, acidosis;

  - intra-operative CVA.

- *Intermediate (days)*

  - all of the above;

  - sepsis and MOF;

- drug, alcohol or nicotine withdrawal;
- sleep deprivation/return of REM sleep.

■ *Late (weeks)*

- all of the above;
- idiopathic, particularly in the elderly and after cardiac surgery.

The investigation of delirium depends on clinical determination of the most likely cause. Smokers who are confused after thoracic surgery for example are more likely to have a respiratory cause for their delirium. Routine investigations may include FBC, urea and electrolytes, glucose and ABGs. Chest X-ray may prove technically difficult.

Treatment depends on the cause. Postoperative oxygen should be administered for at least 72 h after major surgery, because REM sleep is re-established towards the end of this period, and is associated with hypoxaemia due to early morning troughs in respiratory function. Thiamine should be administered to chronic alcoholics. Drug withdrawal may be treated by careful reintroduction of the drug, if it had been stopped, or cautious titration of a parenteral preparation of the drug. For idiopathic cases, the patient should be moved to a monitored, well-lit side-room. Relatives and nursing staff have an important role to play in calming the patient. If reassurance fails, or the patients are at risk to themselves, a titrated dose of haloperidol (2.5–5 mg i.v.) or a benzodiazepine (midazolam 1–2 mg i.v.) may be given.

19

20

Miscellaneous topics

Tables of useful values and formulae

It should be noted that the figures quoted below may vary slightly from the normal values quoted in your hospital, depending on which machines/programmes/assays are used for analysis.

All values given are for adults. Note that sex differences do occur (women have lower RBC, Hb and haematocrit levels).

Blood chemistry

Urea and electrolytes

Sodium	135–145 mmol/l
Potassium	3.5–5.5 mmol/l
Chloride	95–105 mmol/l
Urea	2.5–6.5 mmol/l
Creatinine	50–120 μmol/l

Liver function tests (LFTs)

Aspartate aminotransferase (AST)	6–42 U/l
Alkaline phosphatase (ALP)	100–350 U/l
Gamma glutamyltransferase (GGT)	7–50 U/l
Bilirubin	5–17 μmol/l
Albumin	35–50 g/l

Arterial blood gasses (ABGs) (room air)

pH	7.35–7.45
$PaCO_2$	4.5–6 kPa
PaO_2	11–14.5 kPa
Bicarbonate	22–32 mmol/l
Base deficit	−2 to +2
Lactate	0.3–1.3 mmol/l

Miscellaneous

Amylase	70–300 U/l
Calcium	2.25–2.65 mmol/l
Cholesterol	3.1–6.5 mmol/l
Glucose (fasting)	3.9–6.2 mmol/l
Magnesium	0.7–1.1 mmol/l
Creatinine kinase (CK)	<200 U/l
CK-MB	<3.5% of total CK
Troponin complex	0–0.04 ng/ml >0.1 ng/ml is diagnostic

Haematology

Full blood count

Hb	12–18 g/dl or 120–180 g/l
RBC count	$4–6 \times 10^{12}$/l
WCC	$4–11 \times 10^9$/l
Platelet count	$150–400 \times 10^9$/l
Neutrophil count	$2.5–7.5 \times 10^9$/l
Mean corpuscular volume (MCV)	78–98 fl
Haematocrit	35–55%

Coagulation

Bleeding time	Up to 9 min
aPTT	26–38 s
INR	<2 required for surgery
D-dimers	<200 ng/ml

Miscellaneous

Serum B_{12}	0.15–1 mg/l
ESR	0–6 mm/h > 20 mm/h is abnormal
Total iron-binding capacity	45–72 μmol/l

20

Electrolyte concentrations of some body fluids

All values are mean values in mmol/l.

Fluid	Na$^+$	K$^+$	Bicarbonate	Chloride	H$^+$
Bile	130	6	40	80	0.005
Diarrhoea	70	30	50	70	
Gastric	60	80	0	90	50
Small intestine	110	5	30	100	0.5
Urine	150	50		200	
Sweat	50	10		45	

Cerebrospinal fluid

Glucose	2.2–5.5 mmol/l
Protein	150–400 mg/l
Pressure	7–15 cmH$_2$O
Lymphocytes	0–5 × 10^6/l

Pulmonary function tests

Vital capacity	55–65 ml/kg
Forced expiratory volume in 1 s	75% of vital capacity
PEFR	400–600 l/min

Circulatory values

Regional blood flow

Organ	Blood flow in ml/min	Percentage of cardiac output
Brain	750	15
Heart	250	5

(Continued)

20

(Continued)

Liver	1500	30
Kidneys	1200	24
Rest of body	1400	28
Cardiac output	5000	100

Average cardiovascular pressures (mmHg)

Anatomical site	Systolic pressure	Diastolic pressure	Mean pressure
Right atrium (central venous pressure)			2
Right ventricle	25	2	15
Pulmonary artery	25	8	12
Left atrium			8
Left ventricle	120	5	50
Aortic arch	120	80	90

Glasgow Coma Scale

Record the best response. Glasgow Coma Scale (GCS) <8 on admission *may* require intubation, in order to protect the airway. The GCS is of most use in detecting fluctuations in the level of consciousness.

	Score
Eye opening	
Spontaneous	4
To speech	3
To pain	2
None	1
Best motor response	
Obeys	6
Localises	5
Withdraws	4
Abnormal flexion	3
Extensor	2
None	1
Best verbal response	
Orientated	5
Confused	4
Inappropriate words	3
Incomprehensible sounds	2
None	1
Total	15 (minimum 3)

Multiple choice questions

Explanation for the vast majority of the answers to the following questions can be found in this book. Those that cannot have been included to stimulate further (but not extensive) additional reading.

Suggested time for completion of the questions is 100 min. Complete the paper before checking the answers. Good luck!

1. Drugs may cross membranes via:
   A. Transmembranal ion pumps
   B. Micropores
   C. Passive diffusion against a concentration gradient
   D. Pinocytosis
   E. Facilitated diffusion

2. The following statements are true about the autonomic nervous system:
   A. Atropine increases HR
   B. Norepinephrine increases splanchnic blood flow
   C. Atropine causes miosis
   D. Adrenaline is a bronchoconstrictor
   E. Adrenaline is an ino/chronotrope

3. The following equations are true:
   A. Cardiac output
   $$= \frac{\text{mean arterial pressure}}{\text{systemic vascular resistance}}$$
   B. Volts = amps × resistance
   C. Cardiac output
   = stroke volume × heart rate
   D. Resistance to fluid flow ∝ radius (of a tube)^4
   E. Compliance = volume × pressure

4. Valid consent to surgery:
   A. Should be given voluntarily
   B. Requires that the patient sign a consent form
   C. Cannot be given by a person detained under Section 2 of the Mental Health Act, 1983
   D. Must be obtained before all surgical procedures
   E. May be given by the relative of an unconscious adult patient

5. Normal plasma values for an adult include:
   A. Sodium 135 mmol/l
   B. Potassium 5.4 mmol/l
   C. Glucose 3.2 mmol/l
   D. Creatinine 85 mmol/l
   E. Calcium 2.52 mmol/l

6. One litre of Hartmann's solution contains:
   A. 131 mmol of sodium ions
   B. 111 mmol of chloride ions
   C. 5 mmol of potassium ions
   D. 29 mmol lactate
   E. 50 g glucose

7. The primary acid–base disturbance occurring with certain pathologies include:
   A. Metabolic alkalaemia – vomiting
   B. Metabolic acidaemia – COPD

20

C. Metabolic acidaemia – diabetes
D. Respiratory alkalaemia – pain
E. Respiratory acidaemia – opioid overdose

8. NSAIDs such as diclofenac may cause:
   A. Gastric irritation
   B. Bronchodilation
   C. Perioperative haemorrhage
   D. Analgesia
   E. Renal failure

9. Opioid usage is associated with the following problems:
   A. Tachyphylaxis
   B. Itching
   C. Renal failure
   D. Postoperative nausea
   E. Tachypnoea

10. The following conditions are associated with hypercapnia:
    A. Pulmonary oedema
    B. Pulmonary embolism (PE)
    C. Cardiopulmonary arrest
    D. Sodium bicarbonate administration
    E. Prolonged severe asthma

11. Postoperative nausea and vomiting (PONV) is more likely:
    A. In men
    B. In children
    C. In orthopaedic patients
    D. If the patient has had it previously
    E. If opioids are used for analgesia

12. Liver failure results in:
    A. Hyperglycaemia
    B. Coagulation failure
    C. Immune compromise
    D. Jaundice
    E. Hypernatraemia

13. Considering blood transfusion:
    A. People with blood group O-negative are universal donors
    B. People with blood group AB-positive are universal recipients
    C. 1 unit of blood increases blood Hb concentration in an adult by about 1 g/dl
    D. Blood should be given to patients with a blood Hb concentration of <10 g/dl

E. Hypothermia is a complication of blood transfusion

14. A perioperative cardiovascular complication rate of more than 5% is associated with:
    A. Atrial fibrillation (AF)
    B. Carotid endarterectomy surgery
    C. Silent myocardial infarction 3 weeks prior to surgery
    D. Diabetes mellitus
    E. Abdominal aortic aneurysm repair

15. Myocardial ischaemia may be lessened by:
    A. Blood transfusion
    B. Atenolol
    C. Hypocapnia
    D. Polycythaemia
    E. Oxygen administration

16. In advanced life support (ALS):
    A. PE may cause cardiopulmonary arrest
    B. Lidocaine is an effective anti-dysrhythmic in ventricular fibrillation (VF)
    C. 1 mg adrenaline is administered every minute in VF
    D. 3 mg atropine is administered every 3 min in asystole
    E. Sodium bicarbonate administration may cause hypernatraemia

17. Status epilepticus is associated with:
    A. Alcohol withdrawal
    B. Rhabdomyolysis
    C. Metabolic alkalosis
    D. Increased cerebral metabolic rate
    E. Hyperthermia

18. Perioperative cerebral protection strategies may include administration of:
    A. Paracetamol
    B. Nimodipine
    C. Phenytoin
    D. 5% dextrose solution
    E. Correction of anaemia

19. The following statements are true concerning the side-effects of neuro-psychiatric medications:
    A. Antidepressants – cardiac dysrhythmia
    B. Anti-psychotics – cardiac dysrhythmia

20

C. Anti-psychotics – hypothermia
D. Anti-psychotics – hyperthermia
E. Phenelzine – hypertension

20. The following may cause confusion postoperatively;
    A. Hypoxia
    B. Pain
    C. Opioid analgesia
    D. CVA
    E. Ranitidine

21. The following statements are true concerning antibiotics:
    A. Fluconazole is effective against *Staphylococcus aureus*
    B. Gentamicin is effective against *Staphylococcus aureus*
    C. Vancomycin is effective against MRSA
    D. Gentamicin is associated with hearing loss
    E. Gentamicin is effective against *Escherischia coli*

22. Acute alcohol intoxication:
    A. Is a contraindication to surgical exploration of an open tibial fracture
    B. Increases the risk of perioperative gastric aspiration
    C. Is associated with coagulopathy
    D. May obscure the clinical signs of subarachnoid haemorrhage
    E. Can cause seizures

23. Concerning cigarettes:
    A. Smoking increases the risk of perioperative bronchospasm
    B. Nicotine is a CNS stimulant
    C. Nicotine improves myocardial oxygen balance
    D. Cessation of smoking for 8 h preoperatively reduces improves perioperative oxygen transport
    E. Smoking increases the risk of postoperative chest infection

24. The incidence of DVT may be reduced by:
    A. Administration of fractionated heparin
    B. Administration of unfractionated heparin
    C. Early postoperative mobilisation

D. Fluid restriction
E. Perioperative use of graduated compression stockings

25. Pulse oximetry may be problematic:
    A. In Afro-Caribbean males
    B. In house-fire victims
    C. In hypovolaemic patients
    D. In anaemic patients
    E. In patients with haemoglobinopathies

26. Bupivacaine:
    A. Has a chemical structure identical to Marcaine
    B. Is cardiotoxic in overdose
    C. Has an upper toxic dose limit of 4 mg/kg body weight
    D. May be used for epidural analgesia
    E. Exerts its analgesic effects by blocking sodium channels in A-β nerve fibres

27. Adrenaline:
    A. Is chemically identical to epinephrine
    B. Is synthesised in the adrenal medulla
    C. Is both an α- and β-adrenergic agonist
    D. Causes bronchospasm
    E. May decrease diastolic BP

28. The following doses are identical to each other:
    A. 1 mg = 10 ml of a 1:10,000 solution
    B. 100 mg bupivacaine = 10 ml of a 0.5% solution of bupivacaine
    C. 1% solution = 10 mg/ml of solute
    D. 1 l of a 0.9% solution of sodium chloride contains 90 g sodium chloride
    E. 1 ml of 1:1000 adrenaline contains 1 μg adrenaline

29. Postoperative epidural analgesia is associated with:
    A. Hypotension
    B. Deep vein thrombosis (DVT)
    C. Itching
    D. Leg weakness
    E. Headache

30. Patient-controlled analgesia (PCA) is associated with:
    A. Hypotension
    B. DVT

20

C. Itching
D. Respiratory depression
E. Withdrawal phenomena

31. A blood-gas sample, breathing air of pH 7.35, $PaCO_2$ 5.4 kPa, PaO_2 6.5 kPa, bicarbonate 22 mmol/l, is consistent with the following diagnoses:
    A. Acute left-ventricular failure
    B. Asthma
    C. Pulmonary oedema
    D. Venous blood sampling
    E. Chronic obstructive pulmonary disease (COPD)

32. Acute Renal Failure is associated with:
    A. Hypertension
    B. Plasma potassium concentration of 6.2 mmol/l
    C. Plasma creatinine concentration of 232 μmol/l
    D. Gentamicin therapy
    E. Oliguria

33. The following increase myocardial oxygen demand:
    A. Pain
    B. Shivering
    C. Adrenaline
    D. Glyceryl trinitrate (GTN)
    E. Atenolol

34. Acute left-ventricular failure may occur:
    A. After myocardial infarction
    B. With sepsis syndrome
    C. As a result of epidural analgesia
    D. After administration of β-blockers
    E. After administration of GTN

35. Compared to younger patients, elderly patients:
    A. Have reduced immune function
    B. Are more likely to comply with medical treatment
    C. Have a more sensitive autonomic nervous system
    D. Are more likely to experience postoperative confusion
    E. Are less sensitive to the side-effects of opioid analgesia

36. Compared to non-diabetic patients, insulin-dependent diabetic patients:
    A. Are more likely to suffer adverse perioperative cardiovascular events
    B. Are less prone to perioperative infections
    C. Have a less sensitive autonomic nervous system
    D. Are more prone to gastric aspiration
    E. Exhibit more rapid wound healing

37. Perioperative management of bradycardia may include the following:
    A. Transthoracic pacing
    B. Isoprenaline
    C. Oxygen
    D. Atenolol
    E. Lidocaine

38. Diagnostic criteria for adult respiratory distress syndrome (ARDS) include:
    A. Pleuritic chest pain
    B. Kerly B lines
    C. Wedge-shaped pulmonary opacities
    D. Bilateral diffuse infiltrates on the chest radiograph
    E. $PaO_2 < 8$ kPa

39. Signs of oxygen toxicity include:
    A. Retrosternal chest pain
    B. Dizziness
    C. Nausea and vomiting
    D. Convulsions
    E. Atelectasis

40. Complications of central venous line insertion include:
    A. Femoral artery puncture
    B. Haemothorax
    C. Cardiac tamponade
    D. Hiccoups
    E. Horner's syndrome

41. Capnography may provide information about:
    A. Respiratory rate
    B. Cardiac output
    C. Arterial PaO_2
    D. Carboxy-haemoglobinaemia
    E. Airways resistance

20

42. The following may be associated with postoperative hyperthermia:
    A. Sepsis
    B. Intra-operative warming
    C. Paracetamol
    D. Isoflurane
    E. Haloperidol

43. Drugs which should be continued preoperatively include:
    A. Atenolol
    B. Isoniazid
    C. L-dopa
    D. Gliclazide
    E. Carbamazepine

44. The following occur after major surgery:
    A. Natriuresis
    B. Lipolysis
    C. Gluconeogenesis
    D. Hypokalaemia
    E. Insulin resistance

45. Atrial fibrillation:
    A. Is a contraindication to major surgery
    B. May be converted to sinus rhythm by DC cardioversion
    C. Is associated with hyperthyroidism
    D. Is diagnosed by the absence of T-waves on the ECG
    E. May be converted to sinus rhythm by carotid sinus massage

46. Acute pancreatitis:
    A. May present with neutropaenia
    B. Is a cause of ARDS
    C. Serum amylase may be normal
    D. Is associated with hypercalcaemia
    E. Has a high perioperative mortality

47. Gelofusin
    A. Is a colloid
    B. Has a half-life of 24 h
    C. Interferes with blood cross-matching
    D. Interferes with coagulation
    E. Carries a risk of transmitting Jacob–Creutzfeldt disease (JCD)

48. Contraindications to major elective gastrointestinal surgery include:
    A. Haemoglobin concentration of 9.5 g/dl
    B. Severe bilateral carotid stenoses

C. Complete heart block seen on preoperative ECG
D. M.I. in last 3 months
E. Patient not competent to sign consent form

49. TURP syndrome:
    A. May cause cerebral oedema
    B. Occurs in up to 25% of TURPs
    C. May produce a metabolic alkalosis
    D. May cause hyponatraemia
    E. May cause chest pain

50. Constipation may resolve following:
    A. i.v. fluid administration
    B. Oral erythromycin administration
    C. Rectal lactulose administration
    D. Resumption of cigarette smoking postoperatively
    E. Postoperative mobilisation

Multiple choice answers

Question	A	B	C	D	E
1	T	F	F	T	T
2	T	F	F	F	T
3	T	T	T	F	F
4	T	F	F	F	F
5	T	T	F	F	T
6	T	T	T	T	F
7	T	F	T	T	T
8	T	F	T	T	T
9	T	T	F	T	F
10	F	F	T	T	T
11	F	T	F	T	T
12	F	T	T	T	F
13	T	F	T	F	T
14	F	F	T	F	T

20

Question	A	B	C	D	E
15	T	T	F	F	T
16	T	F	F	F	T
17	T	T	F	T	T
18	T	T	T	F	T
19	T	T	T	T	T
20	T	T	T	T	F
21	F	F	T	T	T
22	F	T	F	T	T
23	T	T	F	T	T
24	T	T	T	F	T
25	F	T	T	F	F
26	T	T	F	T	F
27	T	T	T	F	T
28	T	F	T	F	F
29	T	F	T	T	T
30	F	F	T	T	F
31	T	T	T	T	T
32	T	T	T	T	T

Question	A	B	C	D	E
33	T	T	T	F	F
34	T	T	F	T	F
35	T	F	F	T	F
36	T	F	F	T	F
37	T	T	T	F	F
38	F	F	F	T	F
39	T	T	T	T	T
40	T	T	T	T	T
41	T	T	F	F	T
42	T	T	F	T	T
43	T	T	T	F	T
44	F	T	T	F	T
45	F	T	T	F	F
46	F	T	T	T	T
47	T	F	F	F	F
48	F	T	T	F	F
49	T	F	F	T	T
50	T	T	F	T	T

Basic statistical concepts and their application in perioperative care

Aims

The aims of this chapter are to understand the

- basic statistical concepts relevant to the practice of perioperative medicine;

- 'stochastic approach', probability, significance, null hypothesis, Type-1 and Type-2 errors;

- 'observational method', diagnostic and prognostic tools, the receiver operator characteristic (ROC) curve;

- 'interventional method', study design and interpretation;

- concepts of 'descriptive' and 'inferential' statistics;

- concepts of 'normal' distribution, samples and populations;

- role of evidence-based medicine.

Objectives

21

- To facilitate objective understanding and criticism of published studies, and the place of evidence-based medicine in clinical decision-making.

Introduction

Most working clinicians have a basic aversion to mathematics in general, and statistical method in particular. However, the rigorous discipline of modern clinical practice mandates an ability to both articulate and apply the principles of 'evidence-based medicine'.

The aim of this chapter is not to teach either 'in-depth' statistical method or relevant mathematical theory. The aim is rather to provide a (very) basic conceptual framework relevant to the practice of perioperative medicine on which to hang the various theoretical elements of statistical science. Thus, the busy practising clinician may later choose to examine these elements in detail, on an 'as required basis', by consulting the relevant texts.

'Probability' – the basic language of statistical science

Elsewhere in this volume we consider the problem of the acute phase response. In that context, through the application of the principles of 'teleology' (the explanation of phenomena by the purposes they serve, rather than by postulated causes), we seek to establish a certain chain of 'cause' and 'effect'; this is the basis of the so-called *deterministic approach.*

In considering the problem of clinical decision-making with reference to an 'evidence base', we must apply a wholly different concept called the *stochastic approach.*

The deterministic system establishes cause and effect as a certainty, the stochastic system is very different, it is not governed by the laws of *cause and effect*, but rather by the laws of *probability* where certainty becomes 'probability', and cause and effect become 'association'. Phenomena occurring in such a system are basically classified as either *random*, occurring by chance, or *non-random*, occurring with 'significance'.

Thus, statistical analysis never seeks to establish cause and effect, but simply in the first instance to identify relationships between variables, and in turn the significance of those observed relationships. Further, statistical analysis is applicable to groups of patients, be they populations or samples, not to individual patients.

These two fundamental conceptual limitations to statistical method should always be borne in mind when applying the conclusions of 'evidence-based medicine' to individual patients.

In essence, statistical analysis looks at the incidence of variables within a population (via sampling), compares the relative incidence of a given variable between populations, and/or examines the potential relationship between variables. Potential differences in incidence of a single variable (between populations), or potential relationships between two or more variables (within a population) may be collectively referred to as 'statistical events'.

Statistical analysis aims to determine if these 'events' occurring in a continuum, be it time or space, are occurring in either a random fashion (by chance) or in a non-random fashion (with significance); significance being defined as the absence of chance.

Accounting for chance

Poisson distribution

Fundamental to all statistical analysis is the ability to calculate the probability of an observed 'event' of given magnitude occurring randomly (by chance).

In the teleological approach, we rely on 'nature' to provide the necessary explanation in terms of the laws of physics, chemistry and evolutionary biology.

In the stochastic approach, we rely on 'artifice', namely the construction of a hypothetical *probabilistic model*, into which we feed the observed values for a given 'event', which then in turn generates a probability of those observed values occurring randomly (by chance).

The simplest form of probabilistic model is the *frequency distribution*, an example of which is the *Poisson distribution*.

Consider, in a **non-random** process, events occur at an expected rate '*R*', there is a direct relationship between each successive event. In a **random** process, events occur without any discernable underlying rate, there being no direct relationship between the occurrence of one event and the next. However, in a **random** process events are occurring at an expected *mean* rate 'μ'. The continuum, along which these events are occurring, can be time or space. Each mean value 'μ' has a corresponding frequency distribution about the mean – the Poisson dribution.

Thus, the basis of statistical analysis begins by assigning a numerical value to a given 'event'. Typically on repeated measurements a range of values for that event will be obtained. From this range of values one can determine a mean value μ and model its corresponding frequency distribution (Fig. 21.1).

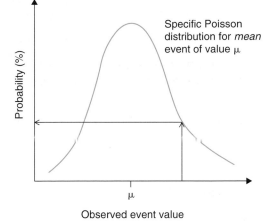

Fig. 21.1 Poisson distribution.

Characteristics of the Poisson distribution

- Is discrete, only assigning probability values to integer (whole number) outcomes.

- The peak probability always occurs at the mean value.

- The spread (dispersion) increases as the volume of 'μ' increases. Because, as the mean increases, the spread of plausible outcomes correspondingly increases, and given that the total probability must always equal 1, that probability must be distributed across a greater number of outcomes, and hence the typical probability of any specified value (including the mean) must diminish.

- The curve becomes more symmetrical (less skewed) as the mean μ value increases.

- **Each mean value has its own Poisson distribution.**

Using the Poisson distribution we can construct a model about an observed mean 'event' rate. We can then plot any observed individual 'event' value on the curve and determine the probability of that 'event' value occurring by chance. By convention, if a given 'event' value generates a probability '*P*' value = 5% (0.05), it is deemed not to have occurred by chance and is thus non-random/significant (Fig. 21.2).

The assumed distribution (of the 'event' values) is termed the 'null distribution'; it is

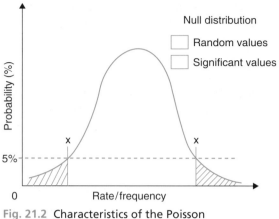

Fig. 21.2 Characteristics of the Poisson distribution.

based, in this case, on the Poisson distribution – the 'null hypothesis' suggests that the data conform to the Poisson distribution with a specific mean. If we observe a value for the 'event' whose calculated probability is <5% (0.05), then we conclude that that occurrence of that event is unlikely to conform to the Poisson distribution, and is thus occurring non-randomly, i.e. not by chance.
Thus, disproving the null hypothesis.

Other common examples of probabilistic models used as null distributions are

- binomial distribution,

- exponential distribution,

- normal distribution, see later,

- Chi-squared distribution, see later.

The 'null hypothesis', Type-1 and Type-2 errors

An hypothesis is defined as a 'tentative explanation that accounts for a set of facts and that can be tested by further investigation'. The starting point in any statistically based investigation is the construction of a 'null hypothesis'.

In essence, the null hypothesis is a clear *testable* statement about chance occurrences, assuming no relationship (difference or association) between variables. Any observed relationship is purely artefact occurring by chance.

In attempting to establish significant relationship between variables through investigation, it is necessary to first disprove this hypothesis (through assessing the fit between observed data, and a given null distribution/probabilistic model, as above).

This leads to the possibility of statistical error:

- Type 1 error = *rejecting the null hypothesis when in fact it is true.* (There being no significant statistical 'event'/false positive.)

- Type 2 error = *accepting the null hypothesis when in fact it is false.* (A significant statistical 'event' actually exists/false negative.)

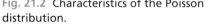

The null hypothesis

	Actually true	Actually false
Accepting the null hypothesis	No error	Type 2 error (β)
Rejecting the null hypothesis	Type 1 error (α)	No error

We will return to the concept of statistical error later when considering study design.

The application of statistical method to the practice of perioperative medicine

Introduction

To understand the relevance of statistical science to the practice of clinical perioperative medicine, we need only to look so far as the three questions commonly addressed when obtaining informed consent from a patient prior to surgery, namely:

1. What is actually wrong with me doctor? *(Establishing a diagnosis.)*

2. What is the natural outcome of my disease process? *(Establishing a prognosis.)*

21

3. What are the chances of your proposed treatment achieving a cure? *(Establishing efficacy of intervention.)*

These three questions together frame the fundamentals of statistical analysis. Questions 1 and 2 relate to the application of *observational* statistical method. Question 3 relates to the application of *interventional* statistical method. Together they provide useful anchor-points on which to construct a broad overview of statistical application.

Observational statistical method in perioperative medicine

Introduction

Let us consider the first stage in the process of 'informed' consent, namely formulating both a diagnosis and a prognosis (questions 1 and 2), i.e. establishing the natural history of the underlying disease process.

Statistical method provides us with both diagnostic tools and prognostic tools. Like all tools they require calibration. Calibration involves the concepts of both *sensitivity* and *specificity* which we will explore later.

> In *observational* statistics the key statistical 'event' is establishing a *dependent relationship* between two or more variables.

Within the context of observational statistics there are essentially two types of variables examined, namely independent (predictor/input) variables and dependent (outcome) variables:

- *An independent variable:* Independent variables have values that are autonomous of dependent or outcome variables; they are also termed 'predictor' variables, 'input variables' or 'risk factors'. Examples of independent variables are age, sex and height.

- *A dependent variable:* Dependent variables have values or 'outcomes' that are dependent on independent/input variables.

Examples of dependent variables are life expectancy and peak expiratory flow.

Diagnostic tools

The Chi-squared test

Clinical diagnosis involves identifying a series of signs and symptoms and equating these with a specific underlying disease process. The question then arises – does the presence of these signs and symptoms always mean that the patient has the disease?

To support the diagnosis, one may apply a series of 'screening tests'; again the question arises – does a positive test always predict disease? Or conversely, does a negative test always exclude disease?

The statistical test commonly applied in this situation is the Chi-squared test. The Chi-squared test applies to categorical (non-numerical) variables, and is thus termed *non-parametric* (see later).

Further, the Chi-squared test examines the relationship between *one* independent/predictor variable, and *one* dependent/outcome variable, and is thus termed *univariate*.

The first step in performing a Chi-squared test is the construction of a '2 × 2' table:

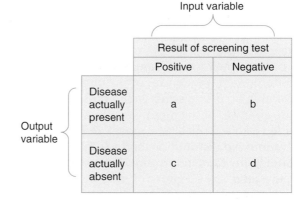

$$\text{sensitivity} = \frac{a}{a + b} \times 100$$
(percentage of subjects with disease who have a positive-test result)

$$\text{specificity} = \frac{d}{c + d} \times 100$$
(percentage of subjects without the disease who have a negative-test result)

$$\text{positive-predictive value} = \frac{a}{a + c} \times 100$$

(likelihood that a positive-test result indicates disease)

$$\text{negative-predictive value} = \frac{d}{b + d} \times 100$$

(likelihood that a negative-test result exclude disease)

likelihood ratio for positive result

$$= \frac{a/(a + b)}{c/(c + d)}$$

(odds of a positive test result in a patient with disease versus odds of a positive result in patient without the disease)

likelihood ratio for a negative result

$$= \frac{b/(a + b)}{d/(c + d)}$$

(odds of a negative test result in a patient with disease versus odds of a negative result in patient without the disease)

The '2 × 2' table above is a simple example of a contingency table, each numerical entry in the table (in this case a, b, c and d) is a frequency. It is not within the remit of this chapter to detail the computation of the 'Chi-squared statistic' from these numerical values. Broadly speaking, computation involves obtaining an observed value for the difference in frequencies of the output variable occurring either in the presence, or the absence, of the input variable. That value is fed into a probabilistic model, in this case a Chi-squared distribution, and a level of probability (and in turn significance) is generated.

However, in essence, the Chi-squared statistic simply indicates whether there is, or is not, a *significant* association between the two variables. In this case, between a positive screening test result and an underlying disease process. *What the Chi-squared test does not do, is indicate the strength of that association.*

Is the Chi-squared test a test of association or difference? Confusion arises in understanding the practical application of the Chi-squared test because some text books classify it as a test of statistical *association*, others as a test of statistical *difference*. The truth is that it can be applied both ways. In the above context, the test is applied to demonstrate that there is a significant *difference* in the incidence of the disease process between the 'screening test positive' and 'screening test negative' groups, with the higher incidence occurring in the 'screening test positive' group. We, therefore, conclude that there is a significant *association* between a positive screening test and the presence of the disease process.

Fisher's exact test

The Chi-squared test is only applicable to large samples. For samples of <20, or an expected frequency of <5 in any one of the four cells, then Fisher's exact test is the appropriate investigation.

Prognostic tools

As discussed above, the Chi-squared test applies only to *categorical* data, and simply indicates the *significance* of an observed association between variables, but does not indicate the *strength* of that association. The strength of association is an important factor in that it allows us to consider the *relative* contribution of a number of variables to an ultimate outcome, and in turn make predictions about that outcome from the presence or absence of those variables.

In any consideration that seeks to establish significant dependent relationships between *numerical* variables, account must be taken of the 'mean' and inherent 'variability' of each variable. Useful prognostic tests should establish both *significance* and *strength* of association. For variables assumed to be *normally distributed* (see later) the following *parametric* tests of dependency may be applied:

■ For *linear* relationships

1. Regression.

2. Correlation/bivariate.

3. Correlation/multivariate.

21

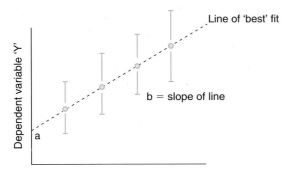

Fig. 21.3 Regression and line of best fit.

■ For *non-linear* relationships

4. Logistic regression.

Regression

Regression examines the relationship between an independent (input/predictor) variable and a single dependent (outcome/response) variable. The outcome variable is assumed to be normally distributed with respect to mean and dispersion. The underlying relationship is assumed to be linear, and can be determined either by the 'line of best fit' or 'least squares' methods. The test is by definition *univariate* (Fig. 21.3).

Any straight line conforms to the equation $y = a + bx$, 'a' equals the 'intercept' and 'b' equals to 'slope' or in this particular case the 'regression coefficient'. The quoted statistic is thus the regression coefficient, a value of '0' for the regression coefficient indicates no dependent relationship, a value of '± 1' represents maximal dependency (Fig. 21.4).

Values may be obtained at any point on the intervening range, either positive or negative, representing, respectively, positive or negative regression of *y* on *x*. Thus, the regression coefficient is an expression of *strength* of association. Observed values for regression coefficient are then fed into a probabilistic model, and their probability and in turn their *significance* generated.

Correlation/bivariate

Correlation examines the relationship between *two* dependent variables. Each are

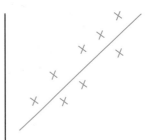

Positive regression Y on X

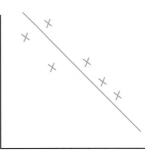

Negative regression Y on X

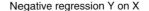
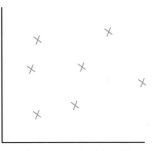

No regression Y on X

Fig. 21.4 Regression lines.

assumed to be normally distributed. The relationship is assumed to be linear (Fig. 21.5).

The quoted statistic derived from this test is the 'correlation coefficient ', sometimes known in this specific case of bivariate analysis, as the 'Pearson *r*' coefficient. As in regression, a value of 0 denotes no correlation, a value of ± 1 denotes perfect correlation, the value of the coefficient denoting *strength* of relationship. Again observed values are fed into a probabilistic model and their *significance* obtained.

Note: Occasionally in the literature correlation coefficients are quoted as their squared value, which is then termed the coefficient of determination.

21

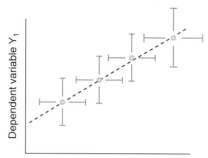

Fig. 21.5 Relationship between two dependent variables.

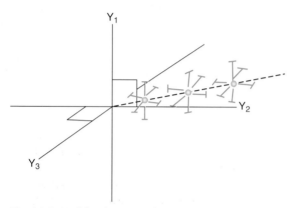

Fig. 21.6 Multivariate correlation.

Correlation/multivariate

Correlation/multivariate examines the relationship between *three or more* dependent variables, each assumed to be normally distributed. Again the relationship is assumed to be linear. Again, the quoted statistic is a correlation coefficient with its attached probability (Fig. 21.6).

Logistic regression

Logistic regression is a multivariate technique that is commonly applied to medical research. Again the variables are assumed to be normally distributed, but their relationship does not necessarily need to be linear.

When outcome is recorded in two categories, such as 'survivors' versus 'non-survivors', logistic regression is an effective way to examine the independent contribution of more than one 'predictor' variable to ultimate outcome.

After the predictor variables are mathematically weighted (according to their relative contribution), logistic regression attempts to predict outcome from the presence or absence of those variables, based on the model.

Non-parametric tests of dependency/association

These tests seek to establish dependency between variables not 'normally' distributed in the population. Firstly, the variables are ranked between two outcomes, e.g. survivors versus non-survivors. Analysis is then applied to the *distribution of ranks* (between the two groups) rather than to the variables themselves. Examples of such tests are given below.

Spearman rank coefficient

This determines *significance* but not *strength* of a dependent relationship between variables. This is, basically, the numerical equivalent of the Chi-squared test.

Kendal rank coefficient

This determines both *significance* and *strength* of a dependent relationship between variables not 'normally' distributed in the population.

Note: It is a point worth remembering that neither regression nor correlation can be interpreted as establishing cause and effect. They can only indicate how and to what extent variables are related to each other.

Bayes' theorem modelling

Risk modelling using Bayes' theorem assumes that inferences can be made about future events based on the analysis of past events. In perioperative medicine this is useful as predictions on outcome of patients undergoing various procedures can be generated using data derived from outcomes of patients who have previously undergone those procedures. In its simplest form, statistical prediction may be expressed as an 'odds ratio'.

The odds ratio

The odds ratio measures the odds of having a particular risk factor in one population compared to another population. An odds ratio of 1 suggests that there is no difference in the incidence of a given risk factor between the two populations being examined. The odds ratio is normally presented with 95% confidence limits indicating to the reader the limits between which they can be assured with 95% confidence of the true relative risk of the population. A relative risk may be much higher than 1.0, but if the 95% confidence intervals overlap the value of 1.0 then the relative risk is probably not significant.

Predictive scoring systems using weighted variables

The relative risk attached to variables can be converted to a 'weighted' score. A cumulative score of risk can then be generated by summing the values of the risk factors (variables) present in a given patient. Examples of such scoring systems are the APACHE 2 scoring system in critical care, and the Parsonet score in cardiac surgery.

Calibration of predictive tools, the Receiver Operator Characteristic

In considering the 'diagnostic' Chi-squared test, the concepts of *sensitivity*, *specificity*, *true-positive fraction* and *true-negative fraction* were all considered as indices of diagnostic accuracy. In calibrating more advanced 'prognostic' tests, such as predictive scoring systems based on weighted variables, a single expression combining all four elements of diagnostic accuracy is used – the receiver operator characteristic (ROC).

This odd term 'ROC' is, in fact, historical, alluding to the fact that much of the mathematics underlying its computation derives from 'signal detection theory'. The general theory of signal detection, based on a combination of probability theory and decision theory, was developed through the 1950s during the development of radar, where it was used as a tool to systematically analyse the ability of radar operators to distinguish between 'true signals' and 'noise'.

Thus, the ROC provides a single index of accuracy. The concept of sensitivity and

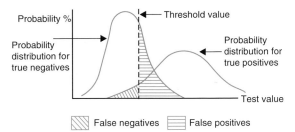

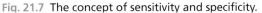

Fig. 21.7 The concept of sensitivity and specificity.

specificity can be summarised diagrammatically (Fig. 21.7).

In principle, for most prognostic tests that yield a single value, the distribution of result values in actually positive and actually negative patients overlap, as above. No single 'threshold' or decision criterion can be found that absolutely separates the two populations clearly, otherwise the test would be perfect!

Usually a threshold value will be chosen arbitrarily, and different choices will yield different frequencies for the various kinds of correct and incorrect decision.

Consider, e.g. a test in which high results values tend to predict say non-survival (e.g. APACHE 2), but the distribution of test result values between true negatives (survivors) and true positives (non-survivors) has considerable overlap. Setting a high value for the decision threshold will make both false-positive and true-positive decisions less frequent, but will make both true-negative and false-negative decisions more frequent. Thus, a threshold value must be selected that is believed to yield an appropriate compromise among these gains and losses.

Each time the threshold value is varied arbitrarily, a different set of decision fractions is obtained.

Decision matrix

		Observation	
		+	−
R **e** **a** **l** **i** **t** **y**	+	True +	False −
	−	False +	True −

21

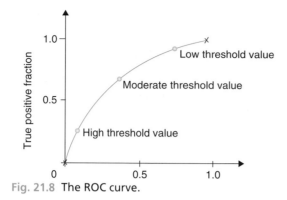

Fig. 21.8 The ROC curve.

These four decision options can be resolved into two fractions which can then be plotted as *x* and *y* co-ordinates namely:

true-positive fraction = *sensitivity*

false-positive fraction = 1 − *specificity*

These fractions are measured at a number of different threshold values and plotted on a curve, the so-called 'ROC curve' (Fig. 21.8).

The curve is termed the ROC curve for the diagnostic test, since it describes the inherent detection characteristics of the test and since the 'receiver' of the test information can 'operate' at any selected point on the curve by applying the appropriate decision threshold.

The area under the curve (AUC) is taken to represent the probability that the risk predictor, e.g. the APACHE 2 score, accurately discriminates between patients who die in hospital following surgery, and patients who survive. An AUC of 0.5 indicates that there is no discrimination, i.e. that patients whose outcome is correctly predicted are allocated purely by chance. An area of 1.0 indicates perfect discrimination – all patients are correctly allocated. Thus, the normal range for AUC is 0.5–1.0 (Fig. 21.9).

Consider, the typical ROC curve must pass through two points:

x, *y* = 0

x, *y* = 1

if:

true-positive fraction

$= \dfrac{\text{number of true test positives}}{\text{number of actual true negatives}}$

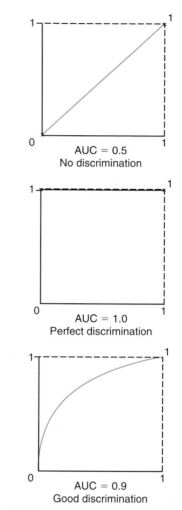

Fig. 21.9 ROC curves.

and

false-positive fraction

$= \dfrac{\text{number of false test positives}}{\text{number of actual true negatives}}$

false-positive fraction = number of false test positives/number of actual true positives

By setting the decision threshold well *below* any of the observed values, then all results will read test positive. Thus,

number of true-test positives
= number of actual positives TPF = 1 (*y* = 1)

number of false-test positives
= number of actual negatives FPF = 1 (*x* = 1)

By setting the decision threshold well *above* any of the observed values, then all results will read test negative. Thus,

number of true-test positives = 0 TPF = 0 ($y = 0$)

number of false-test positives = 0 FPF = 0 ($x = 0$)

Interventional statistics in perioperative medicine

Consider again the final question to be addressed when obtaining informed consent. What is the chance of the proposed treatment achieving a cure? – establishing efficacy of a given therapeutic intervention.

> In *interventional* statistics, the key statistical event is establishing a **significant difference** in the mean values for a dependent variable between test and control populations.

Here interventional statistics gives us the means to objectively assess the efficacy or impact of a given intervention.

Whether planning an interventional study to test a new treatment, or assessing a previously published piece of work, the same sequential approach to critical evaluation of methodology applies with respect to

- a clear and concise statement of the problem;
- the formulation of an hypothesis;
- design of the study;
- collection of the data;
- analysis of the data and conclusions drawn.

It is a point worth remembering that medical journals are mainly written by medical school clinicians. In addition to their altruistic desire to promote medical knowledge and practice, they may also be motivated by concerns about establishing a reputation, obtaining research grants and sustaining employment.

The proper sequence of analysis resolves into six simple questions:

- Why? – Is the hypothesis clearly stated?
- How? – What is the research design?

- Who? – Is the target population clearly defined?
- What? – How was the therapy administered and the data collected?
- How many? – Are the test statistics convincing?
- So what? – Is it clinically relevant to my practice?

A clear and concise statement of the problem

The aims of the study (intervention) should be easily readable and concise. The investigator should aim to provide a clear and concise statement of the purpose of the study in a single sentence, ideally setting it within the relevant clinical context. Published conclusions presented at the end of the study should simply be a restatement of the original intent either in the negative or the affirmative. Deviation from original goals, and the drawing of conclusions relating to matters only indirectly relating to the issues outlined in the initial hypothesis always invokes suspicion.

This may be a particular problem in meta-analysis – conclusions drawn from pooled data may not be pertinent to the problems as stated in the original individual investigations.

Formulation of an hypothesis

As alluded to above, an hypothesis is defined as a tentative explanation that accounts for a set of facts and that can be tested by further investigation.

In statistical terms, the correct hypothesis – the 'null' hypothesis is that no significant difference exists between outcomes in test and control groups. The purpose of the investigation is to disprove this hypothesis.

Study design

The aim of study design is to *minimise error* and *maximise power*. The precise design of the study will depend on the type of variables (data) being analysed.

- *Sampling error*: The amount by which size of the 'difference' between the two groups

21

'test' and 'control' as measured within the sample, differs from the actual difference exiting in the underlying population as a whole. *Sampling error is minimised by increasing sample size.*

■ *Type-1 error (α-error):* Wrongly rejecting the 'null' hypothesis and in turn drawing falsely positive conclusions. The problem of Type-1 error thus depends on two factors:

● the chosen level of significance and

● the actual existence of a difference in outcome variable between 'test' and 'control' groups.

● *Type-1 error is reduced, by increasing the level of significance, e.g. from 5% to 1%.*

■ *Type-2 error (β-error):* Wrongly accepting the 'null' hypothesis, and in turn missing a significant difference. The problem of Type-2 error depends on four factors:

1. The chosen level of significance.

2. The size of the difference that actually exists.

3. The inherent variability within the population being examined.

4. The size of the sample relative to the population from which it was drawn. *Thus, Type-2 error can be minimised by*

– *decreasing the chosen level of significance;*

– *increasing the sample size;*

– *the inherent variability of the population may be reduced by using 'self' controls.*

■ *Power:* The power of a significance test is a measure of how likely that test is to produce a statistically significant result for a population difference of any given magnitude. It thus depends on the size of the sample in relation to the parent population, and on the size of the difference to be detected. *Power is increased by increasing sample size.*

Types of variable in interventional statistics

There are three distinct types of variable (data) that determine methodology in interventional statistics:

■ *Categorical data:* Here variables or individuals are 'categorised' into different classes, these classes may have no numerical relationship to each other, e.g. gender, colour, etc.

■ *Discrete numerical data:* Refers to data arising from numerical 'measurement', the values being expressed as whole numbers (integers), e.g. number of individuals in a particular group.

■ *Continuous numerical data:* Refers to data arising from numerical 'measurement', but measured values can assume any value within a range or scale, e.g. height and weight.

Parametric tests of significant difference

Parametric statistics are the usual choice in the analysis of numerical data, both discrete and continuous. The purpose of such analysis is to test the hypothesis that there is no significant difference in the mean value for a given variable between the 'test' population and the 'control' population. The population means being unknown and being estimated from the sample means. The two commonly used tests are

■ the Student's *t*-test,

■ analysis of variance (ANOVA).

The Student's t-test

The most common use of the Student's *t*-test is to compare the means of two populations. A modification of the test – the 'paired *t*-test' applies when each subject in the investigation has two measurements taken, e.g. one before and one after a drug. Each control measurement taken before drug administration is paired with a measurement in the same patient after drug administration. Thus, this is a 'self-controlled' experiment. This pairing of measurements in the same patient reduces variability and increases statistical power.

Table 21.1 **Appropriate tests used in order to calculate the significance of differences between sets of data**

	Type of data		
	Parametric	**Non-parametric**	**Nominal**
Two treatments in different groups	Unpaired *t*-test	Mann–Whitney *U*-test	Chi-squared test
Two treatments in a single group	Paired *t*-test	Wilcoxon signed routes test	McNemar
>Two treatments in different groups	ANOVA	Kruskal–Wallis test	Chi-squared test
>Two treatments in a single group	ANOVA	Friedman	Cochrane *Q*-test

Analysis of variance

Typically, in acute medicine it is common to follow a variable longitudinally with time, making sequential measurements at specified intervals in both treatment and control groups. One option would then be to apply the Student's *t*-test to each pair of variables (treatment and control) occurring at a given time point. A more appropriate method of comparing sequential sets of variables occurring between two groups is the ANOVA.

The statistic generated by these tests is in the form of a ratio, that ratio is then fed into a probabilistic model to generate a level of significance. The particular model used here is the '*t*-distribution', the *t*-distribution is built on a single variable – the number of 'degrees of freedom', which is computed from the number of individuals within the sample.

Non-parametric tests of significant difference

These tests involve using statistics that do not require any assumptions about probability distributions within the population. Non-parametric tests are the tests of choice for 'categorical' data. Again the categorical data is 'ranked' and it is the distribution of ranks between treatment and control groups that is examined. The difference between the sum of the ranks is fed into a binomial distribution, and its probability computed. There are two commonly used tests:

■ Mann–Whitney rank-sum test, the non-parametric equivalent of the paired *t* test;

■ Krusal–Wallis one-way analysis of variance, the non-parametric equivalent of the unpaired *t* test.

See Table 21.1 for an overview of the type of statistical tests, which can be performed on different types of data and treatment groups. Not all the tests are described in the text.

Collection of data

Organisation of data collection should be directed to *minimising bias* and there are basically three types of bias to avoid:

■ *Selection bias:* Refers to a systematic difference between people, who are selected from a given population for a study, and those who are not. Selection bias can be caused by referral patterns, survival differences or loss to follow up.

■ *Response bias:* Refers to a systematic difference between responders and non-responders, e.g. compliance with test medication.

■ *Information bias:* Refers to a systematic difference between measurements

21

recorded in different study groups, e.g. the response variable may be more carefully tested for in the treatment group.

Analysis of the data and conclusions drawn

Difficulties in data collection and integrity are sometimes alluded to in the final analysis, e.g.:

■ *Intention to treat analysis:* Here comparison is made between a control group – no treatment offered, and a test group – those offered treatment; this latter group will include those who accepted treatment and those who declined.

■ *On treatment analysis:* Here comparison is between 'control' group – no treatment and 'treated' group – those actually treated.

However, the basic underlying principle is to analyse according to the original hypothesis and experimental design. Other results that look interesting can only be the subject of future studies. The conclusions will obviously depend on the study itself but must reflect the intentions of the original problem statement on which the study was based.

Descriptive and inferential statistics, populations and samples

In the forgoing consideration, we have considered the two basic relationships between variables, namely significant correlation and significant difference, and the relevance of these relationships to the practice of clinical medicine. Statistical methods used to examine these relationships *between* variables are referred to as 'inferential statistics'.

How about the variables themselves? – statistics examining the intrinsic properties of a *single* variable are referred to as 'descriptive statistics'. The most important set of descriptive statistics in clinical medicine are associated with the concept of the 'normal distribution'.

The normal distribution

For any outcome variable determined by a single input variable, one would intuitively expect the observed value for the outcome variable to remain constant if the size of the input variable remained unchanged.

In contrast, most biological outcome variables are each determined by a multiplicity of input variables, both genetic and environmental; the environmental input variables particularly, being subject to constant shifts and changes in value. Plotting a frequency distribution for a single given biological output variable (e.g. systolic BP), one consistently obtains the typical symmetrical bell-shaped curve referred to as the 'normal distribution'. The word 'normal' here is used in the sense that when examining biological output variables (or any output variable determined by a large number of input variables) this is the frequency distribution of observed values that is 'normally' obtained.

The normal distribution displays some inviolate characteristics, and as such may be regarded as the fundamental law governing the functional outcome of complex biological systems, in the same way that Newton's laws of motion govern the transfer of energy in inanimate systems. The normal distribution is thus characterised by a unique set of descriptive statistics and properties. Descriptive statistics elude to two aspects of the normal (frequency) distribution, namely 'centralisation' and 'dispersion'; observed values for a biological outcome variables tend to cluster around a central value; however, about this central point there is a degree of dispersion.

The descriptive statistics that describe the degree of 'centralisation' are the mean, the mode and the median.

■ *The mean:* the arithmetic mean of all the observed values of the variable.

■ *The mode:* The most commonly occurring value for a given variable.

■ *The median:* The central value of the distribution, such that 50% of the observed values lie above and 50% of the observed values lie below it.

The first unique property of the normal distribution is that the mean, the mode and the median are all equal.

21

The descriptive statistics that describe the degree of 'dispersion' (about the mean) are the standard deviation and the variance from which it is derived. The variance is in essence the arithmetic mean of the values of the difference between each observed value and the calculated mean value. The standard deviation is computed from the square root of the variance.

The second unique property of the normal distribution is that 95% of all the observed values will occur within ±2 standard deviations from the mean.

Samples, populations and the normal distribution

The fundamental problem in exploring relationships between variables in a population or between populations is that practical logistics preclude examination of every individual within a defined population and thus require that the examination is confined to a representative sample drawn from the parent population.

However, given the inviolate and ubiquitous nature of the normal distribution and assuming that all sources of bias are eliminated in the process of sampling, then precisely the same fundamental principles governing the frequency distribution of observed values for a given biological variable, will pertain to the sample as pertain to the parent population. Thus, both parent and sample frequency distributions will conform to the same 'normal' distribution (Fig. 21.10). The defined parent population itself, being, in point of fact, just a much larger 'sample' drawn from a population of potentially infinite size extending within a limitless continuum in time.

Thus, the same ±2 standard deviations will embrace both 95% of the values observed for the variable in both sample and parent population. It is precisely because the frequency distributions of a given variable in both sample and parent population conform to the same normal distribution, that valid conclusions can be drawn from the sample and applied to the parent population as a whole.

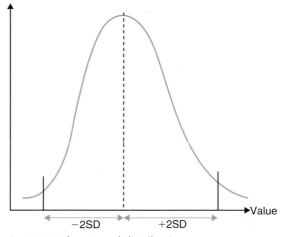

Fig. 21.10 The normal distribution.

Further, the stochastic approach identifies a threshold probability of 5% as defining whether or not an observed value is occurring as a random or non-random event. Thus, for a given variable, any observed value occurring in the *parent population* that lie beyond the ±2 standard deviation limit (derived from the *sample*) is occurring with a probability of <5%, and is thus deemed not to have occurred by chance.

The concept of *descriptive* and *inferential* statistics is best summarised visually in the two basic standard notations used to illustrate significant difference and significant association, namely, the 'Box and Whisker plot' and the 'odds ratio', respectively.

Visual notation of significant difference, the 'Box and Whisker plot'

This notation is basically a visual presentation of the Student's *t* test, and as such is the simplest way to present the typical results of an *interventional* study. Essentially, the aim of such a study is to demonstrate a significant difference in the values for a given outcome variable between the test and control study groups. The function of the Box and Whisker plot is to display data location and spread for each population being compared. Each Box and Whisker represents the descriptive statistics relevant to the occurrence of the specified outcome variable in each

21

303

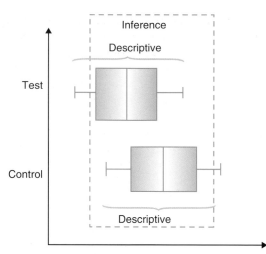

Fig. 21.11 Box and Whisker plot showing non-significant overlap of confidence intervals.

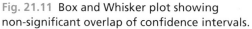

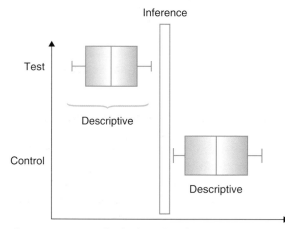

Fig. 21.12 Box and Whisker plot showing significant overlap of confidence intervals.

population. Thus,

- the Box = the spread of the central 50% of the data around the median;

- the Whisker = the range delineated by ±2 standard deviations about the mean.

In Fig. 21.11 there is significant overlap between the confidence intervals specified by the ± 2 standard deviations in test and control populations. The *inference* drawn is that there is *no* significant difference between the occurrence of the measured outcome variable between test and control populations.

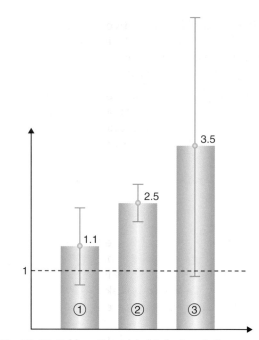

Fig. 21.13 Odds ratios and risk factors 1–3 (for explanation, see text).

In Fig. 21.12, there is no significant overlap between the confidence intervals specified by the ± 2 standard deviations in test and control populations. The *inference* drawn is that there *is* significant difference between the occurrence of the measured outcome variable between test and control populations.

Visual notation of significant association (correlation), the 'odds ratio'

The odds ratio is the simplest way to present the results of an *observational* study, illustrating which potential risk factors are significant to the development of a disease and which are not. Any factor having a relative risk of 1 (unity) between the population with the disease, and the population without the disease is thus not deemed a significant risk factor for the disease.

In Fig 21.13:

- *Risk factor 1* has a relative risk calculated at 1.1; however, its confidence interval crosses the threshold of unity, and is thus deemed not to be a significant risk factor.

- *Risk factor 2* has a relative risk calculated at 2.5, its confidence limits lie above the threshold of unity, thus it is deemed to be a significant risk factor.

- *Risk factor 3* has a relative risk calculated at 3.5; however, its confidence interval crosses the threshold of unity, and is thus deemed not to be a significant risk factor.

The role of evidence-based medicine in perioperative care

The primary aim of 'evidence-based medicine' is to effect a shift from the process of opinion-based decision-making to evidence-based decision-making, aiming to separate conclusion from preconception, and in turn to apply the concept of significance not in an subjective sense but in a mathematical sense.

The basic advantage in constituting anything into a mathematical form is that it can be scrutinised in a way that subjective clinical experience cannot. Although the basic aims of the evidence-based approach are inherently correct, there are both inherent flaws and dangers in the concept.

Meta-analysis

The basic foundation of the evidence base lies in the statistical method of meta-analysis, which can simply be defined as the combination of several (primary) studies to provide a single (common) estimate. The process of meta-analysis, although widely deployed, is not universally accepted as sound by all statisticians. The basic problem lies not in the actual mechanics of meta-analysis as a statistical method, but in the quality of the data analysed, particularly with reference to *homogeneity of data*.

The process of meta-analysis first involves checking that all the studies to be included derive from the same population by looking at the homogeneity of the odds ratios generated in different studies. If this is satisfactory, then the second stage of the analysis is to calculate a common odds ratio.

The problem comes in selecting the primary studies for processing. Firstly, in ensuring that all the studies included address precisely the same question and examine *exactly identical outcome variables*. Secondly, one must ensure that *all* relevant work is included. There is a tendency to only publish studies, which demonstrate a significant difference in outcome, studies demonstrating no significant difference in outcome, although statistically equally valid (particularly in subsequent meta-analysis) are not regarded as interesting enough for publication. This problem is referred to as 'publication bias'.

In selecting the 'best' available evidence, the following classification of data is used:

- Class 1 data – prospective randomised controlled trials;

- Class 2 data – cohort studies;

- Class 3 data – case–control studies;

- Class 4 data – cross-sectional studies;

- Class 5 data – case reports.

In acceding to the relentless demands for an evidence base for every therapeutic intervention, the clinician runs the very real risk of surrendering control of the clinical decision-making process to a non-clinical statistician or (even worse) financial manager!

It is worthwhile remembering that, paradoxically, there is as yet no 'evidence' for an 'evidence base' in comparison to the historical practice of intuitive medicine. So, by the standards of its own demands, there remains no hard clinical evidence for its use as a clinical tool!

It is timely to remind ourselves of Rutherford's often quoted but nonetheless extremely pertinent observation – 'If you need statistics to show your results are relevant, then what you really need is a better experiment.'

In closing this chapter, it is useful to revisit two points made in the introduction: firstly, that statistical method cannot be applied to individual patients, and that secondly, and most importantly, statistical method does not offer proof but only probability.

Index

307